Vitiligo

Editor

JOHN E. HARRIS

DERMATOLOGIC CLINICS

www.derm.theclinics.com

Consulting Editor
BRUCE H. THIERS

April 2017 • Volume 35 • Number 2

ELSEVIER

1600 John F. Kennedy Boulevard • Suite 1800 • Philadelphia, Pennsylvania, 19103-2899

http://www.theclinics.com

DERMATOLOGIC CLINICS Volume 35, Number 2
April 2017 ISSN 0733-8635, ISBN-13: 978-0-323-52404-9

Editor: Jessica McCool
Developmental Editor: Alison Swety

Dermatologic Clinics (ISSN 0733-8635) is published quarterly by Elsevier Inc., 360 Park Avenue South, New York, NY 10010-1710. Months of publication are January, April, July, and October. Business and editorial offices: 1600 John F. Kennedy Blvd., Suite 1800, Philadelphia, PA 19103-2899. Customer service office: 11830 Westline Drive, St. Louis, MO 63146. Periodicals postage paid at New York, NY, and additional mailing offices. Subscription prices are USD 377.00 per year for US individuals, USD 655.00 per year for US institutions, USD 434.00 per year for Canadian individuals, USD 799.00 per year for Canadian institutions, USD 505.00 per year for international individuals, USD 799.00 per year for international institutions, USD 100.00 per year for US students/residents, and USD 240.00 per year for Canadian and international students/residents. International air speed delivery is included in all *Clinics* subscription prices. All prices are subject to change without notice. **POSTMASTER:** Send address changes to *Dermatologic Clinics*, Elsevier Health Sciences Division, Subscription Customer Service, 3251 Riverport Lane, Maryland Heights, MO 63043. **Customer Service: 1-800-654-2452 (U.S. and Canada); 314-447-8871 (outside U.S. and Canada). Fax: 314-447-8029. E-mail: journalscustomerservice-usa@elsevier.com (for print support); journalsonlinesupport-usa@elsevier.com (for online support).**

Reprints. For copies of 100 or more, of articles in this publication, please contact the Commercial Reprints Department, Elsevier Inc., 360 Park Avenue South, New York, New York 10010-1710. Tel.: 212-633-3874; Fax: 212-633-3820; Email: reprints@elsevier.com.

The *Dermatologic Clinics* is covered in *MEDLINE/PubMed (Index Medicus), Current Contents/Clinical Medicine, Excerpta Medica, Chemical Abstracts,* and *ISI/BIOMED.*

Contributors

CONSULTING EDITOR

BRUCE H. THIERS, MD
Professor and Chairman, Department of Dermatology and Dermatologic Surgery, Medical University of South Carolina, Charleston, South Carolina

EDITOR

JOHN E. HARRIS, MD, PhD
Associate Professor, Department of Dermatology, University of Massachusetts Medical School, Worcester, Massachusetts

AUTHORS

GENEVIEVE H.L. ANDERSEN, BS
Human Medical Genetics and Genomics Program, University of Colorado School of Medicine, Aurora, Colorado

STANCA A. BIRLEA, MD, PhD
Associate Professor, Department of Dermatology, University of Colorado Anschutz Medical Campus, Aurora, Colorado

STEPHEN CHU-SUNG HU, MBBS, MPhil
Department of Dermatology, College of Medicine, Kaohsiung Medical University Hospital, Kaohsiung Medical University, Kaohsiung, Taiwan

NADA ELBULUK, MD, MSc
Assistant Professor, Ronald O. Perelman Department of Dermatology, NYU Ambulatory Care Center, NYU Langone Medical Center, New York, New York

SAMIA ESMAT, MD
Phototherapy Unit, Dermatology Department, Faculty of Medicine, Cairo University, Egypt

KHALED EZZEDINE, MD, PhD
Professor, Department of Dermatology, EpiDermE, Henri Mondor Hospital, Université Paris-Est Créteil Val-de-Marne, Créteil, France

BOON-KEE GOH, MD
Medical Director, Skin Physicians Pte Ltd, Visiting Consultant, National Skin Centre, Singapore, Singapore

NATHANIEL B. GOLDSTEIN, BA, MA
Lead Professional Research Assistant, Department of Dermatology, University of Colorado Anschutz Medical Campus, Aurora, Colorado

PEARL E. GRIMES, MD
Director, Vitiligo & Pigmentation Institute of Southern California, Clinical Professor, Division of Dermatology, David Geffen School of Medicine, University of California, Los Angeles, Los Angeles, California

ILTEFAT H. HAMZAVI, MD, FAAD
Senior Staff Physician, Department of Dermatology, Henry Ford Hospital, Detroit, Michigan

JOHN E. HARRIS, MD, PhD
Associate Professor, Department of Dermatology, University of Massachusetts Medical School, Worcester, Massachusetts

REHAB A. HEGAZY, MD
Phototherapy Unit, Dermatology Department, Faculty of Medicine, Cairo University, Egypt

CHENG-CHE E. LAN, MD, PhD
Professor, Department of Dermatology, College of Medicine, Kaohsiung Medical University Hospital, Kaohsiung Medical University, Kaohsiung, Taiwan

JULIETTE MAZEREEUW-HAUTIER, MD, PhD
Centre de Référence des Maladies Rares de la Peau Hôpital Larrey - Service de Dermatologie 24, Toulouse, France

TASNEEM F. MOHAMMAD, MD
Clinical Research Fellow, Department of Dermatology, Henry Ford Hospital, Detroit, Michigan

RAMA NASHAWATI, BS, MSGM
Research Associate, Vitiligo & Pigmentation Institute of Southern California, Los Angeles, California

JAMES J. NORDLUND, MD
Professor and Chairman Emeritus, Department of Dermatology, University of Cincinnati College of Medicine, Cincinnati, Ohio; Professor of Dermatology, Boonshoft Wright State College of Medicine, Dayton, Ohio

DAVID A. NORRIS, MD
Professor and Chair, Department of Dermatology, University of Colorado Anschutz Medical Campus, Aurora, Colorado; Denver Department of Veterans Affairs Medical Center, Denver, Colorado

AMIT G. PANDYA, MD
Professor, Department of Dermatology, University of Texas Southwestern Medical Center, Dallas, Texas

THIERRY PASSERON, MD, PhD
Professor, Department of Dermatology and INSERM U1065, Team 12, C3M, Archet 2 Hospital, University Hospital of Nice, Nice, France

MEHDI RASHIGHI, MD
University of Massachusetts Medical School, Worcester, Massachusetts; Department of Dermatology, Tehran University of Medical Sciences, Tehran, Iran

MICHELLE RODRIGUES, MBBS (Hons), FACD
Dermatologist, Department of Dermatology, St Vincent's Hospital, The Royal Children's Hospital, Skin and Cancer Foundation, Inc, Fitzroy, Victoria, Australia

JULIEN SENESCHAL, MD, PhD
Service de Dermatologie Adulte et Pédiatrique, Centre de Référence des Maladies Rares de la Peau, Hôpital Saint André, INSERM 1035, University of Bordeaux, Bordeaux, France

SUZAN SHALABY, MD
Phototherapy Unit, Dermatology Department, Faculty of Medicine, Cairo University, Egypt

REINHART SPEECKAERT, MD, PhD
Department of Dermatology, Ghent University Hospital, Ghent, Belgium

RICHARD A. SPRITZ, MD
Professor and Director, Human Medical Genetics and Genomics Program, University of Colorado School of Medicine, Aurora, Colorado

ALAIN TAÏEB, MD, PhD
Service de Dermatologie Adulte et Pédiatrique, Centre de Référence des Maladies Rares de la Peau, Hôpital Saint André, INSERM 1035, University of Bordeaux, Bordeaux, France

NANJA VAN GEEL, MD, PhD
Department of Dermatology, Ghent University Hospital, Ghent, Belgium

Contents

Preface: Optimizing Vitiligo Management: Past, Present, and Future xi

John E. Harris

The Medical Treatment of Vitiligo: An Historical Review 107

James J. Nordlund

Discolorations of the skin, such as vitiligo, were recognized thousands of years ago. White spots caused by vitiligo and other disorders have caused significant social opprobrium to those disfigured by these pigmentary disorders, throughout history and still in the present day. Treatments have been desperately sought with only partial success. Recent advances suggest that vitiligo and other pigmentary disorders might soon be curable.

Quality of Life, Burden of Disease, Co-morbidities, and Systemic Effects in Vitiligo Patients 117

Nada Elbuluk and Khaled Ezzedine

Vitiligo is a complex, systemic disease associated with many autoimmune and autoinflammatory conditions. Additionally, the cutaneous changes of vitiligo have significant effects on quality of life and self-esteem. Further efforts are needed to increase our understanding of vitiligo comorbidities as well as to increase awareness of the psychological effects of vitiligo.

Skin Cancer Risk (Nonmelanoma Skin Cancers/Melanoma) in Vitiligo Patients 129

Michelle Rodrigues

The relative genetic and immune protection against melanoma and nonmelanoma skin cancers in those with vitiligo is reassuring. The results of recent studies allow us to be cautiously optimistic when discussing the risk of skin cancer caused by therapeutic exposure to narrow-band ultraviolet B light. However, we should continue to recommend sun protection at all other times to avoid burning in vitiliginous skin and to decrease incidental ultraviolet exposure. It is also important to perform full skin checks regularly in light of the prolonged courses of phototherapy required to repigment vitiliginous skin and maintain repigmentation thereafter.

Presentations, Signs of Activity, and Differential Diagnosis of Vitiligo 135

Boon-Kee Goh and Amit G. Pandya

Vitiligo has a variety of presentations, including focal, acrofacial, segmental, and generalized forms. Thorough knowledge of these presentations is important to make the correct diagnosis. Signs of activity are important to recognize so that treatment is optimized. Clinical findings of confettilike depigmentation, trichrome and inflammatory vitiligo, and the Koebner phenomenon should alert the clinician that a patient's disease is likely to worsen. These patients may require systemic treatment to stabilize their disease. Many other skin disorders present with hypopigmentation or depigmentation and must be distinguished to determine the right diagnosis, advise the patient on prognosis, and prescribe the correct treatment.

Segmental Vitiligo 145

Nanja van Geel and Reinhart Speeckaert

Segmental vitiligo is characterized by its early onset, rapid stabilization, and unilateral distribution. Recent evidence suggests that segmental and nonsegmental vitiligo could represent variants of the same disease spectrum. Observational studies with respect to its distribution pattern point to a possible role of cutaneous mosaicism, whereas the original stated dermatomal distribution seems to be a misnomer. Although the exact pathogenic mechanism behind the melanocyte destruction is still unknown, increasing evidence has been published on the autoimmune/inflammatory theory of segmental vitiligo.

Chemical-Induced Vitiligo 151

John E. Harris

Chemical-induced depigmentation of the skin has been recognized for more than 75 years, first as an occupational hazard but then extending to those using household commercial products as common as hair dyes. Since their discovery, these chemicals have been used therapeutically in patients with severe vitiligo to depigment their remaining skin and improve their appearance. Because chemical-induced depigmentation is clinically and histologically indistinguishable from nonchemically induced vitiligo, and because these chemicals appear to induce melanocyte autoimmunity, this phenomenon should be known as "chemical-induced vitiligo," rather than less accurate terms that have been previously used.

Medical and Maintenance Treatments for Vitiligo 163

Thierry Passeron

Medical treatments alone, or in combination with phototherapy, are key approaches for treating nonsegmental vitiligo and, to a lesser extent, segmental vitiligo. The treatments are useful for halting disease progression and have been proven effective for inducing repigmentation and decreasing risk of relapses. Although the treatments have side effects and limitations, vitiligo often induces a marked decrease in quality of life and in most cases the risk:benefit ratio is in favor of an active approach. Systemic and topical agents targeting the pathways involved in loss of melanocytes and in differentiation of melanocyte stem cells should provide more effective approaches in the near future.

Phototherapy and Combination Therapies for Vitiligo 171

Samia Esmat, Rehab A. Hegazy, Suzan Shalaby, Stephen Chu-Sung Hu, and Cheng-Che E. Lan

Vitiligo is a disease characterized by disappearance of melanocytes from the skin. It can negatively influence the physical appearance of affected individuals, and may profoundly affect a person's psychosocial function and quality of life. Therefore, vitiligo should not be considered as merely a condition that affects a patient's appearance, but needs to be actively treated in patients who seek medical help. Phototherapy has been used as the main treatment modality for patients with vitiligo. Different forms of phototherapy for vitiligo include broadband UVB, narrowband UVB, excimer light and excimer laser, and psoralen plus UVA.

Surgical Therapies for Vitiligo 193

Tasneem F. Mohammad and Iltefat H. Hamzavi

Surgical management is a safe and effective treatment modality for select patients with vitiligo. Many techniques of vitiligo surgery exist, each with unique advantages and disadvantages. Preoperative screening for appropriate candidates, selection of surgical technique, and postoperative management are all key elements in enabling patients to achieve maximal repigmentation.

Repigmentation through Melanocyte Regeneration in Vitiligo 205

Stanca A. Birlea, Nathaniel B. Goldstein, and David A. Norris

Repigmentation in vitiligo is the process that replaces, in the epidermal basal layer of vitiligo skin, the mature melanocytes that have been killed by cytotoxic T cells specific for melanocyte antigens. It consists of mobilization of melanocyte precursors in the hair follicle bulge and infundibulum to proliferate, migrate, and differentiate into mature melanocytes, moving from the hair follicle bulge to the interfollicular epidermis. The most common clinical presentation of repigmentation in vitiligo is the perifollicular pattern. The most potent stimulus for repigmentation is the UV light.

Depigmentation Therapies for Vitiligo 219

Pearl E. Grimes and Rama Nashawati

The general goals of medical management of vitiligo are to repigment vitiliginous areas of skin and to stabilize the progression of depigmentation. However, for some patients with vitiligo affecting extensive body surface areas who are unresponsive to repigmentation therapies, depigmentation of the remaining normal skin may be a better choice. Candidates for depigmentation therapy should be carefully screened and patient education is essential. Permanent topical therapies used for depigmentation include monobenzyl ether of hydroquinone, 4-methoxyphenol, and 88% phenol. Physical modalities, such as cryotherapy and lasers, are also being used successfully.

Special Considerations in Children with Vitiligo 229

Alain Taïeb, Julien Seneschal, and Juliette Mazereeuw-Hautier

Childhood vitiligo differs from adult-onset vitiligo for several features including increased incidence of the segmental variant, higher prevalence of halo nevi, and more common family history for autoimmune diseases and atopic diathesis. The major differential diagnoses are the postinflammatory hypomelanoses for nonsegmental vitiligo and nevus depigmentosus for segmental vitiligo. From a therapeutic standpoint, early awareness of the diagnosis seems to correlate with a good treatment outcome in this age group.

The Role of Diet and Supplements in Vitiligo Management 235

Pearl E. Grimes and Rama Nashawati

Vitiligo is an autoimmune disorder that involves the interplay between oxidative stress and the immune system. Preliminary observations suggest that the presence of gluten in the diet may play a role in vitiligo development in some patients, but to date vitiligo-specific diets have not been studied. The role of oral supplements, including vitamins, minerals, and botanicals, is increasingly being investigated as adjuncts to conventional medical treatment due to their antioxidant and immunomodulatory activity. Studies suggest that many of these agents may have some efficacy as monotherapy, but more often as adjuncts to topical agents and phototherapy.

Genetics of Vitiligo **245**

Richard A. Spritz and Genevieve H.L. Andersen

Vitiligo reflects simultaneous contributions of multiple genetic risk factors and environmental triggers. Genomewide association studies have discovered approximately 50 genetic loci contributing to vitiligo risk. At many vitiligo susceptibility loci, the relevant genes and DNA sequence variants are identified. Many encode proteins involved in immune regulation, several play roles in cellular apoptosis, and others regulate functions of melanocytes. Although many of the specific biologic mechanisms need elucidation, it is clear that vitiligo is an autoimmune disease involving a complex relationship between immune system programming and function, aspects of the melanocyte autoimmune target, and dysregulation of the immune response.

Vitiligo Pathogenesis and Emerging Treatments **257**

Mehdi Rashighi and John E. Harris

The pathogenesis of vitiligo involves interplay between genetic predisposition, environmental triggers, intrinsic melanocyte defects, innate immune inflammation, and T-cell–mediated melanocyte destruction. The goal of treatment is to not only halt disease progression but also promote repigmentation through melanocyte regeneration, proliferation, and migration. Treatment strategies that address all aspects of disease pathogenesis are likely to have greatest efficacy, a strategy that may require combination therapies. Current treatments generally involve nontargeted suppression of autoimmunity, whereas emerging treatments are likely to use a more targeted approach based on in-depth understanding of disease pathogenesis, which may provide higher efficacy with a good safety profile.

Index **267**

DERMATOLOGIC CLINICS

FORTHCOMING ISSUES

July 2017
Atopic Dermatitis
Jonathan I. Silverberg and Nanette Silverberg, *Editors*

October 2017
Non-Invasive Technologies for the Diagnosis of Skin Cancer
Darrell S. Rigel and Aaron S. Farberg, *Editors*

January 2018
Cosmetic Dermatology for Men
Neil S. Sadick, *Editor*

RECENT ISSUES

January 2017
Basic Science Insights into Clinical Puzzles
John J. DiGiovanna, *Editor*

October 2016
Confocal Microscopy
Jane M. Grant-Kels, Giovanni Pellacani, and Caterina Longo, *Editors*

July 2016
Practice Gaps in Dermatology
Murad Alam, *Editor*

ISSUE OF RELATED INTEREST

Pediatric Clinics, April 2014 (Volume 61, Issue 2)
Pediatric Dermatology
Kara N. Shah, *Editor*
Available at: http://www.pediatric.theclinics.com

Preface
Optimizing Vitiligo Management: Past, Present, and Future

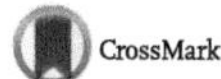

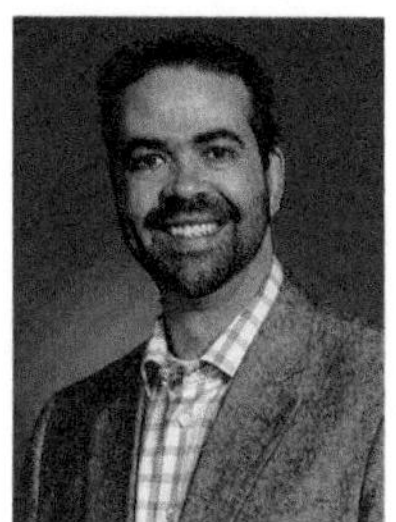

John E. Harris, MD, PhD
Editor

Vitiligo is a very common disease that significantly affects our patients' quality of life. In fact, the mental anguish of patients with vitiligo is comparable to those with psoriasis and other skin diseases. However, compared with psoriasis, our understanding of disease pathogenesis is probably more advanced, while our progress in treatment is far behind. This is likely because psoriasis patients benefit from new biologics and other targeted therapies developed for a wide range of other diseases, yet these treatments are largely ineffective for vitiligo. However, recent advances in our understanding of vitiligo pathogenesis promise to deliver new targeted treatments in the near future.

We have found that many vitiligo patients who attend our clinics have previously seen other dermatologists who told them that vitiligo "wasn't a big deal" or that there was "nothing that could be done for it." In addition, concerns about patients' risk of developing skin cancer, especially from UV-B therapy, have needlessly hampered their treatment. Current topical immunosuppressants, phototherapy, and combined approaches reportedly result in over 75% repigmentation in the majority of patients, with minimal risk. New surgical approaches result in excellent outcomes for most patients with the segmental variant of vitiligo and other stable forms of disease. However, the management strategy must be optimized to achieve the best results.

Our goal in this issue of *Dermatologic Clinics* was to summarize current "best practices" in the management of vitiligo, and also to make recent advances in research accessible to clinicians who are confronted daily with distraught vitiligo patients. Indeed, there is much we can do for these patients, and there is even more on the horizon that should soon make treating this population easier and, yes, even fun! To achieve this goal, clinicians and researchers who are at the forefront of advancements in vitiligo were invited to offer their expertise, advice, and thoughts on future developments in vitiligo. This team effort has resulted in an exciting resource for anyone with an interest in helping the large number of vitiligo patients that seek their advice and entrust themselves to their care.

John E. Harris, MD, PhD
Department of Dermatology
University of Massachusetts Medical School
225 LRB, 364 Plantation Street
Worcester, MA 01605, USA

E-mail address:
John.Harris@umassmed.edu

Dermatol Clin 35 (2017) xi
http://dx.doi.org/10.1016/j.det.2017.01.001
0733-8635/17/© 2017 Published by Elsevier Inc.

The Medical Treatment of Vitiligo: An Historical Review

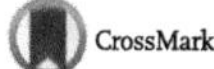

James J. Nordlund, MD[a,b,*]

KEYWORDS

• Vitiligo • Medical treatments • Psoralens • Ultraviolet light

KEY POINTS

- Vitiligo and other disorders causing white spots on the skin have been recognized for thousands of years.
- Vitiligo carries a heavy social burden resulting in banishment, inability to marry, and embarrassment.
- Investigators have sought treatments that range from burning to blistering to tattooing to relieve the suffering of those affected.
- Phototherapy, especially psoralens and exposure to ultraviolet A, have had a modicum of success in treating vitiligo.
- Many other oral and topical agents are used to minimize the scourge of vitiligo.
- Results of new research promise the possibility of a cure that would stop the progression of depigmentation and permit repigmentation in those affected.

You are not just white, but a rainbow of colors. You are not just black, but golden. You are not just a nationality, but a citizen of the world.

— Suzy Kassem, Rise Up and Salute the Sun: The Writings of Suzy Kassem

The color of human skin is remarkable for its breadth of color and fascinating for its science and biology.[1] It ranges from white, to yellow, to brown and even a dark, almost black.[2] Humans have used skin color to distinguish their nation, tribe, and even their family from other peoples, skin color often a designation of friend or foe. The science and biology of skin color remained a mystery until the early twentieth century when melanocytes were described and the chemistry of formation of melanin within the epidermis was worked out.[1]

HISTORY OF LEUKODERMA, WHITE SPOTS, AND VITILIGO

Perfect, flawless skin color is desired by everyone for its beauty and attractiveness. However, like all biologic systems, pigmentation can be abnormal. There can be dark spots or light spots, both of which are disfiguring. These problems have caused distress to people for millennia. Already in 1500 to 1000 BCE, Indian writers described "kilas" and "palita," translated as white or yellowish white spots.[3] The Ebers Papyrus describes people with white spots. In these early writings, the precise condition being described is not known, although leprosy and vitiligo are just two of many possible candidates. There are numerous references to white spots in the Old Testament. Typically these were considered leprosy but it is plausible that much of what was considered to be leprosy was vitiligo or other disorders of skin color.[4] In the Far East prayers known as Makatominoharai dating from 1200 BCE recognized white skin, possibly vitiligo.[5]

In the sixteenth century, Hieronymus Mercurialis[6] published his book on diseases of the skin. In it he devotes an entire chapter, entitled "On Leuce and Alphos," to disorders of abnormal skin color. He cites early Arabic, Greek, and Latin scholars about white spots and notes that the word

Disclaimer: The author has no financial interests or conflicts with any part of this article.

[a] Department of Dermatology, University of Cincinnati College of Medicine, Medical Sciences Building Room 7066, 231 Albert Sabin Way, PO Box 670592, Cincinnati, OH 45267-0592, USA; [b] Department of Dermatology, Boonshoft Wright State College of Medicine, 725 University Boulevard, Fairborn, OH 45234, USA
* Corresponding author. 1156 Riverside Drive, Cincinnati, OH 45202.
E-mail address: jjnordlund@fuse.net

Dermatol Clin 35 (2017) 107–116
http://dx.doi.org/10.1016/j.det.2016.11.001
0733-8635/17/

"...'vitiligo' is a Latin word derived from either 'vitium' (blemish) or 'vitulum' (small blemish)..." The word vitiligo might have been first used by Celsus.[7] Mercurialis suggests that phlegm accumulating under the skin was the source of leukoderma, a theory that he confirms from the writings of "...divine Plato...that white phlegm has two effects in the body....if it begins to vent through the exterior of the body, it will cause ...vitiligo."[6] Herodotus in Greece noted white spots on foreigners and suggested they be banished immediately, their having sinned against the sun.[5]

In China and Korea, writers discussed white spots and white skin. In Korea vitiligo and other pigmentary disorders, such as nevus depigmentosus or tinea versicolor, were described in Doney Bogam, published in the seventeenth century.[5] A portrait of Chang-Myeong Song, a high ranking official of the Yi dynasty of Korea, was painted about this time that shows the typical depigmentation of vitiligo.[5]

In the seventeenth century, William Byrd[8] described "An Account of a Negro-Boy that is, dappel'd in several places of his Body with White Spots." The depigmentation began at age 3 years and continued to spread. Byrd conjectures that in time the boy would become all white. The leukoderma was obviously mysterious in origin.

Brito[9] in the nineteenth century discussed vitiligo. He emphasized the social stigma of white spots and their capacity to disfigure. "The appearance of the unfortunate victims of vitiligo is striking, and scarcely fails to evoke a feeling of horror and pity for the afflicted,...The picture of otherwise dark person,...marked with spots perfectly white,...to even eyes familiarized to the sight, appears repugnant."[9]

The worldwide distribution of these reports dating back thousands of years attests that vitiligo was and is ubiquitous. The comments of some of the previously quoted authors confirm its deleterious effects on those who suffer from it. It is often said that vitiligo is only a cosmetic problem. It is not entirely true that vitiligo does not affect the physical functioning of the body in any detrimental way. There are pigment cells in organs and tissues other than skin, such as the eye, inner ear, and leptomeninges.[10] Vitiligo can affect choroidal melanocytes and retinal pigment epithelium causing iritis and chorioretinitis.[11–13] Vogt-Koyanagi syndrome is characterized by unilateral vitiligo, poliosis, meningitis, and dysacusia, probable manifestations of melanocyte destruction in each of these organs and tissues.[11] These extracutaneous manifestations of vitiligo rarely cause loss of visual acuity or hearing. Regardless vitiligo like albinism causes immense social, emotional, and personal pain and disability. Even today in the middle east, young people with vitiligo find it an impediment to finding a marriageable partner. The plethora of treatments (**Table 1**) proposed and tried for thousands of years attest to its significance in all cultures and societies. Its detrimental effects on quality of life have now been thoroughly studied and are well characterized.[14,15]

STUDY OF SKIN COLOR AND WHITE SPOTS

Skin color was a mystery until modern times after the invention of the microscope, the techniques

Table 1
Historical treatments for vitiligo

ACTH	Levamisole
Agaric, turpeth, and colocynth	Mefloquin
Anapsos	Melaginina
Anthralin	Methotrexate
Arsenic	Minigrafting autografts
Aspirin	Minoxidil
Bergamot	Monoamine oxidase inhibitors
Bavachee seeds	Monobenzyl ether of hydroquinone
Bitter almonds in vinegar	Mustard
Byzantine syrup	Oxymel
Cantharidin	Pimecrolimus
Carmustine (BCNU)	Phenylalanine-ultraviolet A
Clofazimine	Psoralens + sunlight
Chloroquine	Psoralens + ultraviolet A
Copper	Pseudocatalase
Corrosive sublimate	Quinacrine
Cosmetics	Resorcin paste
Crude coal tar	Rose-flavored honey
Cryotherapy	Selective diets
Cyclophosphamide	Steroids oral or topical
Cyclosporine	Surgical excision
Dapsone	Syrup of betony
Dermabrasion	Tacrolimus
Dopa oral and topical	Tattooing
Escharotics	Thermal and caustic blistering
Finsen lamp	Tincture of nux vomica
Fluorouracil	Tretinoin
Fluphenazine enanthate	Ultraviolet B narrow band
Folic acid	Vesicants
Hydrochloric acid	Vibrapuncture
Hydrogen peroxide	Vitamin B_6
Injections of silver nitrate	Vitamin B_{12}
Iron	Vitamin C
Isoprinosine	Vitamin D
Khellin oral and topical	Vitamin E

Adapted from Montes LF. Vitiligo: current knowledge and nutritional therapy. 3rd edition. Buenos Aires: Westhoven Press; 2006.

of biopsy, and the discovery of histochemical stains. Before the seventeenth century, the origin of skin color was based on myths, folklore, and religious theories. Explanations attempted to explain the origin of dark skin color, not why some skin was very light. Jean Roland in 1618 separated the epidermis from the dermis of a black individual. He was able to observe the upper layer of skin (epidermis) was pigmented, the lower dermal layer not pigmented.[16] He proposed that sunlight and heat caused dark skin, a theory that might explain dark skin at the equator but not why Europeans remained white when traveling to southern climes. Another scientist, Thomas Browne, noted this discrepancy and decided skin color was a genetic trait carried within the sperm.[16]

Theories about the mechanism for production of skin color came and went. Many famous investigators, such as van Leeuwenhoek, John Hunter, Immanuel Kant, and Marcello Malpighi, all studied skin color usually in deeply pigmented Ethiopians, often on cadavers but occasionally in living subjects. However, without proper instruments and techniques, the origins of pigmentation remained a mystery. More mysterious back then were the mechanisms for loss of skin color. Benjamin Rush suggested that black skin of Negroes was a form of leprosy and that vitiligo was an indication of spontaneous cure.[16]

HISTORY OF TREATMENT OF VITILIGO

The treatment of white spots or vitiligo has been tried for as long as white spots and/or vitiligo have been recognized. A partial list of therapies tried over the centuries is presented in **Table 1**. Detailed descriptions of methods, mostly ineffective, are found in ancient texts.[17] The stigma of white spots in ancient times was frightening. In the Old Testament, those with white spots/vitiligo were considered unclean from leprosy or sinful, the spots a punishment from God. They were rejected from society.[7] Herodotus noted that those affected had sinned against the sun and were to be driven from Greece.[5] In the sixteenth century Mercurialis acknowledged that the appearance of those with white spots was objectionable. He stated white spots were so offensive that if blistering medications applied topically were not helpful, then fire itself (the actual cautery) was to be applied on the parts involved with care taken to avoid scarring if possible.[6] Even in the nineteenth century, the mechanism for skin color, for white spots, and their treatment were unknown.[9] Brito[9] made a list of therapeutic possibilities for treatment that included escharotics; surgical excision; grafts; injections of dark substances, such as silver nitrate into the dermis; tattooing, or administration of silver salts by mouth.

Early phototherapy was recorded in the Atharva Veda. Black colored seeds combined with other herbs were prepared in an attempt to make the skin an even color as described in this poem.

Born by night art thou, O plant,

Dark, black, sable, do thou,

That art rich in color,

Stain this leprosy and white gray spots.

Even color is the name of thy mother,

Even color is the name of thy father,

Thou O plant produces even color

Render this even color.[4]

The black seeds probably were from the plant *Bavachee*, which contained psoralens and probably had some success following exposure to sunlight.[18] Other references to use of plants containing psoralens, such as *Psoralea corylifolia*, are found in Buddhist, Chinese, and Egyptian writings.[18] In the early twentieth century the Finsen light seemed to be the first treatment offering some hope to those with vitiligo.[19] The Finsen light was a source of short ultraviolet waves produced by a carbon or mercury arc. These observations were confirmed by Menon[20] who exposed patients to ultraviolet light with visible perifollicular repigmentation occurring after a series of treatments.

Psoralens and exposure to ultraviolet light A (PUVA) was started by an Egyptian physician, Abdel Moneim El-Mofty. He cited Bloch's observations that dopa stains for melanocytes were negative in vitiliginous skin.[21] He described the early use of crude extracts from plants containing psoralen followed by exposure to sunlight until inflammation and vesiculation occurred. After the blisters ruptured and the patch healed pigmentation was often restored. Early forms of PUVA using crude extracts were associated with severe gastrointestinal distress and rarely coma followed by death.[21]

El-Mofty[21] isolated from the *Ammi majus Linn* plant a purified form of psoralen that was safer and more tolerable than the original plant extracts. He tested a topical and oral form of the psoralen and found that together they produced the best repigmentation, although alone they were partially successful. He later purified and identified 8-methoxypsoralen (also termed xanthotoxin) and 4,5,8-trimethylpsoralen.[22] Subsequent studies confirmed his earlier observations that psoralens were capable of producing repigmentation in patches of vitiligo, sometimes totally repigmenting white skin, sometimes inducing only partial repigmentation.[23] Typically repigmentation begins as freckling, a manifestation of melanocyte proliferation within hair follicles and migration to the interfollicular skin (**Figs. 1** and **2**).[24] The pigmentation spreads to produce almost total repigmentation, although the PUVA treatments take a year or more (**Figs. 3** and **4**).

A year later, Lerner and Fitzpatrick,[25] giants in pigment cell biology, published their results from studies using PUVA treatments on nine patients with vitiligo. Three of their patients showed striking improvement (**Figs. 3** and **4** illustrate an excellent response), two showed partial response, and four had no response. Three of the nine also exhibited marked increase in tolerance to the erythromogenic properties of sunlight, an effect of psoralens noted by El-Mofty.[20] The authors also treated three albinos with oral 8-methoxypsoralen for 2 to 3 months and all showed lessened sun sensitivity. Toxicity studies indicated that 8-methoxypsoralen had a good safety profile. They also observed that the absorption spectrum of psoralen was maximal at 3200 Å units.[25]

The safety and efficacy of 8-methoxypsoralen and 4,5,8-trimethylpsoralen were confirmed by Pathak and colleagues[26] in 1984 from a study on 366 Indian subjects with vitiligo treated for up to 2 years. Patients receiving a combination of 8-methoxypsoralen and 4,5,8-trimethylpsoralen did especially well, 45% of them fully repigmenting their faces and 67% regaining most of the color of their faces and necks. Hands and feet (glabrous skin) did not respond, as is well known now because of a missing melanocyte reservoir (see **Figs. 3**A and **4A**).[24] The investigators noted long-term treatments were required for significant repigmentation (see **Fig. 3** and **4**). Very little toxicity was observed. From all these data, PUVA became the standard treatment for vitiligo.

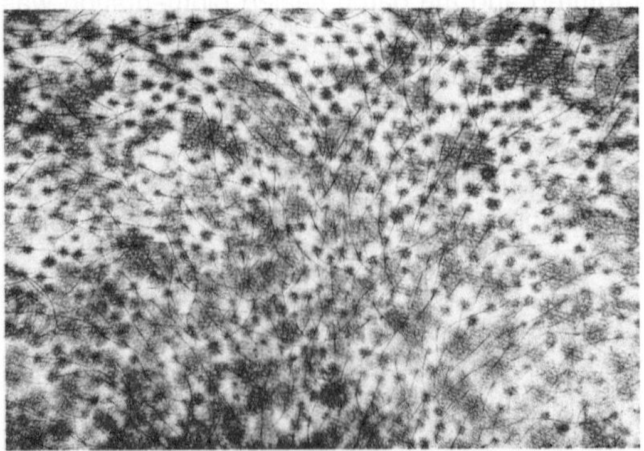

Fig. 1. Early perifollicular repigmentation that is typically observed following successful repigmentation.

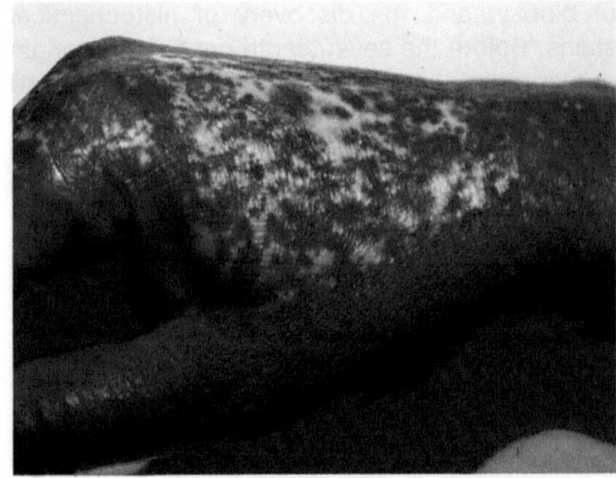

Fig. 2. Perifollicular repigmentation coalescing into large areas of normal skin color.

In other studies investigators demonstrated that PUVA interfered with cell division. From this information, PUVA was shown to be effective for treatment of psoriasis, mycosis fungoides, and other cutaneous disorders.[27] To facilitate the use of PUVA and minimize its photosensitizing capabilities, Fitzpatrick[28] developed the photosensitivity skin reactive scale, which has since been used to classify the depth of skin color. PUVA became the treatment of choice for a wide variety of disorders.

More recently phototherapy has undergone a change. It has been observed that narrow band ultraviolet light B (NBUVB; 311-nm wave length) is as efficacious as PUVA for vitiligo and other conditions.[29–31] NBUVB has been combined with various topical medications, such as calcipotriene,[32–34] with success. A special form of NBUVB, the excimer laser with a 308-nm emission spectrum, has been found to be useful especially in treating localized skin disorders. These topics are discussed in detail elsewhere in this issue.

OTHER ORAL THERAPIES FOR VITILIGO

The need for treatment of vitiligo continues to be great. A long list of suggested treatment has been compiled (see **Table 1**).[35] Phototherapies, such as PUVA, were the first treatments for vitiligo that had at least a modicum of success. Treatments even today are unable to inactivate the vitiliginous pathophysiology and halt progression of the disease or recurrence after successful repigmentation. If there were a safe medication that could be used by children and adults that stopped permanently the progression of depigmentation at its earliest manifestations or after successful treatment, the problem of vitiligo would be mostly solved. Many patients do not respond at all to any treatment and vitiligo often

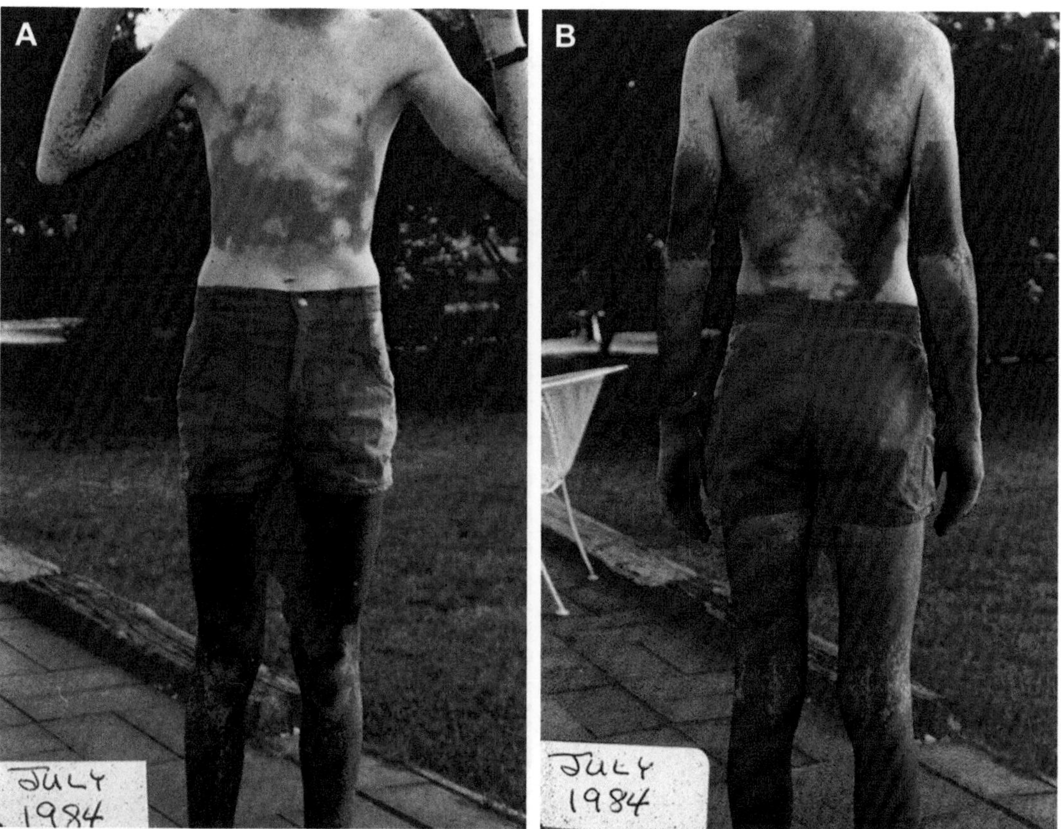

Fig. 3. (*A, B*) Teenage boy with extensive depigmentation from vitiligo before treatment in July 1984.

recurs after the therapy is completed. Other treatments have been developed, some using other oral medications and some topical agents. PUVA has had reasonable success but does carry some risks of skin cancer, cataracts and other ocular dysfunction, and additional problems.[26,27,36–38] More modern alternatives that could be used in lieu or in combination with psoralens have been sought.

Phenylalanine

Phenylalanine is an amino acid found in all proteins. It is a precursor to tyrosine, the substrate for melanin. It has been proposed as a substitute for psoralens in combination with ultraviolet light.[39,40] Recipients have had reasonable success. In particular it has been advocated for children in lieu of psoralens.[41]

Antimalarials

Before PUVA was established as a standard for the treatment of vitiligo, antimalarials were tried including chloroquine and mepacrine[42,43] with slight success.

Khellin

Khellin is a furochrome originally used to dilate cardiac arteries. It is known to be photosensitizing.[44] It has been successfully used to treat patients with vitiligo.[45,46] It is much less photosensitizing to the surrounding skin.

Levamisole

Levamisole, an antihelminthic agent with a wide range of immunomodulatory actions, has been used successfully as monotherapy for a variety of skin diseases.[47] In one study on patients with actively spreading vitiligo, levamisole seemed to halt the progression of the depigmentation.[48] Adverse effects of levamisole are mild and infrequent and include rash, nausea, abdominal cramps, taste alteration, alopecia, arthralgias, and a flulike syndrome. More recently levamisole has been used with illicit narcotics with serious toxicity.[47]

Folic Acid

Folic acid is a vitamin easily available commercially in most drug stores and in many foods. It has been found to be deficient in the blood

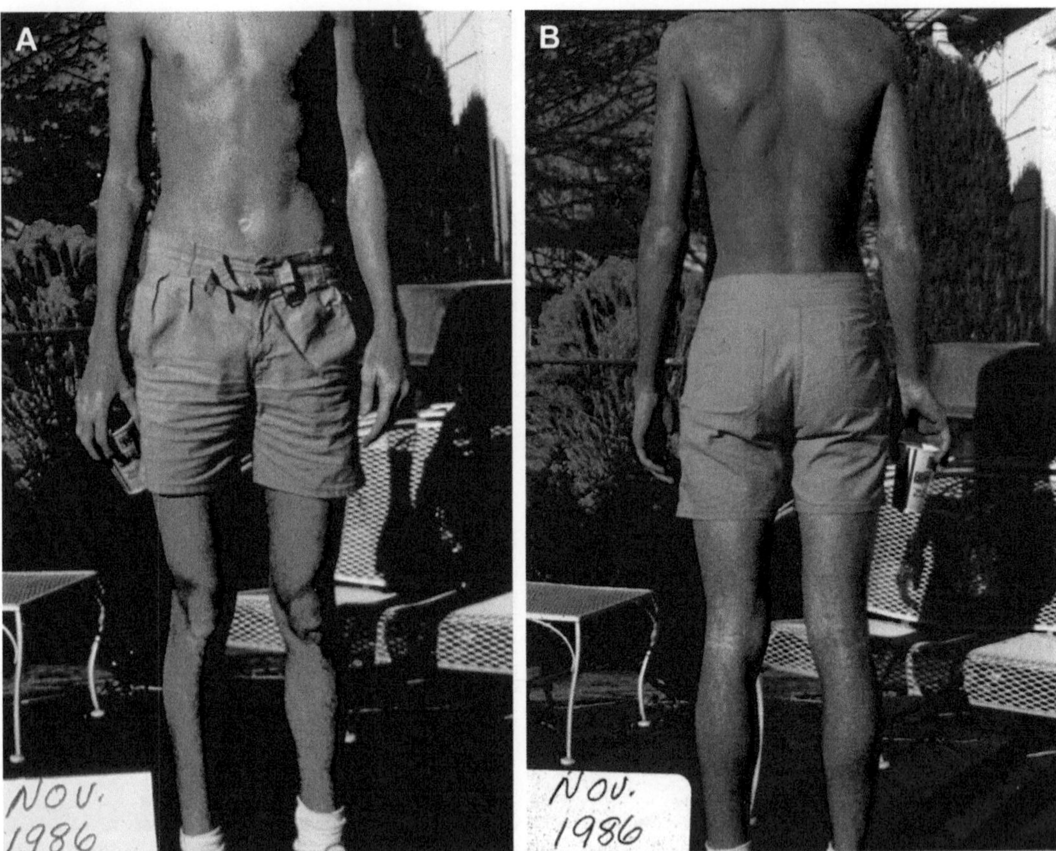

Fig. 4. (*A, B*) Teenage boy with excellent repigmentation from PUVA in November 1986. The prolonged treatment time is typical. Note the hands are not repigmented because glabrous skin lacks a reservoir of melanocytes in the hair follicle.

of some patients with vitiligo.[35] Montes[35] in Argentina has treated and reported on 135 individuals with vitiligo treated with folic acid and exposure to natural sunlight. The dose of folic acid in adults ranged from 5 mg to 10 mg daily for a duration up to 5 years.[35] The folic acid was supplemented with vitamin B_{12} and vitamin C in 60 patients. No toxicity was observed in any patients. Many patients regained significant pigmentation, some totally repigmenting.[35]

Clofazimine

Clofazimine is best known for its efficacy in treating leprosy. However, it has been used for other conditions including lupus and vitiligo. Bor[49] reported from South Africa that clofazimine was effective when combined with sun exposure for repigmenting nine patients with vitiligo.

TOPICAL THERAPIES FOR VITILIGO

Topical Steroids

Vitiligo has been considered an immune-mediated disorder. Medications, such as topical steroids, that alter immune function in the skin have been proposed as possible treatment for vitiligo. They have had success as monotherapies and in combination with various forms of phototherapy or other topical agents, such as calcipotriene.[50–52] Topical steroids seem safer for treatment of children than PUVA, especially because the long-term deleterious effects of PUVA are now known.

Calcineurin Inhibitors

Calcineurin inhibitors, tacrolimus and pimecrolimus, have been tried alone and with NBUVB for treatment of various forms of vitiligo.[4,53–55] Both agents have shown reasonable success, although the role of ultraviolet light seems more important.[56]

Vitamin D Derivatives

Various forms of vitamin D derivatives (calcipotriene and calcipotriol) have been tried for treatment of vitiligo. It is known that melanocytes contain vitamin D receptors within their cytoplasm and their growth is promoted by this vitamin.[4,57]

Applied topically, the vitamin D derivatives seemed to enhance and accelerate repigmentation[32,34,58] but their overall effects were minimal.[33,59]

5-Fluorouracil

Topical application of 5% 5-fluorouracil has been reported by two investigators to produce repigmentation in patches of vitiligo.[60,61]

Pseudocatalase

It has been suggested that melanocytes are particularly sensitive to the effects of H_2O_2 and their cytoplasm has low levels of catalase to catalyze its destruction.[62] A topically applied pseudocatalase has been reported to be effective in eliminating the peroxide thereby permitting in combination with ultraviolet light melanocyte proliferation and repigmentation of vitiliginous spots.[62,63] However, subsequent studies from several countries around the world fail to confirm the original results.[64–67]

Cosmetics

Depigmented macules on the face, neck, and hands, visible to everyone, are cosmetically very distressing. Cosmetics are helpful[68,69] but are not the real solution. For men or young children using cosmetics that are visible to others is socially unacceptable. Cosmetics can rub off in more intimate situations. The patient, who must spend long times daily applying them, still is subject to his/her own feelings of disfigurement underlying the cover up paints. They help but are not the solution.

Depigmentation

Vitiligo can destroy much or most of the pigmentation on the face, neck, hands, forearms, and other areas. Hands and feet are glabrous skin, that is, have no hair follicles from which melanocytes can be recruited for repigmentation.[24] It is possible to remove the remaining pigment from these areas with application of monobenzone (monobenzyl ether of hydroquinone). The most famous example of a person using depigmentation therapy is the singer Michael Jackson. Although the process takes time it is successful in making the person one color, albeit not the original and more desirable normal skin color. However, for those who choose this approach, their lives are greatly improved and they are universally pleased. In my personal experience of having depigmented more than 200 carefully selected patients over the years, it has been most successful.

SUMMARY

That any type of depigmented skin can cause social problems is a real problem even today. People especially in the middle east afflicted with vitiligo might have a difficult time finding employment and often are not marriageable. Jawaharlal Nehru, the first prime minister of India, indicated that vitiligo was one of the major hurdles retarding the modernization of India because of its deleterious social effects.

Albinism is less common than vitiligo although its prevalence in Africa is 10 times greater than that in European and American countries. Albinism is an autosomal-recessive genetic disorder. There are seven genetic types of albinism in which the epidermis, eyes, ears, and meninges retain their melanocyte population but the melanocytes are incapable of producing melanin. All people with albinism have type 1 skin color.[28] Living in sun-drenched countries of Africa, about 50% get skin cancers, almost all squamous cell carcinomas (**Fig. 5**). Basal cell carcinomas and melanomas are rare in albino skin for reasons not known. In contrast, people with vitiligo almost never get skin cancers on their depigmented skin, although they also have type 1 skin color. Melanomas by definition cannot arise in vitiligo skin devoid of melanocytes. In contrast, individuals with metastatic melanoma develop a vitiligo-like depigmentation that seems to herald a prolonged survival.[70] Like people with vitiligo, those with albinism even today are the brunt of severe social abuse, ostracism, and sometimes mutilation and death.

Although treatments for vitiligo have improved, there still is no cure or a medication to stop its advancing to new areas of skin. Were there a

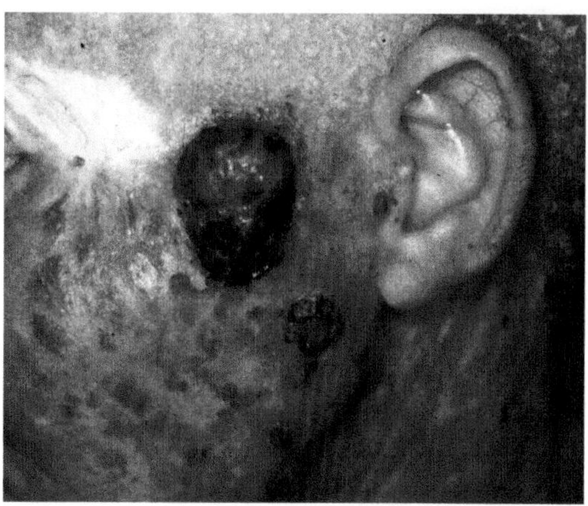

Fig. 5. Squamous cell carcinoma and sun damage on the cheek of an albino woman (OCA [oculocutaneous albinism] 2) living in Tanzania. Note scar from a prior squamous cell carcinoma successfully treated.

safe medication that could halt the progression of vitiligo permanently, the clinical and social problems arising from vitiligo would be mostly solved. To my disappointment, that goal was not achieved during my professional career. However, the advances and new science outlined in this issue bring real hope that such a cure is near at hand.

REFERENCE

1. Nordlund J, Boissy RE, Hearing VJ, et al. The pigmentary system: physiology and pathophysiology. 2nd edition. Oxford (England): Blackwell Scientific Publishers; 2006.
2. Greenwood M. Varfor Grater Puman? Tryckt i Belgien: Bra Bocker; 1984.
3. Berger BJ, Rudolph RI, Leyden JJ. Leyden. Vitiligo in ancient Indian medicine. Arch Dermatol 1974; 109:913.
4. Goldman L, Moraites R, Kitzmiller RW. White spots in biblical times. Arch Dermatol 1966;93:744–53.
5. Kopera D. History and cultural aspects of vitiligo. In: Hann S-K, Nordlund J, editors. Vitiligo: a monograph on the basic and clinical science. Oxford (England): Blackwell Scientific Publishers; 2000. p. 13–7.
6. Mercurialis H. Mercurialis on disease of the skin. In: Sixteenth century physician and his methods. Kansas City (MO): Lowell Press; 1572. p. 226.
7. Ortonne JP. Vitiligo. In: Ortonne JP, Mosher DB, Fitzpatrick TB, editors. Vitiligo and other hypomelanoses of hair and skin. New York: Plenum Medical Book Company; 1982. p. 652.
8. Byrd W. An account of a negro-boy that is dappel'd in several places of his body with white spots. Phil Trans 1695–1697;19:781–2.
9. Brito PS. On leucoderm, vitiligo, ven kuttam (Tamil) or cabbare (Singhalese), and several new methods of treatment. Br Med J 1885;1(1269):834–5.
10. Boissy R, Hornyak TJ. Extracutaneous melanocytes. In: Nordlund JJ, Hearing VJ, King RA, et al, editors. The pigmentary system: physiology and pathophysiology. 2nd edition. Oxford (England): Blackwell Scientific Press; 2006. p. 91–107.
11. Albert DM, Nordlund JJ, Lerner AB. Ocular abnormalities occurring with vitiligo. Ophthalmology 1979;86(6): 1145–60.
12. Albert DM, Wagoner MD, Pruett RC, et al. Vitiligo and disorders of the retinal pigment epithelium. Br J Ophthalmol 1983;67:153–6.
13. Nordlund JJ, Taylor NT, Albert DM, et al. The prevalence of vitiligo and poliosis in patients with uveitis. J Am Acad Dermatol 1981;4(5):528–36.
14. Olsen JR, Gallacher J, Finlay AY, et al. Quality of life impact of childhood skin conditions measured using the children's dermatology life quality index (CDLQI): a meta-analysis. Br J Dermatol 2016; 174(4):853–61.
15. Porter J, Beuf AH, Lerner A, et al. Response to cosmetic disfigurement: patients with vitiligo. Cutis 1987;39(6):493–4.
16. Klaus S. The history of the science of pigmentation. In: Nordlund JJ, Hearing VJ, King RA, et al, editors. The pigmentary system: physiology and pathophysiology. 2nd edition. Oxford (England): Blackwell Publishing; 2008. p. 5–18.
17. Benedetto A. The psoralens: an historical perspective. Cutis 1977;20:469–71.
18. Fitzpatrick TB, Pathak MA. Historical aspects of methoxsalen and other furocoumarins. J Invest Dermatol 1959;31:229–31.
19. Ormsby O. Pigment anomalies. In: Diseases of the skin. Philadelphia: Lea and Febiger; 1927. p. 585–9.
20. Menon AN. Ultra-violet therapy in cases of leucoderma. Ind Med Gaz 1945;80:612–4.
21. El-Mofty AM. A preliminary clinical report on the treatment of leucodermia with *Ammi majus Linn.* J Egypt Med Assoc 1948;31:651–65.
22. El-Mofty AM. Further study on treatment of leucodermia with *Ammi mafus Linn.* J Egypt Med Assoc 1952;35(1):1–2.
23. El-Mofty AM. Observations on the use of *Ammi majus Linn.* In vitiligo. Br J Dermatol 1952;64(12):431–41.
24. Cui J, Shen LY, Wang GC. Role of hair follicles in the repigmentation of vitiligo. J Invest Dermatol 1991; 97(3):410–6.
25. Lerner AB, Denton CR, Fitzpatrick TB. Clinical and experimental studies with 8-methoxypsoralen in vitiligo. J Invest Dermatol 1953;20(4):299–314.
26. Pathak MA, Mosher DB, Fitzpatrick TB. Safety and therapeutic effectiveness of 8-methoxypsoralen, 4,5',8-trimethylpsoralen, and psoralen in vitiligo. Natl Cancer Inst Monogr 1984;66:165–73.
27. Pathak MA, Fitzpatrick TB. The evolution of photochemotherapy with psoralens and UVA (PUVA): 2000 BC to 1992 AD. J Photochem Photobiol B 1992;14(1–2):3–22.
28. Fitzpatrick TB. The validity and practicality of sun-reactive skin types I through VI. Arch Dermatol 1988; 124:869–71.
29. Parsad D, Kanwar AJ, Kumar B. Psoralen-ultraviolet A vs. narrow-band ultraviolet B phototherapy for the treatment of vitiligo. J Eur Acad Dermatol Venereol 2006;20(2):175–7.
30. Njoo MD, Bos JD, Westerhof W. Treatment of generalized vitiligo in children with narrow-band (TL-01) UVB radiation therapy. J Am Acad Dermatol 2000; 42(2 Pt 1):245–53.
31. Scherschun L, Kim JJ, Lim HW. Narrow-band ultraviolet B is a useful and well-tolerated treatment for vitiligo. J Am Acad Dermatol 2001;44(6):999–1003.
32. Arca E, Tastan HB, Erbil AH, et al. Narrow-band ultraviolet B as monotherapy and in combination with topical calcipotriol in the treatment of vitiligo. J Dermatol 2006;33(5):338–43.

33. Ada S, Sahin S, Boztepe G, et al. No additional effect of topical calcipotriol on narrow-band UVB phototherapy in patients with generalized vitiligo. Photodermatol Photoimmunol Photomed 2005;21(2):79–83.
34. Kullavanijaya P, Lim HW. Topical calcipotriene and narrowband ultraviolet B in the treatment of vitiligo. Photodermatol Photoimmunol Photomed 2004; 20(5):248–51.
35. Montes LF. Vitiligo: current knowledge and nutritional therapy. 3rd edition. Buenos Aires (Argentina): Westhoven Press; 2006.
36. Abdullah AN, Keczkes K. Cutaneous and ocular side-effects of PUVA photochemotherapy: a 10-year follow-up study. Clin Exp Dermatol 1989; 14(6):421–4.
37. Wildfang IL, Jacobsen FK, Thestrup-Pedersen K. PUVA treatment of vitiligo: a retrospective study of 59 patients. Acta Derm Venereol 1992;72(4):305–6.
38. Park SH, Hann SK, Park YK. Ten-year experience of phototherapy in Yonsei Medical Center. Yonsei Med J 1996;37(6):392–6.
39. Beretti B, Grupper D, Bermejo B, et al. PUVA 5-MOP + phenylalanine in the treatment of vitiligo. Study of 125 patients: preliminary results. In: Fitzpatrick TB, Forlot P, Pathak M, et al, editors. Psoralens: past, present and future of photochemoprotection and other biological activities. 1st edition. Paris: John Libbey Eurotext; 1989. p. 103–8.
40. Cormane RH, Siddiqui AH, Westerhof W, et al. Phenylalanine and UVA light for the treatment of vitiligo. Arch Dermatol Res 1985;277(2):126–30.
41. Schulpis CH, Antoniou C, Michas T, et al. Phenylalanine plus ultraviolet light: preliminary report of a promising treatment for childhood vitiligo. Pediatr Dermatol 1989;6(4):332–5.
42. Pegum JS. Vitiligo treated with mepacrine. Br J Dermatol 1953;65(9):324–5.
43. Christiansen J. Vitiligo treated with chloroquine: a preliminary report. Acta Derm Venereol 1955;35(6): 453–6.
44. Vedaldi D, Caffieri S, Dall'Acqua F, et al. Khellin, a naturally occurring furochromone, used for the photochemotherapy of skin diseases: mechanism of action. Farmaco Sci 1988;43(4):333–46.
45. Abdel-Fattah A, Aboul-Enein MN, Wassel GM, et al. An approach to the treatment of vitiligo by khellin. Dermatologica 1982;165(2):136–40.
46. Carlie G, Ntusi NB, Hulley PA, et al. KUVA (khellin plus ultraviolet A) stimulates proliferation and melanogenesis in normal human melanocytes and melanoma cells in vitro. Br J Dermatol 2003;149(4):707–17.
47. Scheinfeld N, Rosenberg JD, Weinberg JM. Levamisole in dermatology: a review. Am J Clin Dermatol 2004;5:97–104.
48. Pasricha JS, Khera V. Effect of prolonged treatment with levamisole on vitiligo with limited and slow-spreading disease. Int J Dermatol 1994; 33(8):584–7.
49. Bor S. Clofazimine (lamprene) in the treatment of vitiligo. S Afr Med J 1973;47(32):1451–4.
50. Kwinter J, Pelletier J, Khambalia A, et al. High-potency steroid use in children with vitiligo: a retrospective study. J Am Acad Dermatol 2007;56(2):236–41.
51. Bleehen SS. The treatment of vitiligo with topical corticosteroids. Light and electronmicroscopic studies. Br J Dermatol 1976;94(Suppl 12):43–50.
52. Hann SH. Steroid treatment for vitiligo. In: Nordlund J, editor. Vitiligo: a monograph on the basic and clinical science. Oxford (England): Blackwell Science; 2000. p. 173–81.
53. Sardana K, Bhushan P, Kumar Garg V. Effect of tacrolimus on vitiligo in absence of UV radiation exposure. Arch Dermatol 2007;143(1):119 [author reply: 20].
54. Dawid M, Veensalu M, Grassberger M, et al. Efficacy and safety of pimecrolimus cream 1% in adult patients with vitiligo: results of a randomized, double-blind, vehicle-controlled study. J Dtsch Dermatol Ges 2006;4(11):942–6.
55. Grimes PE, Soriano T, Dytoc MT. Topical tacrolimus for repigmentation of vitiligo. J Am Acad Dermatol 2002;47(5):789–91.
56. Ostovari N, Passeron T, Lacour JP, et al. Lack of efficacy of tacrolimus in the treatment of vitiligo in the absence of UV-B exposure. Arch Dermatol 2006; 142(2):252–3.
57. Abdel-Malek Z, Kadekaro AL. Human pigmentation: its regulation by ultraviolet light and by endocrine, paracrine and autocrine factors. In: Nordlund J, Boissy RE, Hearing VJ, et al, editors. The pigmentary system: physiology and pathophysiology. 2nd edition. Oxford (England): Blackwell Scientific; 2006. p. 394–409.
58. Chiaverini C, Passeron T, Ortonne JP. Treatment of vitiligo by topical calcipotriol. J Eur Acad Dermatol Venereol 2002;16(2):137–8.
59. Baysal V, Yildirim M, Erel A, et al. Is the combination of calcipotriol and PUVA effective in vitiligo? J Eur Acad Dermatol Venereol 2003;17(3):299–302.
60. Szekeres E, Morvay M. Repigmentation of vitiligo macules treated topically with Efudex cream. Dermatologica 1985;171(1):55–9.
61. Tsuji T, Hamada T. Topically administered fluorouracil in vitiligo. Arch Dermatol 1983;119(9): 722–7.
62. Schallreuter K, Moore J, Wood J. Pseudocatalase in the treatment of vitiligo. In: Hann S-K, Nordlund J, editors. Vitiligo: monograph on basic and clinical science. 1st edition. Oxford (England): Blackwell Science Ltd; 2000. p. 182–92.
63. Schallreuter KU, Wood JM, Lemke KR, et al. Treatment of vitiligo with a topical application of pseudocatalase and calcium in combination with

short-term UVB exposure: a case study on 33 patients [see comments]. Dermatology 1995;190(3): 223–9.
64. Naini FF, Shooshtari AV, Ebrahimi B, et al. The effect of pseudocatalase/superoxide dismutase in the treatment of vitiligo: a pilot study. J Res Pharm Pract 2012;1(2):77–80.
65. Gawkrodger DJ. Pseudocatalase and narrowband ultraviolet B for vitiligo: clearing the picture. Br J Dermatol 2009;161(4):721–2.
66. Bakis-Petsoglou S, Le Guay JL, Wittal R. A randomized, double-blinded, placebo-controlled trial of pseudocatalase cream and narrowband ultraviolet B in the treatment of vitiligo. Br J Dermatol 2009;161(4):910–7.
67. Patel DC, Evans AV, Hawk JL. Topical pseudocatalase mousse and narrowband UVB phototherapy is not effective for vitiligo: an open, single-centre study. Clin Exp Dermatol 2002;27(8):641–4.
68. Goldstein E, Haberman HF, Menon IA, et al. Non-psoralen treatment of vitiligo. Part I. Cosmetics, systemic coloring agents, and corticosteroids. Int J Dermatol 1992;31(4):229–36.
69. Boehncke WH, Ochsendorf F, Paeslack I, et al. Decorative cosmetics improve the quality of life in patients with disfiguring skin diseases. Eur J Dermatol 2002;12(6):577–80.
70. Nordlund JJ, Kirkwood JM, Forget BM, et al. Vitiligo in patients with metastatic melanoma: a good prognostic sign. J Am Acad Dermatol 1983;9(5):689–96.

Quality of Life, Burden of Disease, Co-morbidities, and Systemic Effects in Vitiligo Patients

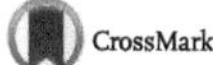

Nada Elbuluk, MD, MSc[a,*], Khaled Ezzedine, MD, PhD[b]

KEYWORDS

• Vitiligo • Comorbidities • Autoimmune diseases • Systemic • Quality of life • Burden • Depression

KEY POINTS

- Vitiligo is a disfiguring systemic disease with a complex and multifactorial pathogenesis.
- Vitiligo is associated with many autoimmune (AI) and autoinflammatory conditions that may be owing to shared AI and genetic susceptibilities.
- Vitiligo has a major impact on quality of life and self-esteem.
- Depression, anxiety, and other psychiatric comorbidities are common in vitiligo patients.
- Increased awareness of quality of life issues will help to ensure that vitiligo is no longer dismissed as a cosmetic or insignificant disease.

Vitiligo is an acquired chronic autoimmune (AI) pigmentation disorder resulting in patchy, white, nonscaly macules and patches. The worldwide prevalence of the disease is estimated to be around 1%.[1] Vitiligo is also a disfiguring disease that, despite its profound impact on quality of life and its frequent association with other comorbid AI diseases, is still considered a cosmetic condition.[2]

COMORBIDITIES AND SYSTEMIC EFFECTS

The etiology and pathogenesis of vitiligo is complex and multifactorial, including theories of AI, genetic, neural, cytotoxic, biochemical, oxidative, melanocyte, inflammatory, and hormonal origin.[3–7] Multiple susceptibility genes and various environmental triggers have also been associated with having a role in the pathogenesis of vitiligo.[8] Studies have also shown that vitiligo patients, including those with an AI or autoinflammatory disease, are more likely to have a family member with an AI disease, supporting the theory of a genetic AI susceptibility.[1,3,9] The AI origin of vitiligo, which includes cellular and humoral immunity, has been widely supported through the presence of circulating antibodies against melanocyte antigens whose levels correlate with disease activity, the immune-mediated destruction of melanocytes from vitiliginous skin, and the increased prevalence of associated AI disorders.[3,9,10]

Multiple studies have shown that individuals with vitiligo have an increased incidence (up to 25%) of other AI and inflammatory conditions.[10–12] These include AI thyroid disease (AITD), type I diabetes mellitus, pernicious anemia (PA), rheumatoid arthritis (RA), alopecia areata (AA), atopic dermatitis (AD), Addison's disease, psoriasis, dermatitis herpetiformis, celiac disease, systemic lupus erythematous (SLE), Sjögren syndrome

Disclosures: The authors have no financial conflicts of interest to disclose.
[a] Ronald O. Perelman Department of Dermatology, NYU Ambulatory Care Center, NYU Langone Medical Center, 240 East 38th Street, 12th Floor, New York, NY 10016, USA; [b] Department of Dermatology, EpiDermE, Henri Mondor Hospital, Université Paris-Est Créteil Val-de-Marne, 51 Avenue du Maréchal de Lattre de Tassigny, Créteil 94010, France
* Corresponding author.
E-mail address: Nada.elbuluk@nyumc.org

Dermatol Clin 35 (2017) 117–128
http://dx.doi.org/10.1016/j.det.2016.11.002
0733-8635/17/

(SS), myasthenia gravis, inflammatory bowel disease, and, more generally, auditory, neurologic, and ocular abnormalities (**Table 1**).[12–16] Vitiligo has also been observed in association with these latter abnormalities in several rare syndromes, including AI polyglandular disease (APG), Alezzandrini syndrome, and Vogt-Koynagi-Harada disease (VKH).[3] Isolated case reports also exist describing patients who have vitiligo with other conditions, including mucous membrane pemphigoid and mycosis fungoides.[17,18]

One reason suggested to account for these associations is a shared underlying genetic susceptibility between vitiligo and the AI diseases associated with it.[19] Genome-wide association studies and candidate gene association studies have been performed in patients with generalized vitiligo and many of the associated genes found in these patients encode immunoregulatory proteins, which were also associated with other AI diseases.[20,21] Many of these AI associations have been studied across varied populations from different regions of the world. The frequencies of AI diseases associated with vitiligo vary, but for several conditions have been found in higher frequencies than those found in the general population.[19] Studies show that these frequencies vary by geographic region and may be influenced by genetic and environmental differences within these regions.[6,20] A retrospective 10-year study by Sheth and colleagues[16] in a US population found that 23% of vitiligo patients had associated comorbid AI conditions. A cross-sectional study by Gill and colleagues[13] also in a US population, found that nearly 20% of vitiligo patients had at least 1 comorbid disease. In this study, older age, later age of onset, and longer duration of vitiligo all seemed to play a role in the development of AI disease. A Turkish study by Akay and colleagues[5] found that up to 55% of vitiligo patients having an associated AI disease, and another Japanese study by Narita and colleagues[19] found that it affected 20.3% of vitiligo patients. Chen and colleagues[22] evaluated comorbidity in a Taiwanese nationwide population-based study and found that 14.4% of the patients had 1 or more associated AI or atopic diseases, with AA being the most commonly associated AI disease.

The frequencies of AI diseases associated with vitiligo can also be affected by other demographic factors, such as race, age, and gender.[3,16,22] Several studies have found that women with vitiligo, compared with men, tend more frequently to have an associated AI disease, particularly thyroid disease.[3,16] A Taiwanese study found that female vitiligo patients were more likely to have thyroid disease, AD, RA, SLE, and SS, whereas male vitiligo patients were more likely to have psoriasis.[22] This study also stratified the data by age and found that older vitiligo patients were more likely to have SLE, SS, and RA, whereas younger vitiligo patients were more likely to have myasthenia gravis.[22] Some studies that have stratified their results by race have found the most common associations with vitiligo in Caucasian and Hispanics to be hypothyroidism and psoriasis, whereas in blacks, it has been RA and lupus, and in Asians, psoriasis.[16] Another study found that AA was less frequent in white patients and psoriasis was less frequent in black patients.[13]

In many of these studies, 15% to 26% of patients also had a positive family history of AI

Table 1
Comorbidities associated with vitiligo

More Common Associations	Less Common Associations
Thyroid disease Hashimoto's thyroiditis Graves' disease Hypothyroidism Hyperthyroidism	HIV/AIDS
Alopecia areata	Lichen sclerosus et atrophicus
Type I diabetes mellitus	Mucous membrane pemphigoid
Pernicious anemia	Mycosis fungoides
Atopic dermatitis	Spondyloarthritis
Rheumatoid arthritis	Scleroderma (including morphea)
Systemic lupus erythematosus	Pemphigus vulgaris
Sjögren syndrome	Rheumatic fever
Myasthenia gravis	Multiple sclerosis
Inflammatory bowel disease	Guillan-Barre syndrome
Psoriasis	Type 2 diabetes mellitus
Halo nevus	Addison's disease
Uveitis[a]	Dermatitis herpetiformis
	Celiac disease
	Sarcoidosis
	Multiple sclerosis
	Discoid lupus
	HIV/AIDS

Abbreviation: HIV, human immunodeficiency virus.
[a] Associated with Vogt-Kayanagi-Harada and Alezzandrini syndrome.

disease. An epidemiologic study done in Caucasian vitiligo patients and their families found that nearly 6% of vitiligo patients with thyroid disease also had family members with thyroid disease.[23] Other diseases, including PA, Addison's disease, and SLE, also occurred in higher frequencies in the family members of vitiligo patients.[23] Vitiligo subtype has also been evaluated in association with AI diseases with varied results. Some studies have found no significantly increased association among those with nonsgemental versus segmental vitiligo, whereas others have found those with nonsgemental vitiligo to be more likely to have an associated AI disease.[13]

Laboratory Evaluation

Various studies have advocated for the routine screening of serologies associated with AI diseases including T3, T4, thyroid-stimulating hormone (TSH), thyroid autoantibodies, antinuclear antibodies (ANA), fasting blood glucose levels, complete blood count, vitamins B_{12} and D, and antiparietal cell antibodies.[3] Ingordo and colleagues[20] evaluated circulating antibodies in vitiligo patients and found that 41.8% of patients had at least 1 circulating antibody with the highest being anti–thyroid peroxidase antibody (25.6%) followed by anti-thyroglobulin (23.4%), ANA (16.8%), and gastric antiparietal cell antibodies (7.8%). Further laboratory screening recommendations are discussed with each appropriate disease.

Ocular and Auditory Abnormalities

Melanocytes exist not only in the skin, but also in mucous membranes, eyes (including the uveal tract and retinal pigment epithelium), inner ears, brain, leptomeninges, heart, hair bulbs, and adipocytes.[6] Ocular and auditory abnormalities can also occur in association with vitiligo owing to the presence of melanocytes in these tissues.

Melanin plays several important roles in creating and maintaining the structure and function of the auditory system as well as affecting the transduction of the auditory stimuli in the inner ear.[5] The heaviest pigmentation is located in the scala vestibuli of the membranous labyrinth of the inner ear, where melanocytes and melanin are responsible for normal function of the stria vascularis, development of the endolymphatic potentials, and preservation of the ion and fluid gradient between the endolymph and perilymph (**Fig. 1**).[24] Vitiligo patients can have profound auditory abnormalities or more subtle findings owing to alteration of melanocytes. Clinical studies show that 12% to 18% of vitiligo patients have sensorineural hearing loss.[24] Gopal and colleagues[4] found mild hearing loss (hypoacusis) to be present in up to 20% of

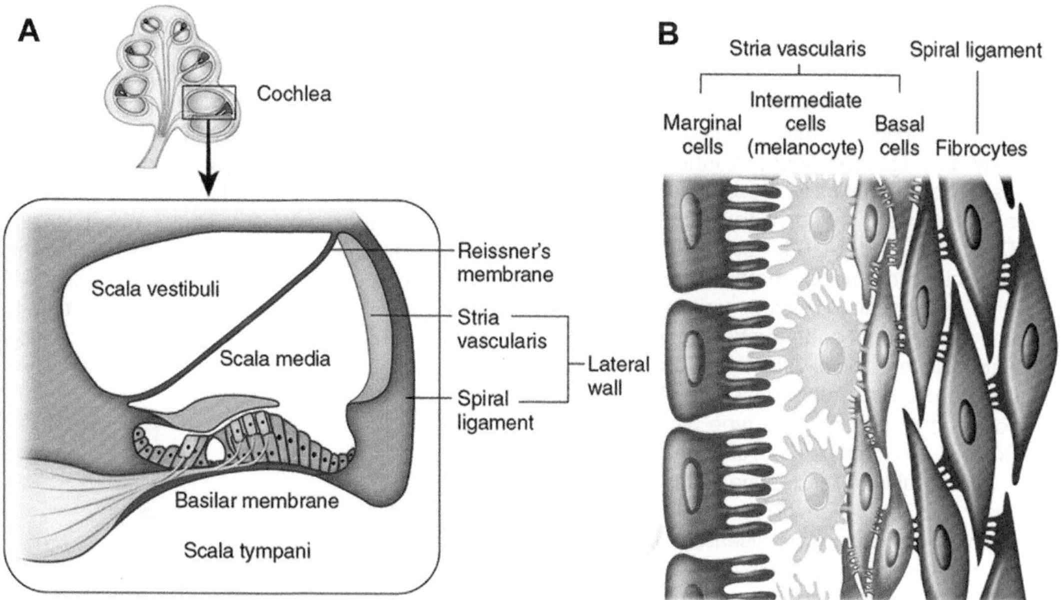

Fig. 1. (*A*) Components of the cochlea (*B*) Components of the lateral wall within the cochlea. Melanocyes and melanin are located in the stria vascularis which, is in the scala vestibuli of the membranous labyrinth of the inner ear. They are responsible for normal function of the stria vascularis, development of the endolymphatic potentials, and preservation of the ion and fluid gradient between the endolymph and perilymph.

vitiligo patients. Other studies have found hypoacusis to occur in 4% to 20% of vitiligo patients, although many of these patients may not have been aware of this loss.[5] A Turkish study found that 37.7% of vitiligo patients had auditory abnormalities, including unilateral and bilateral hearing loss.[5] An Egyptian study found that 60% of vitiligo patients had cochlear dysfunction compared with zero patients in their control group. They did not find the presence of the cochlear dysfunction was affected by vitiligo type (nonsegmental vitiligo vs segmental vitiligo).[24]

Vitiligo patients may also have ocular abnormalities that can affect the iris and retinal pigment epithelium, resulting in uveitis.[25] One study found that 16% of vitiligo patients had ocular abnormalities compared with 5% of the control patients.[4] These ocular abnormalities included uveitis as well as pigmentary changes of the retinal pigmented epithelium and iris. The association of vitiligo with ocular, auditory, and neurologic abnormalities provides further support for vitiligo being a systemic disease.[5,6,24]

Abnormal auditory and ocular findings are also present in association with other AI conditions in unique syndromes, such as VKH, Alezzandrini syndrome, and APG.[4] VKH is an uncommon multisystem, AI disease that affects organs containing melanin and can result in bilateral uveitis, hypoacusis, mengingoencephalitis, poliosis, vitiligo, and alopecia.[26] The disease often begins with neurologic symptoms and then progresses to the ophthalmic phase, and finally the cutaneous manifestations.[27] The etiology is still being investigated, but it is thought to be secondary to a $CD4^+$ T-cell–mediated AI process against melanocytes. The condition is often thought to be triggered by an infectious agent in individuals who are susceptible genetically. Several susceptibility alleles have been linked with VKH, including HLA-DRB1*045, HLA-DR4, and HLA-DR53.[26] Alezzandrini syndrome is another rare condition in which individuals develop unilateral retinal pigment epithelium degeneration and hearing loss with ipsilateral facial vitiligo and poliosis.[28]

Vitiligo can be present in all types of APG, but is most commonly part of APG type 3, specifically type 3C.[21,29] APG consists of AI diseases associated with multiple endocrine gland insufficiencies.[8,29] APG 3C involves AITD plus skin, neural, or neuromuscular disease. The most accepted theory underlying the cause of APG relates to the AI genetic hypothesis involving genes associated with regulation of the immune system.[29] APG has been associated with vitiligo in up to 21% of patients with APG type 1 having vitiligo.[27] Amerio and colleagues[8] found that, among 113 vitiligo patients, 31 had APG (most had the 3C subtype, AITD, and vitiligo), and suggested that in cases positive for antithyroid antibodies, other autoantibodies should be tested for including anti–gastric parietal cell, anti–pancreatic islet cell, and anti–adrenal gland. Vitiligo can also occur as part of AI polyendocrinpathy–candidiasis–ectodermal dystrophy syndrome caused by an *AIRE* gene mutation.[8]

Alopecia Areata

AA has been reported in vitiligo patients with a frequency ranging from 1.2% to 16%.[12,30,31] Vitiligo is also 4 times more common in patients with AA than in the general population.[31] Studies in children with vitiligo have found an association with AA in 1.1% to 2.6%.[32] Although there are antigenic differences between the distinct melanocyte populations that exist in the follicular epithelium and in the epidermis, the 2 conditions also share many similarities.[31] Both conditions share similar pathogenic factors, including autoimmunity, genetic inheritability, and environmental triggers.[9,30,33] From an immune standpoint, the conditions may be related through a shared underlying stimulation of a proinflammatory T helper-1 cell–mediated immunologic response or inactivation of a suppressor T-cell–mediated response.[31] Finally, in a recently published study, Gan and colleagues[34] hypothesized that a common antigen may exist between AA and certain forms of vitiligo, namely follicular vitiligo.

Atopic Dermatitis

Some studies have found AD to occur in higher than expected frequencies in association with vitiligo (**Fig. 2**). A metaanalysis study found higher odds of AD in patients with vitiligo than control patients.[31] Furthermore, early onset vitiligo (<12 years) was associated with significantly greater odds of AD compared with those with late-onset vitiligo,[31,35] even when correcting for potential confounders such as age, gender, vitiligo

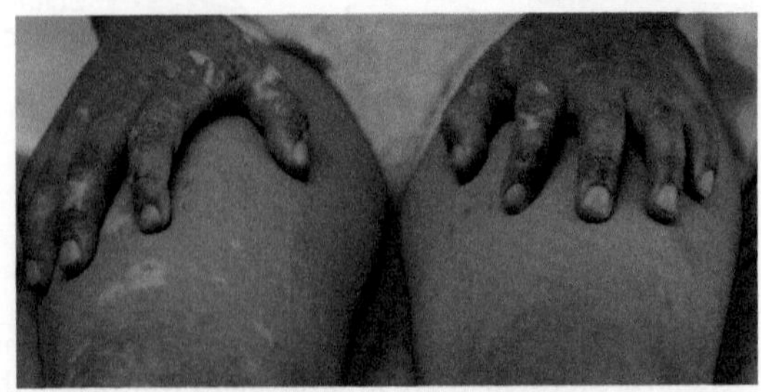

Fig. 2. A 3-year-old boy with vitiligo and atopic dermatitis on his dorsal hands.

severity, and disease duration. In a Korean population-based study, Lee and colleagues[14] found that 5.53% of the vitiligo patients also had AD. Another study found that atopic disease was associated with vitiligo involving a body surface area of at least 76% as well itching or burning of the skin.[36] The authors suggest that a history of atopic disease can be helpful to predict which vitiligo patients will experience progression to extensive disease.[36] The proinflammatory state of AD is thought to be a potential predisposing factor for vitiligo.[6] The association between the 2 conditions may also occur from common pathways activated in both disorders, including thymic stromal lymphopoetin and T helper-17 cells.[31] Pruritus from AD can also lead to scratching and subsequent koebnerization of vitiligo.[31,36] The 2 conditions may also share a common genetic mutation; however, the question of whether atopy predisposes one toward vitiligo or if the 2 conditions coexist remains to be answered.[36]

Celiac Disease

Celiac disease is an immune-mediated enteropathy with a US and European prevalence of about 1%.[37] Several cases in the literature have reported vitiligo patients with celiac disease, some of whom had an improvement in their vitiligo after consuming a gluten-free diet.[34,38] Celiac disease autoantibodies have been found to be more common in some vitiligo patients, suggesting a possible common genetic basis and pathophysiologic pathway for both diseases. Dermatitis herpetiformis, an immunobullous skin disorder also related to gluten sensitivity, has occurred reportedly with vitiligo in several cases.[39] It has been speculated that vitiligo may occur as a koebnerization reaction secondary to the inflammation triggered by dermatitis herpetiformis or the 2 conditions may be correlated pathologically through circulating immune complexes.[39] Further studies are needed to shed light on the strength of the association between vitiligo and these gluten-sensitive disorders, as well as the role that gluten-free diets might play in improving vitiligo in these patients.

Diabetes Mellitus

Type 1 diabetes mellitus and vitiligo are both AI diseases, but there may also be an additional shared inflammatory link between the 2 conditions. A recent study found that vitiligo patients with type 1 diabetes mellitus had higher levels of tumor necrosis factor-α, interleukin (IL)-6, and IL-1β compared with patients with only vitiligo, type 1 diabetes mellitus, or controls.[40] In particular, IL-6 serum levels were significantly higher in patients with both conditions, suggesting that IL-6 may play an important role in the pathogenesis of patients who share both conditions and could be a potential therapeutic target for these patients. The relationship between vitiligo and type 2 diabetes mellitus has also been investigated in several studies as possibly coexisting with vitiligo or having a causal relationship with it. Several small studies have found that nearly 3% to 5% of individuals with type 2 diabetes mellitus have vitiligo.[41] Various pathogenic mechanisms are thought to be involved in this association including oxidative stress, free radicals, and growth factors that have a cytotoxic effect on melanocytes.[41] Larger studies are needed to further elucidate this potential association.

Pernicious Anemia

Several reports have found an increased association between vitiligo and PA.[13,15,42] The incidence of vitiligo in PA has been found to be 4 to 10 times higher than the general population and more common with late-onset vitiligo.[13,15,42] Other studies have failed to find an increased association between the 2 conditions and have not advocated for routine screening of folic acid, vitamin B_{12}, or anti–gastric parietal cells.[16,22,42]

Helicobacter pylori Infection

Various microbial agents through their communication with the environment and the immune system have been suggested to play a role in the pathogenesis of vitiligo including hepatitis C, cytomegalovirus, and human immunodeficiency virus (HIV).[43] These agents are thought to cause AI disease through antibody production, molecular mimicry, high cytokine levels, major histocompatibility complex activation, regulatory T-cell dysfunction, immune complex formation, and chronic inflammatory damage.[44] More recently, studies have evaluated whether *H pylori* may also be a trigger for vitiligo. *H pylori* affects 50% to 80% the world's population and has been linked with various AI and systemic diseases.[43,44] In addition to causing gastric inflammation, including gastric ulceration and carcinogenesis, *H pylori* leads to systemic inflammation through production of tumor necrosis factor-α, IL-6, IL-8, and IL-1β. These systemic effects may lead to a change in the cutaneous microenvironment that subsequently causes melanocyte damage.[44] A recent study found the prevalence of *H pylori* to be 64.7% in vitiligo patients compared with 33.3% in the control group.[43,44] Another study supporting this association advocates for *H pylori* eradication in vitiligo patients with dyspepsia.[44] Further studies are needed to better understand the association between *H pylori* and vitiligo, including whether *H pylori* serves as a trigger for vitiligo and if its eradication affects the disease course of vitiligo.

Human Immunodeficiency Virus Infection and AIDS

A limited number of case reports have found individuals with HIV and AIDS who develop vitiligo; however, studies have not shown whether individuals with HIV have vitiligo at a higher frequency than the general population.[45] HIV-associated vitiligo was first reported in 1987, with the majority of cases resulting in vitiligo onset after the diagnosis of HIV or AIDS.[46] Several mechanisms have been proposed to account for this pathogenesis including immune disequilibrium among cytotoxic, suppressor, and helper T cells, direct HIV activation of melanocytes, and cellular cytotoxicity against melanocytes.[45] Because AI disease occurs when there is a loss of tolerance to autoantigens, HIV may be the stimulus for loss of peripheral tolerance to self-reactive B and T cells. One case report found a 5-fold increase in $CD8^+$ cells in a patient who developed vitiligo after having HIV.[46] This significant increase in $CD8^+$ count may also affect T-cell cytotoxicity in the pathogenesis of vitiligo.

Lichen Sclerosus et Atrophicus and Morphea

Lichen sclerosus et atrophicus and morphea have also been associated with vitiligo; however, this association has been mainly in case reports rather than large epidemiologic studies.[14,47,48] Lichen sclerosus et atrophicus is considered by some to be an AI disease based on the presence of antibodies to extracellular matrix protein 1 and its association with other AI diseases. Morphea has also been linked to neurologic, infectious, and immunologic abnormalities, as well as other AI diseases.[49] A recent cross-sectional study done in the United States in 1873 patients found a higher prevalence of linear morphea (0.2%) compared with the general US population (182 cases per 100,000).[13] The presence of lichen sclerosus et atrophicus and morphea in several vitiligo patients has raised speculation about a shared AI basis among these conditions as well as a possible shared decrease in T-regulatory cells, leading to a loss of tolerance.[49]

Psoriasis

Psoriasis, which has significant immune system alterations, has also been associated with vitiligo.[13,16,50] This concomitance could be owing to chance, given that in several epidemiologic studies, the percentage of vitiligo patients with psoriasis has ranged from 1% to 2.2%, which corresponds with the 1.5% to 2% frequency of vitiligo in the general population.[12,13,15] Sheth and colleagues,[16] however, found that the prevalence of psoriasis in their study of vitiligo patients to be higher at 7.3% with psoriasis and hypothyroidism being the most commonly associated AI diseases in Caucasian and Hispanic vitiligo patients. In the majority of case reports (63%), vitiligo occurred first, followed by the development of psoriasis.[50] A common AI origin of the 2 conditions could be IL-17A produced by T-helper 17 cells, which has been implicated in the pathogenesis of psoriasis and has been speculated as having a role in the pathogenesis of vitiligo.[50] Another study found that the strongest predictors of concomitant psoriasis and vitiligo were having inflammatory-type vitiligo and a positive family history of cardiovascular disease.[51] In addition to shared inflammatory pathways and genetic susceptibility, a locus in the MHC region has been identified that is associated with both psoriasis and vitiligo.[52] Similar to AD, the Koebner phenomenon may be another reason to account for the concomitance and colocalization of the 2 conditions.[50]

Rheumatologic Diseases

Rheumatologic diseases including RA, SLE, spondyloarthritis, and SS have also been associated with vitiligo.[13,16,22,53] Sheth and colleagues[16] found that 2.2% of vitiligo patients had SLE and 2.9% had RA. Interestingly, rates of RA and SLE were more common among African Americans than other races. In the same population, 41% of the patients had elevated anti-ANA titers and 66.7% had positive rheumatoid factor. Gill and colleagues[13] found a frequency of 0.2% having SS and 0.3% having SLE with the latter also only occurring in black patients with vitiligo. Chen and colleagues[22] conducted a nationwide population-based study in Taiwan and in their age- and gender-stratified analysis, the risk of SLE and SS was higher in vitiligo subjects ages 60 to 79 years, whereas RA was higher in only females of the same age group. Tumor necrosis factor-α polymorphisms have been associated with susceptibility to both RA and vitiligo.[54] Spondyloarthritis, which includes ankylosing spondylitis, Reiter syndrome, and reactive and psoriatic arthritis, as well as arthritis associated with inflammatory bowel disease, was found in another study to affect 3.4% of vitiligo patients.[53] These studies show that rheumatologic disease in vitiligo patients may be affected by demographic factors such as age, gender, and race.

The prevalence of positive ANA in vitiligo patients has also varied with percentages ranging from 2.5% to 41%.[16,55] Many patients with a positive ANA may have low titers without concomitant SLE or rheumatologic disease.[15] One study found positive ANA levels in 19.57% of the vitiligo patients with no individuals or their family members having SLE.[15] Some studies have cited the presence of circulating antibodies as being associated with a longer duration of vitiligo and an older age of onset of the disease.[20] Other studies that failed to find a higher association of positive ANA titers in vitiligo patients have argued that it should not be screened routinely.[15,16,20,55]

Thyroid Disease

Many vitiligo patients are often found to have thyroid abnormalities resulting in subclinical or clinical thyroid disease.[56,57] The prevalence of thyroid disease is 3 to 8 times higher in vitiligo patients, with AITD being the AI disorder most commonly associated with vitiligo.[10,56–58] Hypothyroidism tends to be the most common of the associated thyroid disease followed by Graves disease.[5,15,16,19,23,25] Vitiligo often precedes thyroid disease with the risk of developing thyroid disease increasing with age and doubling every 5 years.[7,25,56] This increased association with thyroid disease has supported the AI basis of vitiligo and suggested that the 2 diseases may share a common AI etiology.[7,55] This includes a shared existence of T-helper 1 cell–driven AI processes.[59] Other studies have also suggested that oxidative stress and autoimmunity interact and work together in thyroid and vitiligo autoimmunity pathways causing one condition to lead to the other.[60] Studies from across the world have found varying percentages of vitiligo patients with concomitant thyroid disease ranging from 1.3% to 40%.[5,8,15] An Iranian study found the prevalence of AITD to be 21.1%, and found that those with a positive family history of AI diseases had a decreased response to vitiligo treatment.[58] A Belgian study found that patients with vitiligo and thyroid disease, which was 15.4% of their patient population, had a higher affected body surface area as well as a predilection to depigmentation of the joints and acral skin.[3] A Canadian study by Sawicki and colleagues[15] found hypothyroidism in 19.0% of vitiligo patients with twice as many females being affected compared with males. In Turkey, 55% of vitiligo patients have been found to have thyroid disease, and in Brazil, the rate was 22%; Indian studies have shown a range of 3% to 11%.[16]

This reality has led many to advocate for the routine screening of thyroid function tests to discover the development of thyroid disease at an early stage.[12] A Chinese study examined serologies in vitiligo patients and found that elevated free T3 and TSH were the laboratories that differed the most from the control group.[61] Many vitiligo patients (2.2% to 50%) have also been found to have positive antithyroid antibodies against thyroglobulin, thyroid peroxidase, and TSH receptor.[5,20,55,60] In some patients, the presence of positive thyroid antibodies can exist without the presence of thyroid dysfunction. Thyroglobulin antibodies and in particular TPO-antibodies may be helpful in serving as an immune screening marker in vitiligo patients who have subclinical AITD or those who may have not yet developed thyroid disease but are at risk for it.[20,59,61] The risk of these antibodies being increased in vitiligo patients is 5 times higher than the general population, and may be present up to 7 years before development of thyroid disease.[56]

Screening guidelines for thyroid serologies vary, with some researchers recommending routine screening every 1 to 3 years in all vitiligo patients, whereas others recommend it for those who are symptomatic or have higher risk factors for it.[7,10,16,25,56,59] Recommendations of which thyroid tests to perform also vary, with some studies advocating solely for TSH and others supporting additional testing of thyroid antibodies to pick up risk of future development of AITD.[15] One study found that those at higher risk for developing AITD includes female patients, patients with longer duration of disease, and greater body surface area.[7] In another study, the risk of AITD with vitiligo was found to be associated independently with disease duration and the risk of patients with vitiligo developing AITD was found to double every 5 years.[7] These results were corroborated by another study, which recommended screening of women every 2 years owing to an association between AITD and females with long duration of disease.[7] Pediatric studies have also recommended screening in children owing to thyroid hormones playing an important role in normal childhood development.[59] Other studies have advocated for it to be tested in those who have a family history of thyroid disease, those with long disease duration, or those with stressful life events.[10,62] It is this author's opinion that vitiligo patients should be screened for thyroid disease with TSH and thyroid antibody testing at least every 1 to 2 years. For providers who prefer to not order initial laboratory evaluation, at a minimum patients should be questioned annually about thyroid symptoms with a thorough review of systems. Laboratory testing can then be reserved for those with any positive symptoms.

QUALITY OF LIFE AND BURDEN OF DISEASE

The skin plays an important role in our interaction with the world and skin color is an important element of the perception of someone's health. In that sense, any change in the skin may have psychological consequences.[63] Historically, there is an important amount of literature witnessing the social stigma associated with vitiligo throughout the centuries and in different cultural settings. As an example, old Buddhist literature (624–544 BC) declared that patients with vitiligo are not eligible for ordainment.[64] Other religions and cultures have also participated in the social stigmatization of patients with vitiligo. Indeed, Islamic theologians have considered vitiligo a defect in marriage, allowing thus the husband or the wife to divorce. Similarly, in "Rigveda," an Indian book, it is written that "persons suffering from 'switra' [a name for vitiligo][2] and their progeny are disqualified from marrying others."[64]

Quality of life and burden of vitiligo may be measured by generic instruments such as the Dermatology Quality of Life Index (DLQI) or specific instruments such as the Vitiligo Impact Scale,[65] the Vitiligo-specific Health-related Quality of Life Instrument (VitiQoL)[66] or the Vitiligo Impact Patient scale.[67] Although generic instruments such as the DLQI or Short Form-12 may provide a general picture of impaired quality of life, they usually fail to detect nuances in how patients deal with the overall vitiligo burden.[68,69]

In the late 1970s, Porter and colleagues[70] first reported the major impact of vitiligo on patients' quality of life and there is now strong evidence that patients with vitiligo are negatively affected in their sexual relationships.[71,72] Moreover, several studies have shown that adult patients with generalized vitiligo have a comparable decrease in their quality of life as patients with other skin diseases such as eczema[73,74] and psoriasis.[74–77] Indeed, many people are scared and uncomfortable with others who have vitiligo and patients with vitiligo experience discrimination. In addition, these patients complain of not receiving enough support from their physicians.[72,78] More recently, in 2005, a survey was conducted among the members of the United Kingdom Vitiligo Society showing that more than 50% of respondents declared that vitiligo has an important impact on their quality of life.[79] Finding a cure or effective and lasting treatment was the main priority for most affected respondents. Disappointingly, only a small number of respondents acknowledged obtaining information about vitiligo from their dermatologist (12.5%), whereas more than 80% get this information from nonmedical sources.[79]

More generally, several factors may impact quality of life in patients with vitiligo, that is, age of onset, skin phototype, extent and distribution, and impact of treatment, among others. Thus, Nogueira and colleagues[80] found that most vitiligo patients with affected areas on exposed skin (88%) complain of negative emotions as compared with those with lesions in unexposed areas (20%). Among emotions related to the disease, fear of spread of the disease (71%), shame (57%), insecurity (55%), sadness (55%), and inhibition (53%) were the most cited.[80] Another study found that the extent of stigmatization experienced by vitiligo patients was higher in patients with visible lesions.[81]

Similarly, Parsad and colleagues[71] found that lesions involving the face, arms, legs, and hands had a higher impact on the DLQI. In addition, the degree of stigmatization is probably linked to cultural background and may thus explain some of the variations in DLQI observed among countries.[82]

More specifically, self-image of vitiligo patients is also decreased considerably and mood instabilities are common, particularly in teenagers.[83] Moreover, the psychological impact of vitiligo in childhood may be deep and may have a long-lasting effect on personal self-esteem.[84] Parsad and colleagues[71] found that children with vitiligo were prone to avoid or restrict sport activities and miss more school days than controls. In another study conducted in the Netherlands, it has been shown that the impact of childhood vitiligo may persist in adult life with an impact in social development.[85] Of note, a recent review article of quality of life issues in childhood skin disease found that those with vitiligo experience low self-esteem, social stigmatization, shame, avoidance of intimacy, anxiety, depression, adjustment disorder, fear, suicidal ideation, and other psychiatric morbidities.[86] In an Internet-based survey of children aged 0 to 17 years and their families, quality of life impairment increased with age. Indeed, more than 90% of adolescents (15–17 years) were bothered by vitiligo versus 50% of children aged 0 to 14 years. Location of vitiligo on face, arms, and legs was found to be most distressing and associated with teasing and bullying.[83] Finally, depression and anxiety was reported in 26% and 42% of parents and caregivers, respectively, in pediatric vitiligo.[87]

Despite the considerable burden of vitiligo and its consequences on quality of life, there is still limited research done into the efficacy of psychological therapy on patients with vitiligo.[88,89]

Nonetheless, Papadopoulos and colleagues[89] have shown that cognitive–behavioral therapy may benefit patients in terms of coping and living with vitiligo and that psychological therapy itself may limit the progression of the disease.

Vitiligo is a complex disease that also involves patients' relatives and other close contacts. In fact, many vitiligo patients are extremely emotional and are prone to anticipate being rejected. Many report cruel and embarrassing comments from strangers, but also from close friends. Porter and colleagues[90] have studied the way patients cope with the disease. They identified a group of patients they called "poor adjusters," who represented one-third of the group and who were considered extremely depressed. They emphasized the importance of addressing this in patients, considering that severe depression has been clearly linked to suicide. In another cultural setting, Mattoo and colleagues[91] found that vitiligo was also associated with important psychiatric morbidity, that is, depression, adjustment disorders, dysthymia, and other psychiatric comorbidities, because almost 25% of the patients attending their clinic were affected.

Most of the studies evaluating quality of life and burden of vitiligo have used a generic questionnaire, the DLQI. This questionnaire has been used widely in dermatology and allows comparison between different skin disorders. However, there is a need for a vitiligo-specific scale because disease-specific quality of life instruments are more relevant to detect nuances specific to the disease and are a marker for disability. In the last decade, several vitiligo specific scales have been published,[66,67,92] although these scales need to now be validated on larger populations. In addition, when dealing with vitiligo patients, it is of prime importance to consider psychosocial stress and possible psychiatric comorbidity related to the disease because these may have important implications when constructing a work plan for disease management.

In addition to psychiatric comorbidity, other medical comorbidities associated with vitiligo need to be considered. Current research supports vitiligo as a systemic disease that can exist beyond skin to involve other organs. Continued investigation is needed into the shared pathways, genes, molecular markers, and environmental triggers that may underlie vitiligo and associated conditions.

SUMMARY

It is time for physicians to acknowledge the negative psychological impact of vitiligo as well as its disease comorbidities to adequately address their patients' suffering. This is a crucial step because it will allow providers to treat vitiligo patients not only according to the disease "clinical severity," but also by its psychological impact. Increasing awareness of quality of life issues associated with vitiligo as well as improved understanding into the pathogenesis of vitiligo and associated systemic diseases will help to ensure that vitiligo is no longer dismissed as a cosmetic or otherwise unimportant disease, particularly with regard to funding for research and treatments.

REFERENCES

1. Ezzedine K, Eleftheriadou V, Whitton M, et al. Vitiligo. Lancet 2015;386(9988):74–84.
2. Ezzedine K, Sheth V, Rodrigues M, et al. Vitiligo is not a cosmetic disease. J Am Acad Dermatol 2015;73(5):883–5.
3. van Geel N, Speeckaert M, Brochez L, et al. Clinical profile of generalized vitiligo patients with associated autoimmune/autoinflammatory diseases. J Eur Acad Dermatol Venereol 2014;28(6):741–6.
4. Gopal KV, Rama Rao GR, Kumar YH, et al. Srikant. Vitiligo: a part of a systemic autoimmune process. Indian J Dermatol Venereol Leprol 2007;73(3):162–5.
5. Akay BN, Bozkir M, Anadolu Y, et al. Epidemiology of vitiligo, associated autoimmune diseases and audiological abnormalities: Ankara study of 80 patients in Turkey. J Eur Acad Dermatol Venereol 2010;24(10):1144–50.
6. Lee H, Lee MH, Lee DY, et al. Prevalence of vitiligo and associated comorbidities in Korea. Yonsei Med J 2015;56(3):719–25.
7. Gey A, Diallo A, Seneschal J, et al. Autoimmune thyroid disease in vitiligo: multivariate analysis indicates intricate pathomechanisms. Br J Dermatol 2013;168(4):756–61.
8. Amerio P, Di Rollo D, Carbone A, et al. Polyglandular autoimmune diseases in a dermatological clinical setting: vitiligo-associated autoimmune diseases. Eur J Dermatol 2010;20(3):354–8.
9. Walker A, Mesinkovska NA, Boncher J, et al. Colocalization of vitiligo and alopecia areata presenting as poliosis. J Cutan Pathol 2015;42(2):150–4.
10. Saylam Kurtipek G, Cihan FG, Erayman Demirbas S, et al. The frequency of autoimmune thyroid disease in alopecia areata and vitiligo patients. Biomed Res Int 2015;2015:435947.
11. Khurrum H, AlGhamdi KM. The relationship between the serum level of vitamin D and vitiligo: a controlled study on 300 subjects. J Cutan Med Surg 2016; 20(2):139–45.
12. Schallreuter KU, Lemke R, Brandt O, et al. Vitiligo and other diseases: coexistence or true association? Hamburg study on 321 patients. Dermatology 1994; 188(4):269–75.

13. Gill L, Zarbo A, Isedeh P, et al. Comorbid autoimmune diseases in patients with vitiligo: a cross-sectional study. J Am Acad Dermatol 2016;74(2):295–302.
14. Lee H, Kim YJ, Oh SH. Segmental vitiligo and extragenital lichen sclerosus et atrophicus simultaneously occurring on the opposite sides of the abdomen. Ann Dermatol 2014;26(6):764–5.
15. Sawicki J, Siddha S, Rosen C. Vitiligo and associated autoimmune disease: retrospective review of 300 patients. J Cutan Med Surg 2012;16(4):261–6.
16. Sheth VM, Guo Y, Qureshi AA. Comorbidities associated with vitiligo: a ten-year retrospective study. Dermatology 2013;227(4):311–5.
17. Aithal S, Ganguly S, Kuruvila S. Coexistence of mucous membrane pemphigoid and vitiligo. Indian Dermatol Online J 2014;5(4):485–7.
18. Herrmann JL, Syklawer E, Tarrillion M, et al. Concomitant mycosis fungoides and vitiligo: how mycosis fungoides may contribute to melanocyte destruction. Dermatology 2015;230(2):143–9.
19. Narita T, Oiso N, Fukai K, et al. Generalized vitiligo and associated autoimmune diseases in Japanese patients and their families. Allergol Int 2011;60(4):505–8.
20. Ingordo V, Cazzaniga S, Raone B, et al. Circulating autoantibodies and autoimmune comorbidities in vitiligo patients: a multicenter Italian study. Dermatology 2014;228(3):240–9.
21. Spritz RA. Shared genetic relationships underlying generalized vitiligo and autoimmune thyroid disease. Thyroid 2010;20(7):745–54.
22. Chen YT, Chen YJ, Hwang CY, et al. Comorbidity profiles in association with vitiligo: a nationwide population-based study in Taiwan. J Eur Acad Dermatol Venereol 2015;29(7):1362–9.
23. Alkhateeb A, Fain PR, Thody A, et al. Epidemiology of vitiligo and associated autoimmune diseases in Caucasian probands and their families. Pigment Cell Res 2003;16(3):208–14.
24. Anbar TS, El-Badry MM, McGrath JA, et al. Most individuals with either segmental or nonsegmental vitiligo display evidence of bilateral cochlear dysfunction. BR J Dermatol 2015;172(2):406–11.
25. Nordlund JJ, Taylor NT, Albert DM, et al. The prevalence of vitiligo and polisosis in patients with uveitis. J Am Acadm Dermatol 1981;4(5):528–36.
26. Greco A, Fusconi M, Gallo A, et al. Vogt-Koyanagi-Harada syndrome. Autoimmun Rev 2013;12(11):1033–8.
27. Huggins RH, Janusz CA, Schwartz RA. Vitiligo: a sign of systemic disease. Indian J Dermatol Venereol Leprol 2006;72(1):68–71.
28. Gupta M, Pande D, Lehl SS, et al. Alezzandrini syndrome. BMJ Case Rep 2011;2011:1–2.
29. Kasznicki J, Drzewoski J. A case of autoimmune urticaria accompanying autoimmune polyglandular syndrome type III associated with Hashimoto's disease, type 1 diabetes mellitus, and vitiligo. Endokrynol Pol 2014;65(4):320–3.
30. Kumar S, Mittal J, Mahajan B. Colocalization of vitiligo and alopecia areata: coincidence or consequence? Int J Trichology 2013;5(1):50–2.
31. Mohan GC, Silverberg JI. Association of vitiligo and alopecia areata with atopic dermatitis: a systematic review and meta-analysis. JAMA Dermatol 2015;151(5):522–8.
32. Al-Jabri MA-R, Ali A. Childhood vitiligo: a retrospective hospital based study, Jeddah, Saudi Arabia. JSSDDS 2011;15:15–7.
33. Harris JE. Vitiligo and alopecia areata: apples and oranges? Exp Dermatol 2013;22(12):785–9.
34. Gan EY, Cario-Andre M, Pain C, et al. Follicular vitiligo: a report of 8 cases. J Am Acad Dermatol 2016;74(6):1178–84.
35. Ezzedine K, Le Thuaut A, Jouary T, et al. Latent class analysis of a series of 717 patients with vitiligo allows the identification of two clinical subtypes. Pigment Cell Melanoma Res 2014;27(1):134–9.
36. Silverberg JI, Silverberg NB. Association between vitiligo and atopic disorders: a pilot study. JAMA Dermatol 2013;149(8):983–6.
37. Shahmoradi Z, Najafian J, Naeini FF, et al. Vitiligo and autoantibodies of celiac disease. Int J Prev Med 2013;4(2):200–3.
38. Khandalavala BN, Nirmalraj MC. Rapid partial repigmentation of vitiligo in a young female adult with a gluten-free diet. Case Rep Dermatol 2014;6(3):283–7.
39. Karabudak O, Dogan B, Yildirim S, et al. Dermatitis herpetiformis and vitiligo. J Chin Med Assoc 2007;70(11):504–6.
40. Farhan J, Al-Shobaili HA, Zafar U, et al. Interleukin-6: a possible inflammatory link between vitiligo and type 1 diabetes. Br J Biomed Sci 2014;71(4):151–7.
41. Afkhami-Ardekani M, Ghadiri-Anari A, Ebrahimzadeh-Ardakani M, et al. Prevalence of vitiligo among type 2 diabetic patients in an Iranian population. Int J Dermatol 2014;53(8):956–8.
42. Kim SM, Kim YK, Hann SK. Serum levels of folic acid and vitamin B12 in Korean patients with vitiligo. Yonsei Med J 1999;40(3):195–8.
43. Rifaioglu EN, Aydogan F, Bulbul Sen B, et al. Investigation into the frequency of Helicobacter pylori infection with carbon 14 urea breath test in patients with vitiligo. Turk J Med Sci 2014;44(6):1051–4.
44. Dogan Z, Ozdemir P, Eksioglu M, et al. Relationship between Helicobacter pylori infection and vitiligo: a prospective study. Am J Clin Dermatol 2014;15(5):457–62.
45. McGowan JWT, Long JB, Johnson CA, et al. Disseminated vitiligo associated with AIDS. Cutis 2006;77(3):169–73.

46. Duvic M, Rapini R, Hoots WK, et al. Human immunodeficiency virus-associated vitiligo: expression of autoimmunity with immunodeficiency? J Am Acad Dermatol 1987;17(4):656–62.
47. Attili VR, Attili SK. Acral vitiligo and lichen sclerosus - association or a distinct pattern? A clinical and histopathological review of 15 cases. Indian J Dermatol 2015;60(5):519.
48. Lakjiri S, Meziane M, Benani A, et al. Eosinophilic fasciitis, morphea and vitiligo in a single patient. Ann Dermatol Venereol 2014;141(10):598–602 [in French].
49. Yadav P, Garg T, Chander R, et al. Segmental vitiligo with segmental morphea: an autoimmune link? Indian Dermatol Online J 2014;5(Suppl 1): S23–5.
50. Langley AR, Manley P, Asai Y. A case of colocalized vitiligo and psoriasis. J Cutan Med Surg 2016;20(2): 150–2.
51. Arunachalam M, Dragoni F, Colucci R, et al. Non-segmental vitiligo and psoriasis comorbidity - a case-control study in Italian patients. J Eur Acad Dermatol Venereol 2014;28(4):433–7.
52. Zhu KJ, Lv YM, Yin XY, et al. Psoriasis regression analysis of MHC loci identifies shared genetic variants with vitiligo. PLoS One 2011;6(11):e23089.
53. Padula A, Ciancio G, La Civita L, et al. Association between vitiligo and spondyloarthritis. J Rheumatol 2001;28(2):313–4.
54. Lee YH, Bae SC. Associations between TNF-alpha polymorphisms and susceptibility to rheumatoid arthritis and vitiligo: a meta-analysis. Genet Mol Res 2015;14(2):5548–59.
55. Kasumagic-Halilovic E, Ovcina-Kurtovic N, Jukic T, et al. Vitiligo and autoimmunity. Med Arch 2013; 67(2):91–3.
56. Vrijman C, Kroon MW, Limpens J, et al. The prevalence of thyroid disease in patients with vitiligo: a systematic review. Br J Dermatol 2012;167(6): 1224–35.
57. Afsar FS, Isleten F. Prevalence of thyroid function test abnormalities and thyroid autoantibodies in children with vitiligo. Indian J Endocrinol Metab 2013; 17(6):1096–9.
58. Nejad SB, Qadim HH, Nazeman L, et al. Frequency of autoimmune diseases in those suffering from vitiligo in comparison with normal population. Pak J Biol Sci 2013;16(12):570–4.
59. Kroon MW, Vrijman C, Chandeck C, et al. High prevalence of autoimmune thyroiditis in children and adolescents with vitiligo. Horm Res Paediatr 2013;79: 137–44.
60. Colucci R, Dragoni F, Moretti S. Oxidative stress and immune system in vitiligo and thyroid diseases. Oxid Med Cell Longev 2015;2015:631927.
61. Xianfeng C, Yuegen J, Zhiyu Y, et al. Pediatric patients with vitiligo in eastern china: abnormalities in 145 cases based on thyroid function tests and immunological findings. Med Sci Monit 2015;21: 3216–21.
62. Arunachalam M, Pisaneschi L, Colucci R, et al. Autoimmune thyroid disease in Italian patients with non-segmental vitiligo. Eur J Dermatol 2014;24(5): 625–6.
63. Silverberg JI, Silverberg NB. Association between vitiligo extent and distribution and quality-of-life impairment. JAMA Dermatol 2013;149(2):159–64.
64. Gauthier Y, Benzekri L. Historical aspects. Heidelberg (Germany): Springer Verlag; 2010.
65. Krishna GS, Ramam M, Mehta M, et al. Vitiligo impact scale: an instrument to assess the psychosocial burden of vitiligo. Indian J Dermatol Venereol Leprol 2013;79(2):205–10.
66. Lilly E, Lu PD, Borovicka JH, et al. Development and validation of a vitiligo-specific quality-of-life instrument (VitiQoL). J Am Acad Dermatol 2013;69(1): e11–18.
67. Salzes C, Abadie S, Seneschal J, et al. The vitiligo impact patient scale (VIPs): development and validation of a vitiligo burden assessment tool. J Invest Dermatol 2016;136(1):52–8.
68. Ezzedine K, Grimes PE, Meurant JM, et al. Living with vitiligo: results from a national survey indicate differences between skin phototypes. Br J Dermatol 2015;173(2):607–9.
69. Linthorst Homan MW, Spuls PI, de Korte J, et al. The burden of vitiligo: patient characteristics associated with quality of life. J Am Acad Dermatol 2009;61(3): 411–20.
70. Porter J, Beuf AH, Nordlund JJ, et al. Psychological reaction to chronic skin disorders: a study of patients with vitiligo. Gen Hosp Psychiatry 1979;1(1): 73–7.
71. Parsad D, Dogra S, Kanwar AJ. Quality of life in patients with vitiligo. Health Qual Life Outcomes 2003;1:58.
72. Sukan M, Maner F. The problems in sexual functions of vitiligo and chronic urticaria patients. J Sex Marital Ther 2007;33(1):55–64.
73. Holm EA, Wulf HC, Stegmann H, et al. Life quality assessment among patients with atopic eczema. Br J Dermatol 2006;154(4):719–25.
74. Lundberg L, Johannesson M, Silverdahl M, et al. Health-related quality of life in patients with psoriasis and atopic dermatitis measured with SF-36, DLQI and a subjective measure of disease activity. Acta Derm Venereol 2000;80(6):430–4.
75. Shikiar R, Willian MK, Okun MM, et al. The validity and responsiveness of three quality of life measures in the assessment of psoriasis patients: results of a phase II study. Health Qual Life Outcomes 2006;4:71.
76. Wahl A, Moum T, Hanestad BR, et al. The relationship between demographic and clinical variables,

and quality of life aspects in patients with psoriasis. Qual Life Res 1999;8(4):319–26.
77. Wahl A, Hanestad BR, Wiklund I, et al. Coping and quality of life in patients with psoriasis. Qual Life Res 1999;8(5):427–33.
78. Porter J, Beuf AH, Lerner A, et al. Response to cosmetic disfigurement: patients with vitiligo. Cutis 1987;39(6):493–4.
79. Talsania N, Lamb B, Bewley A. Vitiligo is more than skin deep: a survey of members of the Vitiligo Society. Clin Exp Dermatol 2010;35(7):736–9.
80. Nogueira LS, Zancanaro PC, Azambuja RD. Vitiligo and emotions. An Bras Dermatol 2009;84(1):41–5 [in English, Portuguese].
81. Schmid-Ott G, Kunsebeck HW, Jecht E, et al. Stigmatization experience, coping and sense of coherence in vitiligo patients. J Eur Acad Dermatol Venereol 2007;21(4):456–61.
82. Kruger C, Schallreuter KU. Cumulative life course impairment in vitiligo. Curr Probl Dermatol 2013;44: 102–17.
83. Silverberg JI, Silverberg NB. Quality of life impairment in children and adolescents with vitiligo. Pediatr Dermatol 2014;31(3):309–18.
84. Ingordo V, Cazzaniga S, Gentile C, et al. Dermatology life quality index score in vitiligo patients: a pilot study among young Italian males. G Ital Dermatol Venereol 2012;147(1):83–90.
85. Linthorst Homan MW, de Korte J, Grootenhuis MA, et al. Impact of childhood vitiligo on adult life. Br J Dermatol 2008;159(4):915–20.
86. Brown MM, Chamlin SL, Smidt AC. Quality of life in pediatric dermatology. Dermatol Clin 2013;31(2): 211–21.
87. Manzoni AP, Weber MB, Nagatomi AR, et al. Assessing depression and anxiety in the caregivers of pediatric patients with chronic skin disorders. An Bras Dermatol 2013;88(6):894–9.
88. Picardo MT, Alain T, editors. Vitiligo. 1st edition. Berlin - Heidelberg: Springer; 2010. No. 1.
89. Papadopoulos L, Bor R, Legg C. Coping with the disfiguring effects of vitiligo: a preliminary investigation into the effects of cognitive-behavioural therapy. Br J Med Psychol 1999;72(Pt 3):385–96.
90. Porter J, Beuf A, Nordlund JJ, et al. Personal responses of patients to vitiligo: the importance of the patient-physician interaction. Arch Dermatol 1978;114(9):1384–5.
91. Mattoo SK, Handa S, Kaur I, et al. Psychiatric morbidity in vitiligo: prevalence and correlates in India. J Eur Acad Dermatol Venereol 2002;16(6): 573–8.
92. Gupta V, Sreenivas V, Mehta M, et al. Measurement properties of the Vitiligo Impact Scale-22 (VIS-22), a vitiligo-specific quality-of-life instrument. Br J Dermatol 2014;171(5):1084–90.

Skin Cancer Risk (Nonmelanoma Skin Cancers/Melanoma) in Vitiligo Patients

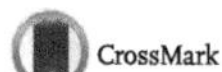

Michelle Rodrigues

KEYWORDS

• Vitiligo • Leukoderma • Skin cancer • Cancer • Melanoma • Basal cell skin cancer • Squamous cell skin cancer • Nonmelanoma skin cancer • Phototherapy • Depigmentation

KEY POINTS

- The risk of skin cancer in vitiligo is still being debated.
- The genetic profile of those with vitiligo seems to be opposite to those with melanoma.
- The autoimmunity seen in vitiligo seems protective against melanoma.
- Current evidence suggests narrow-band ultraviolet B does not increase the risk of cutaneous malignancies, even with long-term therapy, especially in those with skin phototype IV to VI.

INTRODUCTION

Vitiligo affects approximately 0.5% to 2% of the population[1,2] and has no geographic or ethnic boundaries. Vitiligo results in patchy depigmentation of the skin, mucous membranes, and hair owing to a combination of genetic susceptibility, cellular stress, and an autoimmune cytotoxic CD8+-mediated melanocyte attack. Although an absence of melanin in lesional skin and prolonged administration of phototherapy may cause concern about the development of skin cancer in this population, the genetic and autoimmune profiles of vitiligo patients confer a degree of protection against melanoma and nonmelanoma skin cancers (NMSC). A growing body of evidence suggests there is no significant increased risk of melanoma or NMSC in vitiligo, even with prolonged narrow-band ultraviolet (UV) B light therapy. However, well-constructed, prospective studies are a lacking and are clearly needed to substantiate the recent published findings on the topic.

CONTENT

Exposure to UV is an important factor in the development of basal cell carcinoma (BCC), squamous cell carcinoma (SCC), and possibly other skin cancers. In Australia, 2 of 3 people will have skin cancer diagnosed by the time they are 70[3] with melanoma cited as the most common cancer in those between 15 and 44 years of age. High rates of skin cancer, however, are not unique to Australia. One in 5 Americans will have skin cancer in their lifetime,[4] and the estimated annual cost of treating skin cancers in the United States is 8.1 billion dollars.[5]

Those with black skin have an intrinsic sun protection factor of 13.4[6] resulting in lower rates of skin cancer compared with lighter skin types. Those with dark skin, however, are not immune to UV-induced cutaneous malignancies. The incidence of melanoma and nonmelanoma skin cancer is approximately 5% in Hispanics, 4% in Asians, and 2% in blacks.[7] Those with vitiligo

Disclosures: The author has no conflicts of interest to declare.
Department of Dermatology, St Vincent's Hospital, The Royal Children's Hospital, Skin and Cancer Foundation, Inc, 41 Victoria Parade, Fitzroy, Victoria 3065, Australia
E-mail address: michelleannerodrigues@hotmail.com

Dermatol Clin 35 (2017) 129–134
http://dx.doi.org/10.1016/j.det.2016.11.003
0733-8635/17/

lack melanin in affected white patches of skin. It is, therefore, understandable that dermatologists around the world have been concerned about the development of melanoma and nonmelanoma skin cancer secondary to incidental and therapeutic UV light exposure in this subgroup of patients.

Genetic studies found polymorphisms in the TYR gene of vitiligo patients. This gene encodes tyrosinase, which is involved in melanin synthesis. The TYR allele that confers risk for vitiligo is also protective against melanoma.[8,9] In addition, human leukocyte antigen–A2 is the protective allele against melanoma development and was the risk allele for development of vitiligo in a meta-analysis.[10]

Further evidence to support this inverse relationship between vitiligo and melanoma is noted in the melanoma literature. Vitiligo has been reported to confer an enhanced 5-year survival in melanoma patients.[11] Furthermore, treatments used for metastatic melanoma have been reported to induce vitiligo including vemurafenib, a BRAF inhibitor,[12] and therapeutic immune checkpoint inhibitors such as anti–cytotoxic T-lymphocyte–associated protein 4 and anti–programmed cell death protein 1 (PD-1) agents. The development of vitiligo while on such therapy seems to improve treatment response (**Figs. 1** and **2**).[13,14] Inhibition of cytotoxic T-lymphocyte–associated protein 4 and PD-1 reduces regulatory T-cell activity, which may explain why they are associated with the development of autoimmune diseases.[13,15,16] This body of evidence suggests melanoma and vitiligo represent opposite ends of the genetic risk spectrum, which has led to vitiligo being recently labeled *the white armour*.[17]

Although autoimmunity in vitiligo confers protection against melanoma, the lesional skin of those with vitiligo lacks melanin. In normal skin,

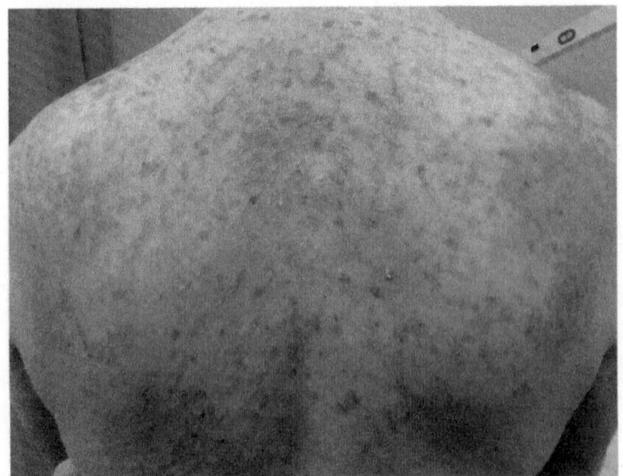

Fig. 1. Back of a patient with metastatic melanoma in whom vitiligo developed while on PD-1 inhibitor, pembrolizumab, with coexistant solar keratoses.

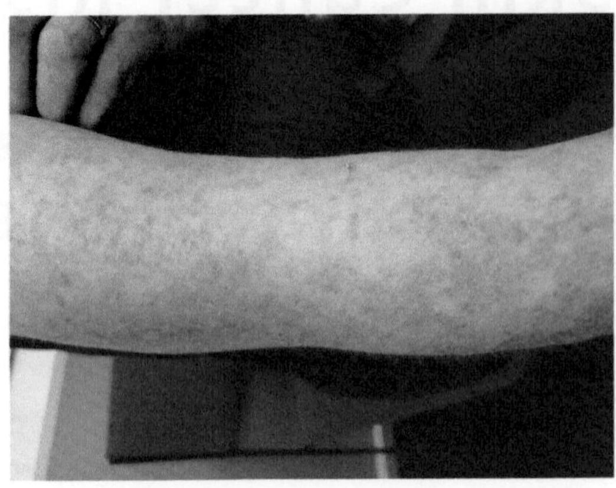

Fig. 2. Right arm of the same patient.

melanin affords an inherent skin protection factor that is proportional to the darkness of the skin. It has been assumed, therefore, that when melanin is reduced in amount or absent, the skin is more photosensitive and susceptible to UV light–induced carcinogenesis. The assumption that vitiliginous skin acts like Fitzpatrick skin phototype (SPT) I, however, has been challenged in the literature. Studies found that photoadaptation and tolerance seem to mirror the patient's normal skin phototype, even in vitiliginous lesions.[18,19] Studies also found that those with darker skin types tolerate higher doses of UVB, suggesting that photobiological properties such as epidermal thickness and chromophores play a more significant role in photoprotection than previously assumed.

Therapeutic exposure to narrow-band UVB light (NB-UVB) (311 nm) is currently the treatment of choice for widespread or progressive vitiligo.[20] NB-UVB was first introduced in the Netherlands in the early 1980s[21,22] and is now a standard therapy for many dermatologic conditions including vitiligo for which it is commonly combined with topical corticosteroid and calcineurin inhibitors for widespread disease. Yones and colleagues,[23] in a randomized double-blind trial, found that NB-UVB had superior efficacy, better color matching of repigmented skin, and fewer side effects compared with psoralen and UV light A (PUVA). This superior safety and efficacy profile was also noted in prior studies.[24,25] Yones and colleagues[23] also found that approximately 6 months of NB-UVB was required to achieve 50% repigmentation and 12 months to regain 75% pigmentation. Studies examining optimal duration of phototherapy for vitiligo are lacking because of heterogeneous study designs, the use of variable outcome measures, and the paucity of prospective trials. What is clear is that prolonged therapy is required to achieve repigmentation (12–24 months), and maintenance therapy may also need to be considered thereafter.

In the past, PUVA was used extensively for both psoriasis and vitiligo. Prolonged therapy with PUVA demonstrates an increased skin cancer risk in white psoriasis patients (especially squamous cell skin cancer). Studies of NB-UVB, however, have not found a significant association between treatment and BCC, SCC, or melanoma.[26,27] In contrast to those with psoriasis, PUVA treatment in vitiligo patients does not seem to be associated with NMSC (although the follow-up periods were short and patient numbers limited in these studies).[28–30]

The long-term risk of carcinogenesis with NB-UVB therapy in vitiligo is assumed by some researchers to be less than those treated for psoriasis because of the lower UVB dose per treatment and the rarity of immunosuppressive medication use in this group. To precisely establish the carcinogenic potential of NB-UVB, a decade-long, large, multicenter trial is needed. In 2008, in the absence of such data, English investigators, using a mathematical model, suggested that those with types I to III should not exceed 200 treatments, but European guidelines published in 2012[1] for the management of vitiligo suggest "phototherapy is usually continued as long as there is ongoing repigmentation or over a maximum period of 1 or 2 years. Maintenance irradiation is not recommended, but regular follow-up examinations are suggested for detecting relapse."

Use of topical tacrolimus for prolonged periods is another area of concern for some prescribers. When first available, the long-term safety of tacrolimus had not been established, and animal studies raised the possibility of immune-mediated malignancies with systemic exposure.[31] A boxed warning was therefore issued in 2006 for tacrolimus use resulting in widespread fear of use. Despite release of a comprehensive review of its safety by the US Food and Drug Administration in September 2010 and May 2011, they concluded that there was still a possibility of associated malignancy but qualified this stating that causality could not be proven.

Although there are currently no studies assessing long-term safety specifically in vitiligo patients, tacrolimus is also used as maintenance in those with atopic dermatitis. A recent Cochrane database review of topical tacrolimus use in those with atopic dermatitis[32] reported that systemic absorption of topical tacrolimus was "rarely detectable, only in low level and this decreased with time." Exceptions were noted in those with severe epidermal barrier dysfunction (eg, Netherton's syndrome). No cases of lymphoma were found in this review.

The baseline incidence of melanoma and NMSC in vitiligo is still debated. Although 2 studies examining the prevalence of vitiligo in patients with melanoma have been published,[33,34] it is more useful to examine the prevalence of melanoma in patients with vitiligo.

Hexsel and colleagues[35] reported, in a retrospective study of 477 patients with vitiligo, that with the exception of BCCs in female patients, the annual incidence rates of NMSC in patients with vitiligo were higher than the incidence rates in the United States. In 2 patients, skin cancer developed in vitiliginous skin. Hammoud and colleagues[36] reviewed this study and calculated an absolute risk of 0.013 (95% confidence interval [CI], 0.0058–0.0272) with a BCC/SCC ratio of 2:1. Of note, these patients were not treated with phototherapy, and the results of this study were not statistically significant.

In contrast to the above-mentioned study, 5 studies have reported lower rates of melanoma and NMSC in those with vitiligo (**Table 1**). In 1998, Lindelof and colleagues,[37] in a retrospective cohort study of 1052 patients, found that patients with vitiligo have a lower risk of melanoma development (only 1 patient had melanoma). No cases of SCC were noted.

In 2002, Schallreuter and colleagues[38] conducted a prospective study of 136 sun-exposed white patients with vitiligo. Photodamage and NMSC were not seen in those with vitiligo. Given the selection bias (white patients only), results from this study may be more significant.

A large retrospective, comparative cohort, Dutch, survey-based study in 2013 assessing 1307 patients found a 3-fold decreased lifetime prevalence of melanoma (adjusted odds ratio, 0.32; 95% CI, 0.12–0.88) and a decreased probability of NMSC (adjusted odds ratio, 0.28; 95% CI, 0.16–0.50) in those with nonsegmental vitiligo compared with nonaffected individuals.[39] All melanomas in patients with vitiligo occurred in unaffected (normally pigmented) skin. Two patients reported development of BCC in vitiliginous skin. Subgroup analyses of patients treated with NB-UVB and PUVA did not find increased age-adjusted lifetime prevalence of melanoma or NMSC. After stratification into subgroups according to cumulative number of phototherapy treatments (NB-UVB and PUVA combined), no trends were found regarding skin cancer prevalence rates. This finding was supported by a prior study undertaken at the University of California, San Fransisco.[40] The Dutch study was a retrospective survey and the control group comprised life

Table 1
Publications examining the risk of melanoma and non-melanoma skin cancer risk in those with vitiligo

Author and Year	Journal	Study	Results	Weakness of Study
Hexsel et al,[35] 2009	*J Am Acad Dermatol*	Retrospective; 477 patients	Overall higher annual incidence of NMSC in those with vitiligo compared with those in the United States	Retrospective; results not statistically significant
Lindelof et al,[37] 1998	*Acta Derm Venereol*	Retrospective cohort; 1052 patients	Lower risk of melanoma in those with vitiligo	Retrospective
Schallreuter et al,[38] 2002	*Dermatology*	Prospective; 136 patients	No photodamage or NMSC in those with vitiligo	Recall bias on questionnaire; study in Northeast Germany—no patients had clinical evidence of sun damage
Park et al,[40] 2012	*J Am Acad Dermatol*	Retrospective chart review; 10 patients	No melanoma or NMSC seen in vitiligo patients who had between 33 and 93 mo of NB-UVB (3 patients also had oral PUVA)	Retrospective; small number of patients
Teulings et al,[39] 2013	*Br J Dermatol*	Retrospective comparative cohort; 1307 patients	Lifetime risk of melanoma decreased 3-fold and decreased probability NMSC in those with vitiligo	Retrospective; controls were life partners of those with vitiligo
Paradisi et al,[41] 2014	*J Am Acad Dermatol*	Retrospective chart review; 10,040 patients	Lower risk of melanoma and NMSC in those with vitiligo; phototherapy markedly increased skin cancer risk	Control group was those seen for vascular surgery and were not age matched

partners of those with vitiligo, which may be considered a weakness of the study.

In 2014, Paradisi and colleagues[41] studied a cohort of 10,040 patients with vitiligo. The study compared the frequency of NMSC in patients who were seen for vitiligo with patients seen for vascular surgery in the institute. Occurrence of NMSC was 3.8% (95% CI, 2.7%–5.2%) among subjects and 19.6% (95% CI, 18%–21.4%) among controls. Occurrence of melanoma was 1.1% (95% CI, 0.5%–2.0%) in patients with vitiligo and 4.5% (95% CI, 3.8%–5.4%) in the control cohort. However, a markedly higher risk was noted in patients treated with phototherapy compared with the control group (14.1% vs 3.2%, respectively). Although this is the largest study examining melanoma and NMSC risk in vitiligo patients, the age range in both groups was different.

None of the studies to date describe how the extent of vitiligo may influence the risk of melanoma and NMSC development. Furthermore, patients who may have succumbed to their melanoma and NMSC could not be included in these studies, creating selection bias and the possibility of higher incidences of skin cancer than described above.

In 2005, a review of the literature suggested chronic use of UVB does not seem to increase the risk of skin cancer and there do not seem to be any indications to limit exposure.[42] This finding was noted despite the higher UV exposure in vitiligo patients. These results, however, need to be substantiated by prospective studies and need to include groups of patients with greater ambient UV light exposure. Further well-constructed prospective studies are clearly required to support the findings of these studies.

The lower risk of melanoma makes sense in the context of possible sun avoidance by those affected, the absence of melanocytes in lesional skin, and the genetic profile and TYR polymorphisms seen in vitiligo. The lower incidence of NMSC, however, may seem counterintuitive at first. The latter observation, however, may relate to the decreased photodamage[43] and increased wild-type p53 expression in keratinocytes in the skin of those with vitiligo.[44–46] The p53 tumor suppressor may protect against actinic damage and the development of keratinocyte cancer. Furthermore, the proinflammatory state noted in vitiligo stimulates production of superoxide dismutase and glutathione peroxidase, which reduces the risk of skin cancer.[47]

SUMMARY

The relative genetic and immune protection against melanoma and NMSC in those with vitiligo is reassuring. If skin cancers do develop, they are most commonly found in nonlesional areas. The results of recent studies allow us to be cautiously optimistic when discussing the risk of skin cancer caused by therapeutic exposure to NB-UVB. However, we should continue to recommend sun protection at all other times to avoid burning of vitiliginous skin and to decrease incidental UV exposure. It is also important to perform full skin checks regularly in light of the prolonged courses of phototherapy required to repigment vitiliginous skin and maintain repigmentation thereafter. Scientific literature examining the risk of skin cancer in this subgroup of patients will be interesting to follow when new targeted biologic therapies (immunosuppression) are available for vitiligo.

REFERENCES

1. Taieb A, Alomar A, Bohm M, et al. Guidelines for the management of vitiligo: the European Dermatology Forum consensus. Br J Dermatol 2013;168:5–19.
2. Kruger C, Schallreuter KU. A review of the worldwide prevalence of vitiligo in children/adolescents and adults. Int J Dermatol 2012;51:1206–12.
3. Staples MP, Elwood M, Burton RC, et al. Non-melanoma skin cancer in Australia: the 2002 national survey and trends since 1985. Med J Aust 2006;184:6–10.
4. Robinson JK. Sun exposure, sun protection, and vitamin D. JAMA 2005;294:1541–3.
5. Guy GP Jr, Machlin SR, Ekwueme DU, et al. Prevalence and costs of skin cancer treatment in the U.S., 2002-2006 and 2007-2011. Am J Prev Med 2015;48:183–7.
6. Jimbow K, Quevedo WC Jr, Fitzpatrick TB, et al. Some aspects of melanin biology: 1950-1975. J Invest Dermatol 1976;67:72–89.
7. Gloster HM Jr, Neal K. Skin cancer in skin of color. J Am Acad Dermatol 2006;55:741–60 [quiz: 61–4].
8. Jin Y, Birlea SA, Fain PR, et al. Variant of TYR and autoimmunity susceptibility loci in generalized vitiligo. N Engl J Med 2010;362:1686–97.
9. Bishop DT, Demenais F, Iles MM, et al. Genome-wide association study identifies three loci associated with melanoma risk. Nat Genet 2009;41:920–5.
10. Liu JB, Li M, Chen H, et al. Association of vitiligo with HLA-A2: a meta-analysis. J Eur Acad Dermatol Venereol 2007;21:205–13.
11. Naveh HP, Rao UN, Butterfield LH. Melanoma-associated leukoderma - immunology in black and white? Pigment Cell Melanoma Res 2013;26:796–804.
12. Alonso-Castro L, Rios-Buceta L, Vano-Galvan S, et al. Vitiligo in 2 patients receiving vemurafenib for metastatic melanoma. J Am Acad Dermatol 2013;69:e28–9.
13. Mochel MC, Ming ME, Imadojemu S, et al. Cutaneous autoimmune effects in the setting of therapeutic immune checkpoint inhibition for metastatic melanoma. J Cutan Pathol 2016;43(9):787–91.
14. Hua C, Boussemart L, Mateus C, et al. Association of Vitiligo With Tumor Response in Patients With Metastatic Melanoma Treated With Pembrolizumab. JAMA Dermatol 2016;152:45–51.
15. Friedline RH, Brown DS, Nguyen H, et al. CD4+ regulatory T cells require CTLA-4 for the maintenance of systemic tolerance. J Exp Med 2009;206:421–34.
16. Postow MA, Callahan MK, Wolchok JD. Immune Checkpoint Blockade in Cancer Therapy. J Clin Oncol 2015;33:1974–82.
17. Taieb A, Ezzedine K. Vitiligo: the white armour? Pigment Cell Melanoma Res 2013. [Epub ahead of print].
18. Hexsel CL, Mahmoud BH, Mitchell D, et al. A clinical trial and molecular study of photoadaptation in vitiligo. Br J Dermatol 2009;160:534–9.
19. Caron-Schreinemachers AL, Kingswijk MM, Bos JD, et al. 311 nm tolerance of vitiligo skin increases with skin photo type. Acta Derm Venereol 2005;85:24–6.
20. Taieb A, Picardo M. Clinical practice. Vitiligo. N Engl J Med 2009;360:160–9.
21. van Weelden H, De La Faille HB, Young E, et al. A new development in UVB phototherapy of psoriasis. Br J Dermatol 1988;119:11–9.

22. Green C, Ferguson J, Lakshmipathi T, et al. 311 nm UVB phototherapy–an effective treatment for psoriasis. Br J Dermatol 1988;119:691–6.
23. Yones SS, Palmer RA, Garibaldinos TM, et al. Randomized double-blind trial of treatment of vitiligo: efficacy of psoralen-UV-A therapy vs Narrowband-UV-B therapy. Arch Dermatol 2007;143:578–84.
24. Westerhof W, Nieuweboer-Krobotova L. Treatment of vitiligo with UV-B radiation vs topical psoralen plus UV-A. Arch Dermatol 1997;133:1525–8.
25. Parsad D, Kanwar AJ, Kumar B. Psoralen-ultraviolet A vs. narrow-band ultraviolet B phototherapy for the treatment of vitiligo. J Eur Acad Dermatol Venereol 2006;20:175–7.
26. Hearn RM, Kerr AC, Rahim KF, et al. Incidence of skin cancers in 3867 patients treated with narrow-band ultraviolet B phototherapy. Br J Dermatol 2008;159:931–5.
27. Weischer M, Blum A, Eberhard F, et al. No evidence for increased skin cancer risk in psoriasis patients treated with broadband or narrowband UVB phototherapy: a first retrospective study. Acta Derm Venereol 2004;84:370–4.
28. Harrist TJ, Pathak MA, Mosher DB, et al. Chronic cutaneous effects of long-term psoralen and ultraviolet radiation therapy in patients with vitiligo. Natl Cancer Inst Monogr 1984;66:191–6.
29. Wildfang IL, Jacobsen FK, Thestrup-Pedersen K. PUVA treatment of vitiligo: a retrospective study of 59 patients. Acta Derm Venereol 1992;72:305–6.
30. Halder RM, Battle EF, Smith EM. Cutaneous malignancies in patients treated with psoralen photochemotherapy (PUVA) for vitiligo. Arch Dermatol 1995; 131:734–5.
31. Carr WW. Topical calcineurin inhibitors for atopic dermatitis: review and treatment recommendations. Paediatr Drugs 2013;15:303–10.
32. Cury Martins J, Martins C, Aoki V, et al. Topical tacrolimus for atopic dermatitis. Cochrane Database Syst Rev 2015;(7):CD009864.
33. Schallreuter KU, Levenig C, Berger J. Vitiligo and cutaneous melanoma. A case study. Dermatologica 1991;183:239–45.
34. Nordlund JJ, Kirkwood JM, Forget BM, et al. Vitiligo in patients with metastatic melanoma: a good prognostic sign. J Am Acad Dermatol 1983;9:689–96.
35. Hexsel CL, Eide MJ, Johnson CC, et al. Incidence of nonmelanoma skin cancer in a cohort of patients with vitiligo. J Am Acad Dermatol 2009;60:929–33.
36. Hammoud SM, Kruis RW, Sigurdsson V. Prediction of the Occurrence of Melanoma and Non-melanoma Skin Cancer in Patients with Vitiligo. Acta Derm Venereol 2016;96:106–7.
37. Lindelof B, Hedblad MA, Sigurgeirsson B. On the association between vitiligo and malignant melanoma. Acta Derm Venereol 1998;78:483–4.
38. Schallreuter KU, Tobin DJ, Panske A. Decreased photodamage and low incidence of non-melanoma skin cancer in 136 sun-exposed caucasian patients with vitiligo. Dermatology 2002;204:194–201.
39. Teulings HE, Overkamp M, Ceylan E, et al. Decreased risk of melanoma and nonmelanoma skin cancer in patients with vitiligo: a survey among 1307 patients and their partners. Br J Dermatol 2013;168:162–71.
40. Park KK, Murase JE, Koo J. Long-term prognosis of vitiligo patients on narrowband UVB phototherapy. J Am Acad Dermatol 2012;66:326–7.
41. Paradisi A, Tabolli S, Didona B, et al. Markedly reduced incidence of melanoma and nonmelanoma skin cancer in a nonconcurrent cohort of 10,040 patients with vitiligo. J Am Acad Dermatol 2014;71: 1110–6.
42. Lee E, Koo J, Berger T. UVB phototherapy and skin cancer risk: a review of the literature. Int J Dermatol 2005;44:355–60.
43. Calanchini-Postizzi E, Frenk E. Long-term actinic damage in sun-exposed vitiligo and normally pigmented skin. Dermatologica 1987;174:266–71.
44. Salem MM, Shalbaf M, Gibbons NC, et al. Enhanced DNA binding capacity on up-regulated epidermal wild-type p53 in vitiligo by H2O2-mediated oxidation: a possible repair mechanism for DNA damage. FASEB J 2009;23:3790–807.
45. Schallreuter KU, Behrens-Williams S, Khaliq TP, et al. Increased epidermal functioning wild-type p53 expression in vitiligo. Exp Dermatol 2003;12:268–77.
46. Nordlund JJ. Nonmelanoma skin cancer in vitiligo patients. J Am Acad Dermatol 2009;61:1080–1.
47. Feily A, Pazyar N. Why vitiligo is associated with fewer risk of skin cancer?: providing a molecular mechanism. Arch Dermatol Res 2011;303:623–4.

Presentations, Signs of Activity, and Differential Diagnosis of Vitiligo

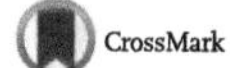

Boon-Kee Goh, MD[a], Amit G. Pandya, MD[b,*]

KEYWORDS

• Vitiligo • Presentations • Clinical activity • Differential diagnosis • Confetti • Trichrome • Koebner

KEY POINTS

- Thorough knowledge of the various presentations of vitiligo is important to make the correct diagnosis.
- Signs of activity in vitiligo patients are important to recognize so that treatment selection is optimized.
- Many skin disorders present with hypopigmentation or depigmentation and must be distinguished from vitiligo to make the correct diagnosis and prescribe the right treatment.

PRESENTATIONS OF VITILIGO

Vitiligo most commonly presents as bilaterally symmetric macules of depigmentation, with a preference for periorificial skin as well as skin prone to trauma. Frequent sites of presentation are the eyelids, nostrils, perioral skin, ears, axillae, elbows, wrists, hand, fingers, areolae, periumbilical skin, inguinal folds, genitals, knees, ankles, feet, and toes.

Generalized Vitiligo

Focal vitiligo

Focal vitiligo is a localized, small depigmented lesion that is isolated, lacks a segmental distribution and has not progressed into generalized vitiligo after 2 years.[1] Sometimes there will be 2 to 3 lesions in 1 area, but if they start to form a linear arrangement it is more likely to be segmental vitiligo. Because vitiligo usually spreads over time, it is important to rule out other diseases in patients with focal vitiligo, such as nevus depigmentosus and trauma-induced leukoderma.

Segmental vitiligo

A unilateral patch of depigmentation is known as segmental vitiligo. This form, comprising 5% to 30% of all cases of vitiligo, does not cross the midline and is often linear or blocklike in shape.[2] Segmental vitiligo usually presents in childhood, with 1 large study reporting a mean age of onset of 15.6 years.[2] Areas of involvement are the face, trunk, neck, extremities, and scalp, in descending order of frequency. Lesions usually progress rapidly over 6 months to 2 years and then stabilize. Rarely, patients develop segmental vitiligo first and then present with generalized vitiligo, which is then called "mixed vitiligo."[3]

Acrofacial vitiligo

Many patients have bilateral, depigmented macules limited to the head and distal extremities. There are too many lesions to make a diagnosis of focal vitiligo but fewer than is typically seen in generalized vitiligo. The term "acrofacial vitiligo" has been used to describe this variant. Although many patients never develop truncal lesions, this

[a] Skin Physicians Pte Ltd, 3 Mount Elizabeth, Suite 11-08 Mount Elizabeth Medical Centre, Singapore 228510, Singapore; [b] Department of Dermatology, University of Texas Southwestern Medical Center, 5323 Harry Hines Boulevard, Dallas, TX 75390-9069, USA
* Corresponding author.
E-mail address: amit.pandya@utsouthwestern.edu

Dermatol Clin 35 (2017) 135–144
http://dx.doi.org/10.1016/j.det.2016.11.004
0733-8635/17/

form may progress to generalized vitiligo over time. Another variant, known as lip-tip vitiligo, only affects the lips, fingers, and toes, and has been described most often in South Asians.[4,5]

SIGNS OF ACTIVITY

Determination of disease activity is important to assess prognosis and select the right treatment. In addition, establishing disease stability is critical when treating patients with surgical therapy, such as noncultured epidermal suspension grafting. The lack of erythema, scale, itching, burning or any other symptom in most patients with vitiligo causes difficulty in determining activity. However, a few clinical findings have been reported to be associated with disease activity and should be looked for during examination of a patient with vitiligo.

Koebner Phenomenon

Also known as an "isomorphic response," the Koebner phenomenon is defined as the development of lesions at the site of traumatized, uninvolved skin.[6] This finding is present in about one-third of patients by history. Those with greater body surface involvement and earlier age of involvement have a higher risk of the Koebner phenomenon.[6] Careful examination for linear macules of depigmentation at sites of scratches, abrasions, and other traumatic occurrences is necessary in all patients with vitiligo to detect this important sign of activity.

Trichrome Lesions

As a lesion of vitiligo progresses, the depigmentation gradually expands, with a sharp line of demarcation between pigmented and depigmented skin. In patients with rapidly progressing vitiligo, however, there is often an intervening zone of hypopigmented skin, known as trichrome vitiligo (**Fig. 1**). A biopsy of the border of these lesions reveals an inflammatory infiltrate and degeneration of the basal layer, which are signs of activity.[7]

Inflammatory Vitiligo

A rare form of vitiligo, known as inflammatory vitiligo, presents as erythema on the areas of depigmentation and/or the border of the lesion. These patients usually give a history of rapid enlargement of their vitiligo lesions. Mild scale may be seen overlying the lesions and pruritus of the affected may areas be a presenting complaint. An infiltrate of lymphocytes and macrophages with concomitant disappearance of melanocytes has been reported in this form of vitiligo.[8]

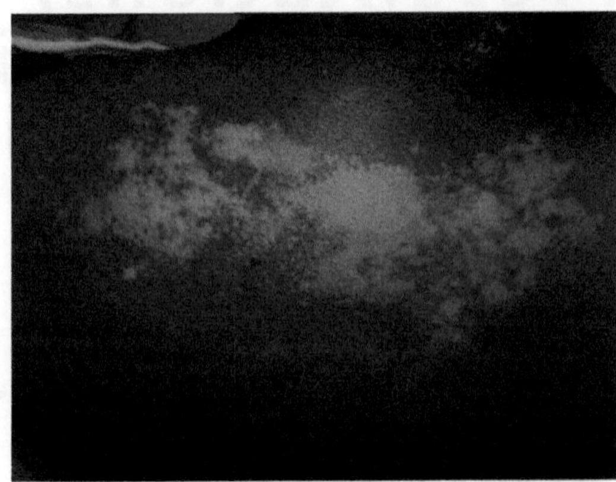

Fig. 1. Depigmented macule on back owing to vitiligo showing confettilike depigmentation, trichrome vitiligo, and the Koebner phenomenon.

Confettilike Lesions

Confettilike macules of depigmentation have been recently reported as a marker of rapidly progressive vitiligo.[9] These patients present with clusters of small, 1- to 5-mm macules, often at the periphery of existing lesions. The small lesions enlarge, and rapidly coalesce and form larger, more typical lesions of vitiligo. Affected patients have a higher Vitiligo Disease Activity Score and Koebner Phenomenon Vitiligo Score, which correlates with disease progression. Biopsy of confetti lesions reveals an inflammatory infiltrate of lymphocytes with $CD8^+$ lymphocytes at the basal cell layer, where melanocytes reside.

Recognition of the signs of vitiligo activity is helpful in selecting therapy. Stable disease can usually be treated with topicals and phototherapy, which may take several months to achieve the first signs of repigmentation. However, patients with active disease may also need to be treated with oral corticosteroids for a period of time to stabilize their disease.[10]

DIFFERENTIAL DIAGNOSIS OF VITILIGO

Many disorders can mimic vitiligo, especially early vitiligo. A useful clinical approach is to classify them based on the extent of the lesions (localized or widespread), the pattern of lesions (eg, guttate/confetti) and the degree of pigment loss (depigmented or hypopigmented).[11] Further clinical differentiation can be made on the basis of associated morphologic signs, including secondary changes of the epidermis (such as scaling and atrophy) and dermis (such as induration and infiltration; **Figs. 2** and **3**).

To differentiate between depigmented and hypopigmented lesions, Wood's light is a useful

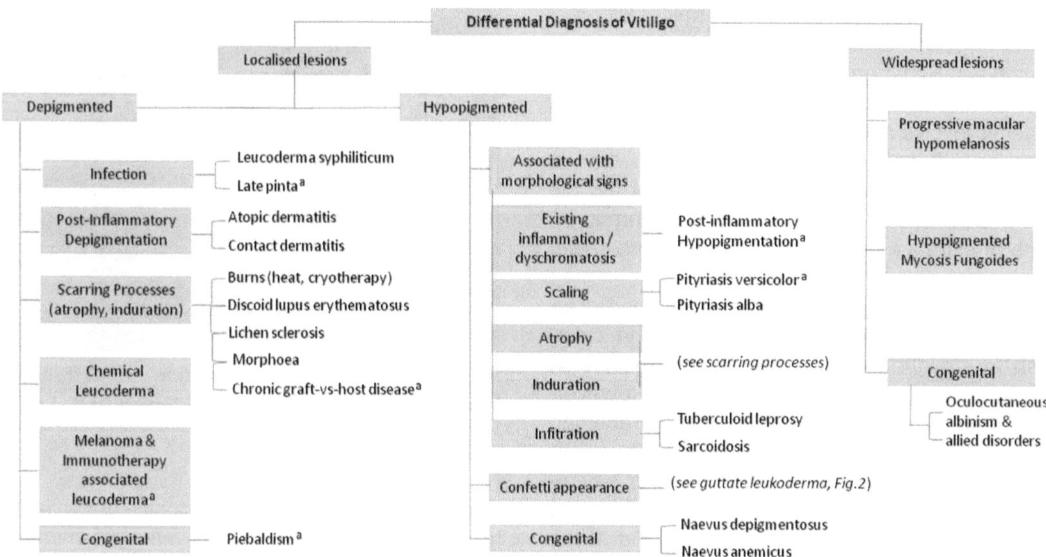

Fig. 2. Clinical approach to the differential diagnosis of vitiligo. [a] Lesions can be widespread.

bedside tool. Wood's light is a form of long-wave ultraviolet radiation (320–400 nm, peak at 365 nm) emitted from a high-pressured mercury arc lamp after passing through a compound filter of barium silicate and 9% nickel oxide. In depigmented lesions, the absence of melanocytes results in a lack of absorption of Wood's light by epidermal melanin causing most of the light to be reflected. A window is also created for autofluorescence of dermal collagen, giving off a small band of blue light. Depigmented lesions therefore appear as bright bluish-white patches under Wood's light. This tool is useful in distinguishing established vitiligo (depigmented) in a dark room from hypopigmented conditions such as naevus anemicus, naevus depigmentosus, pityriasis alba, and postinflammatory hypopigmentation, which fail to accentuate.[12] Wood's light is also useful in evaluating vitiligo in fair-skinned individuals, where the lesion and its margins may be difficult to discern.

Guttate Leucoderma

- Idiopathic guttate hypomelanosis
- Leucoderma en confetti (chemical leucoderma)
- Confetti macules of tuberous sclerosis
- Confetti macules of lichen sclerosis
- Guttate morphoea
- Achromic pityriasis lichenoides chronica
- Guttate leucoderma of Darier's disease
- Amyloidosis cutis dyschromica
- Punctate leucoderma from laser toning

Fig. 3. Differential diagnosis of confetti lesions of vitiligo.

Localized Depigmentation

Many acquired conditions other than vitiligo can present with depigmentation. Depigmented lesions are porcelain white in color because of the complete absence of melanocytes; however, they can be admixed with hypopigmented lesions if the degree of pigment loss is variable. A careful history is of paramount importance in eliciting the precipitating factors and identifying the etiology. The acquired loss of melanocytes and reduction of melanin production can be owing to a variety of mechanisms, including infective, inflammatory, immune, and chemical- and drug-induced causes.

Focal depigmented lesions can occur in Treponemal diseases such as secondary syphilis (leucoderma syphiliticum) and late stage pinta. Although rarely seen, depigmented and hypopigmented macules and patches can present in patients with secondary syphilis.[13,14] Classically described by Hardy in 1854 as leucodermic macules on the neck (necklace of Venus), these lesions can manifest on different parts of the body including the groin and genitalia. Histologic differentiation from vitiligo can be made by detecting lichenoid interface dermatitis, plasma cell infiltrates and endothelial edema.[14,15] Serologic tests for syphilis are confirmatory. It remains controversial if the loss of pigment is a result of postinflammatory changes or a direct effect of spirochetes on melanocytes, because ultrastructural evidence of *Treponema pallidum* has been demonstrated within the leucodermic lesions.[16] Unlike syphilis, pinta is predominantly found in Central and South America and is caused by *T carateum*. The disease is limited only to the skin, without systemic involvement. In late pinta, depigmented lesions have been classically described to appear symmetrically on bony prominences, such as the wrists, elbows, and ankles.[17] Late leucodermic lesions of pinta are not infectious, unlike early pinta, which are teeming with treponemes.

Postinflammatory depigmentation is a particular problem in dark-skinned individuals. The diagnosis is straightforward when the primary lesion and its secondary changes are present. However, it can pose a diagnostic challenge if the preceding inflammatory changes have receded. Depigmentation can occur as a result of chronic or severe inflammation in atopic dermatitis and contact dermatitis, particularly owing to scratching. If the lesions are associated with changes such as epidermal atrophy, dermal sclerosis (induration) and loss of follicular ostia, scarring processes are to be considered, including burns, discoid lupus erythematosus (**Fig. 4**), lichen sclerosus (**Fig. 5**), scleroderma, and rarely, chronic graft-versus-host disease (**Fig. 6**). Patients with systemic sclerosis can present with depigmented patches dotted with perifollicular pigmentation (classically described as "salt and pepper" pattern). This presentation can mimic or be confused with repigmenting vitiligo.[18] Histologically, there is a loss of interfollicular but not follicular melanocytes. The key to distinguishing these dyschromic lesions from vitiligo is the presence of sclerosis (induration), which can be visualized histologically and palpated clinically.

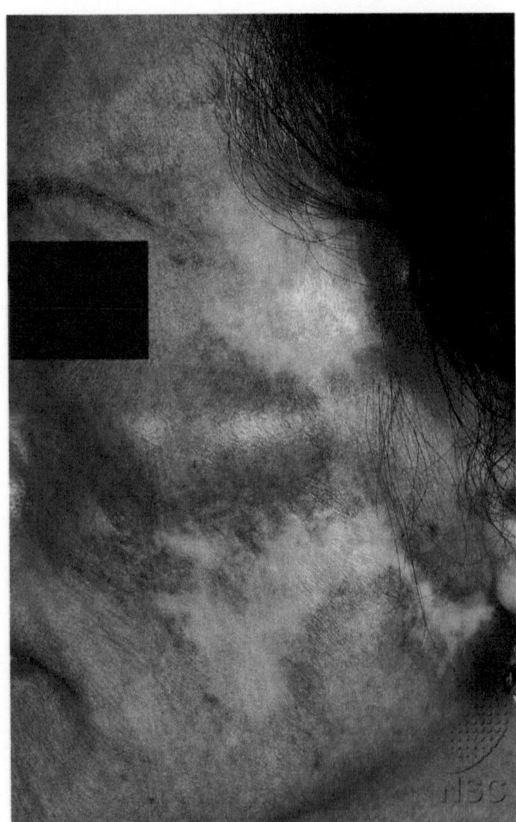

Fig. 4. Atrophic, sclerotic depigmented patches of "burnt out" discoid lupus erythematosus. (*Courtesy of* National Skin Centre, Singapore; with permission.)

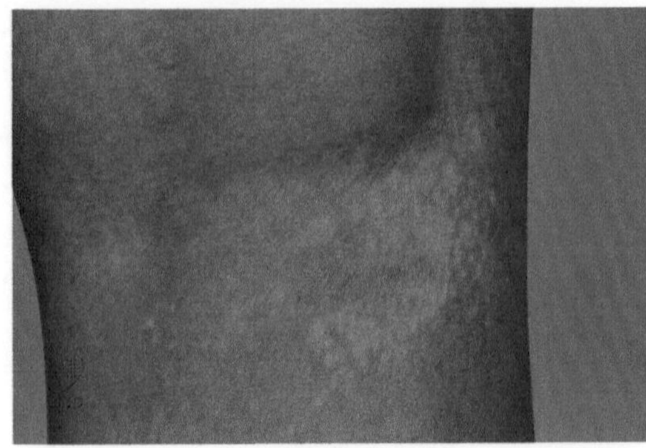

Fig. 5. Macular hypopigmentation of extragenital lichen sclerosus. (*Courtesy of* National Skin Centre, Singapore; with permission.)

Vitiligo-like depigmentation can also occur in patients with melanoma or as a side effect from immunotherapy with interleukin-2, interferon-alpha, or immune checkpoint inhibitors (anti–CTLA-4 and anti–PD1/PD-L1). The depigmentation is a result of antimelanoma immunity that also targets normal melanocytes, owing to shared expression of melanocyte differentiation antigens. Whether this form of depigmentation is considered a subtype of vitiligo remains controversial, although an international consensus had considered it not to be.[1] It is interesting to note that melanoma-associated depigmentation portends a favorable prognostic outcome for patients with advanced disease, and is associated with a clear survival benefit.[19]

Chemical leucoderma denotes an acquired depigmentation or hypopigmentation induced by repeated exposure to specific chemical compounds, notably aromatic and aliphatic derivatives of phenols and catechols (**Fig. 7**). Examples of these compounds are monobenzyl ether of hydroquinone (historically used as an antioxidant in the rubber industry) and para-tertiary butyl phenol and its homologues. The clues to diagnosis of chemical leucoderma include a history of repeated exposure to a depigmenting agent, distribution of lesions corresponding to the primary site of

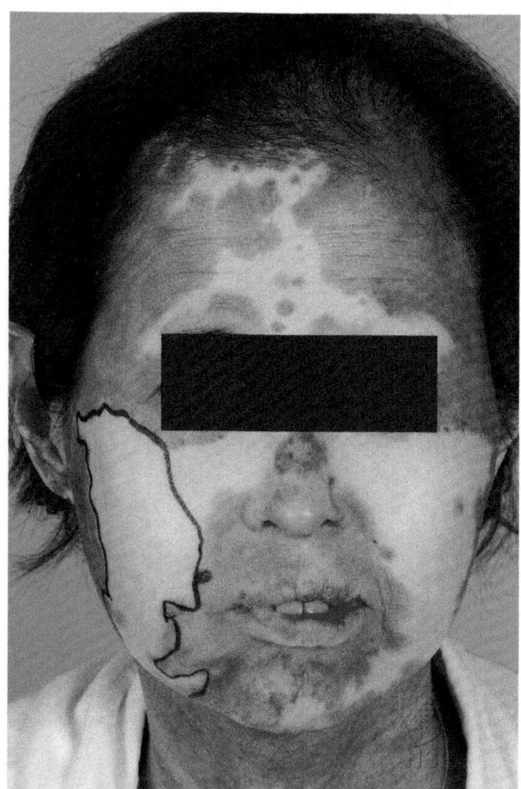

Fig. 6. Leukoderma of chronic graft-versus-host disease. This patient developed chronic graft-versus-host disease after her second bone marrow transplant for acute myeloid leukemia. She had extensive depigmentation, misdiagnosed as vitiligo. Note the microstomia and cutaneous sclerosis. The depigmented patch on right cheek was demarcated for a trial of cellular grafting; the outcome of which was excellent repigmentation. (*Courtesy of* National Skin Centre, Singapore; with permission.)

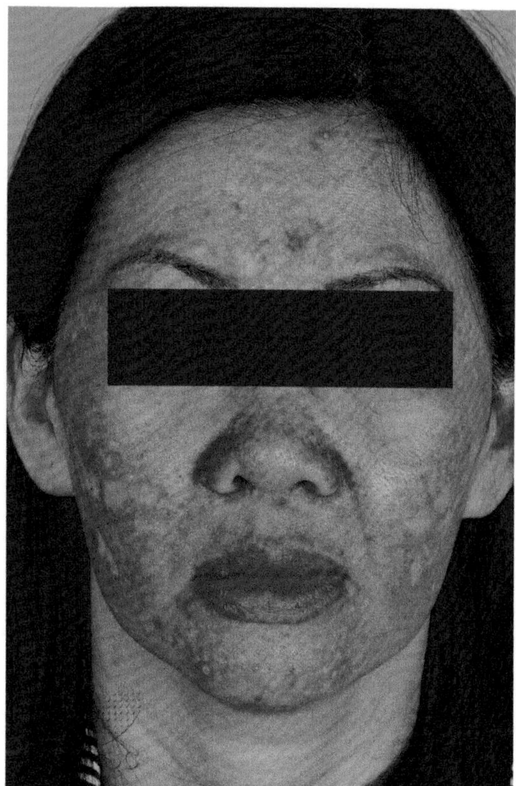

Fig. 7. Chemical leukoderma. This patient developed extensive hypopigmented and depigmented macules and patches on her face after using a skin-lightening cream of unknown source for her melasma. (*Courtesy of* National Skin Centre, Singapore; with permission.)

contact, and confetti appearance of leucodermic macules. In Asia, depigmented macules have been reported on the forehead of Indian women owing to free para-tertiary butyl phenol in "Bindi" adhesives.[20] Confetti leucoderma complicating ochronosis has also been reported in Asian and Hispanic individuals with melasma, owing to long term use of skin-lightening creams containing hydroquinone (and possibly adulteration with other phenolic compounds and mercury).[21,22] Recently an unexpected outbreak of depigmentation was reported in Japan, as a result of a novel phytochemical introduced into skin-lightening creams: Rhododenol or 4-(4-hydroxyphenyl)-2-butanol. This compound is a potent competitive inhibitor of tyrosinase, but its metabolites are melanocytotoxic, resulting in vitiligo-like lesions that are hypopigmented or depigmented (**Fig. 8**). To distinguish this from vitiligo, histopathology is important in demonstrating (i) the presence of melanophages and (ii) perifollicular cellular infiltration.[23]

Piebaldism is often confused with vitiligo. A careful history, however, will distinguish between the two: piebaldism is congenital and familial. Unlike vitiligo, the depigmented lesions in piebaldism are relatively static in shape and size, and have a typical distribution on the ventral surfaces of the torso, limbs and frontal scalp (white forelock). Embryologically, this is owing to the aborted dorsolateral migration of melanocyte precursors from the neural crest. Within these depigmented lesions, leukotrichia is invariable and often islands of hyperpigmentation are present (**Fig. 9**).

Localized Hypopigmentation

Several localized hypopigmented conditions can be confused with vitiligo. If the lesions are associated with epidermal changes such as scaling and dryness, pityriasis alba and tinea versicolor should be considered. Pityriasis alba is predominantly seen in the pediatric age group. The affected child

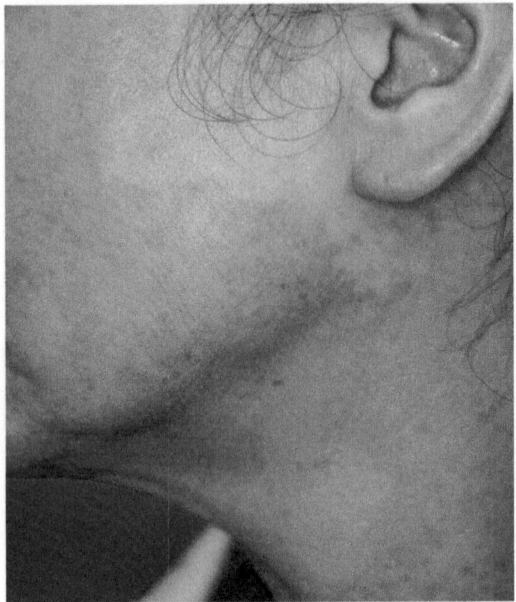

Fig. 8. Chemical leukoderma. Hypopigmented patches as a result of a skin-lightening cream containing Rhododenol. (*Courtesy of* Chikako Nishigori, MD, Phd, Kobe University Graduate School of Medicine, Kobe, Japan.)

usually has an atopic diathesis. The patches of pityriasis alba are hypopigmented and dry, and the borders are diffuse and ill-defined. Scaling, however, may be very subtle (**Fig. 10**). Typically, the lesions are seen on sun-exposed areas like the face and upper limbs, and are often precipitated after a period of tanning. At times, it may be difficult to distinguish pityriasis alba from very early vitiligo.

Tinea versicolor is caused by overgrowth of the commensal yeast found on our skin, *Malassezia furfur*. The yeast invades the stratum corneum

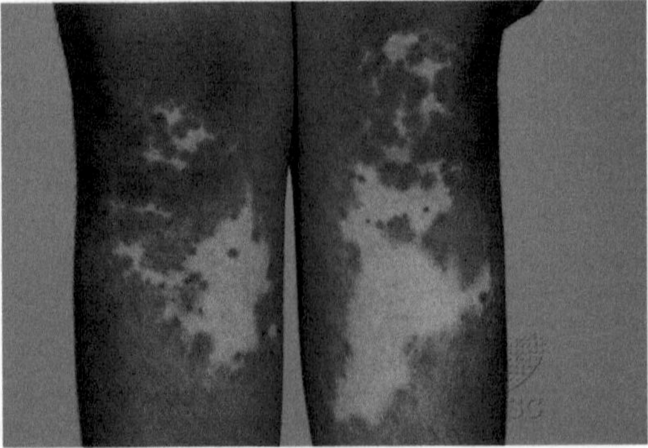

Fig. 9. Piebaldism. Symmetric depigmented patches on the anterior aspects of lower limbs. Note the leukotrichia and islands of pigmentation within the lesions. (*Courtesy of* National Skin Centre, Singapore; with permission.)

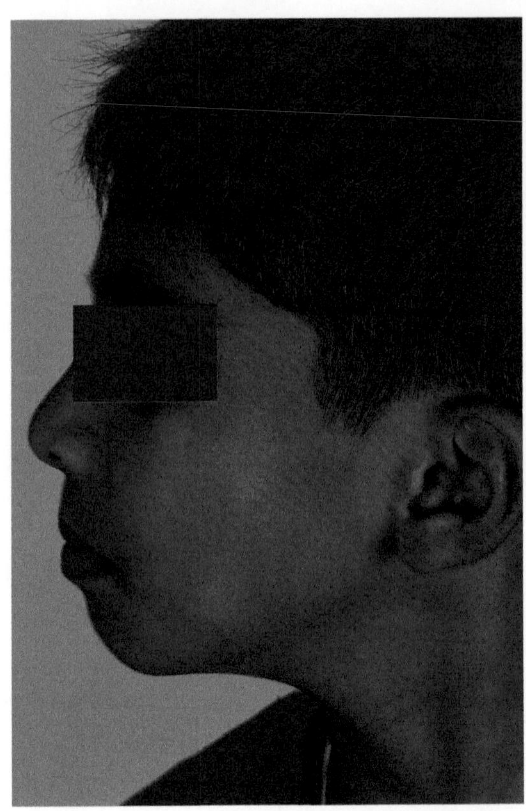

Fig. 10. Pityriasis alba. Ill-defined, hypopigmented, and dry patches on the cheeks of a child. (*Courtesy of* National Skin Centre, Singapore; with permission.)

and induces hypopigmentation through its metabolites, such as azelaic acid, which inhibits tyrosinase. The lesions present as hypopigmented macules or confluent patches, affecting typically the shoulders and back. Stretching the lesions reveals fine powdery scale (**Fig. 11**). During the inflammatory stages, the lesions seem to be pinkish brown, owing to dermatitis caused by the yeast and/or its metabolites. Confirmation of the diagnosis is established after microscopy of skin scrapings; the sample will show typical spores and hyphae. In dark-skinned individuals, resolution of the infection after antifungal therapy results in residual hypopigmentation without epidermal changes, which can be confused with early vitiligo.

If hypopigmented patches are associated with an infiltrated consistency, tuberculoid leprosy and sarcoidosis are to be considered. Hypopigmented patches of tuberculoid leprosy are characterized by hypoaesthesia, accompanied by xerosis and atrichia (**Fig. 12**). In countries where leprosy is endemic, bedside testing for hypoesthesia using a pin or the sharp corner of a folded sheet of paper is mandatory for examining any hypopigmented patches. Sarcoidosis is one of the “great

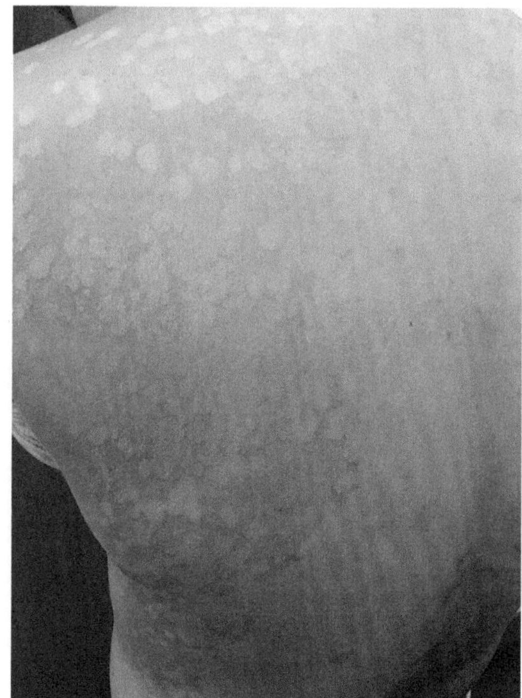

Fig. 11. Hypopigmented patches of tinea versicolor. Note the fine powdery scaling.

mimickers" in dermatology because of its multiform presentations. Hypopigmentation may present as patches, papules, or plaques. The cause of hypopigmentation is not known, but possibly attributed to interface dermatitis or postinflammatory changes.[24] If erythematous papules or plaques are seen within the lesions, diascopy can be useful in obliterating the erythema and revealing the yellowish-brown tinge ('apple-jelly") of underlying granulomas.[25]

Naevus depigmentosus is typically congenital, although it may not be apparent at birth. It presents as a unilateral, solitary patch and is hypopigmented rather than depigmented (hence the title is a misnomer). Borders are often more jagged than typical vitiligo lesions. It can be mistaken for early focal or segmental vitiligo. However, the hairs within naevus depigmentosus are invariably pigmented and the lesion remains relatively static in shape and size (apart from enlarging proportionately with the growing child).

Naevus anemicus is another congenital anomaly that can be mistaken for focal vitiligo. The lesion presents as a localized patch but is not depigmented. Instead, it seems to be paler than the surrounding skin, owing to sustained vasoconstriction as a result of localized hypersensitivity to catecholamines.[26] Pressing the lesional border with a glass slide renders the lesion indistinguishable from the surrounding blanched skin.

Confettilike lesions of vitiligo (**Fig. 13**) can be confused with other causes of guttate leucoderma (see **Fig. 3**). One of them is idiopathic guttate hypomelanosis, which is a benign, acquired condition commonly seen on the limbs of middle-aged to elderly individuals (**Fig. 14**). The lesions appear as hypopigmented to depigmented discrete macules, ranging usually 1 to 3 mm in size (rarely 10 mm or more). The exact etiology of idiopathic guttate hypomelanosis is not fully understood, although photoaging is believed to play an important role.[27] Histologically there is a variable reduction to complete absence of melanocytes. Although treatment of idiopathic guttate hypomelanosis is a challenge, gentle cryotherapy (a short, single-pass freeze of 2–3 seconds) is a simple and inexpensive way of inducing repigmentation (personal experience). Topical calcineurin inhibitors

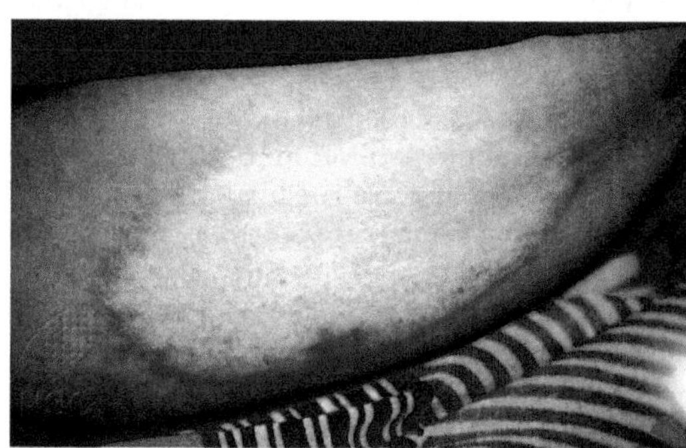

Fig. 12. An anesthetic hypopigmented patch of tuberculoid leprosy. Note the inflamed, infiltrated border. (*Courtesy of* National Skin Centre, Singapore; with permission.)

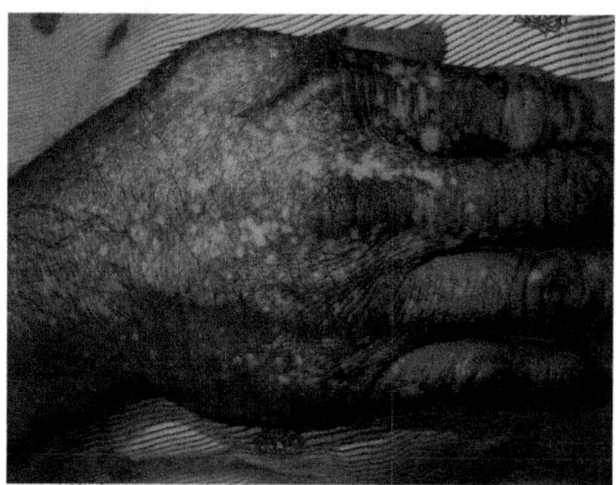

Fig. 13. Confettilike lesions of vitiligo on the dorsal hand and fingers.

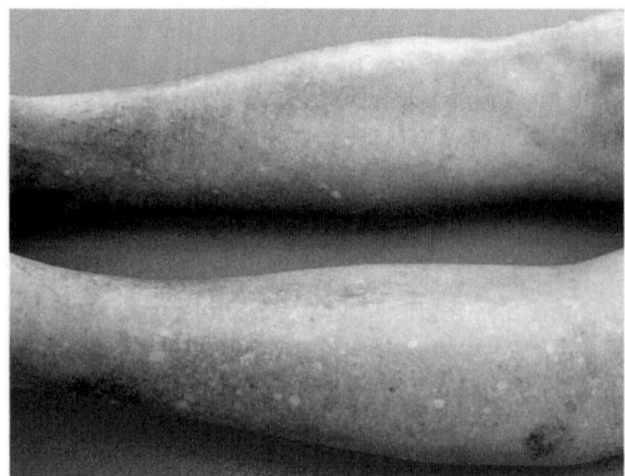

Fig. 14. Idiopathic guttate hypomelanosis. Small hypopigmented round macules on the limbs of an elderly man.

(tacrolimus and pimecrolimus) have been tried, but the repigmentation rates are variable.[28,29]

Widespread Hypopigmentation and Depigmentation

Several leucodermic conditions can be mistaken for extensive vitiligo. Progressive macular hypomelanosis is an idiopathic hypopigmented condition, predominantly seen in young adults. Interestingly, Relyveld and colleagues[30] associated the condition with an undefined species of *Propionibacterium*, rather than *Propionibacterium acnes*, which was previously incriminated. In 2004, Westerhof and colleagues[31] published the detection of follicular red fluorescence within the lesions of progressive macular hypomelanosis and demonstrating, by culture, the presence of the *P acnes* from lesional but not healthy skin. They proposed that a factor produced by this bacterial strain impairs melanogenesis. Progressive macular hypomelanosis has the following distinctive features that differ from vitiligo vulgaris: (i) the lesions are hypopigmented and never depigmented and (ii) the lesions have a characteristic distribution: confined to the trunk, uniformly confluent in the midline with small nummular macules radiating from the margins of this central confluence (**Fig. 15**). No epidermal changes are found in the lesions of progressive macular hypomelanosis, which distinguishes it from tinea versicolor or hypopigmented mycosis fungoides.

Hypopigmented mycosis fungoides (MF) is a variant of cutaneous T-cell lymphoma. Unlike classical cutaneous T-cell lymphoma, this variant affects the younger age group of patients with skin of color. The diagnosis of hypopigmented MF is often missed and mistaken for tinea versicolor, vitiligo vulgaris, or progressive macular hypomelanosis.[32] This leads to a failure of obtaining biopsies and prolongs the latency to definitive treatment. A high index of suspicion is therefore required. Unlike vitiligo, epidermal changes (albeit subtle at times) are a feature in hypopigmented MF. The typical hypopigmented patches in this cutaneous lymphoma are associated with a wrinkled surface (epidermal atrophy) and dryness; scaling may be subtle. The patches vary in shape and size, and may have a pinkish hue owing to telangiectasia (**Fig. 16**). The buttocks should always be examined, because this is a site of predilection (**Fig. 17**). In pediatric cases, it remains a challenge to differentiate hypopigmented MF from achromic pityriasis lichenoides chronica, although remnants of small scaly erythematous papules may be found in the latter on careful examination. It is likely that both conditions represent different manifestations of the same disease.[33]

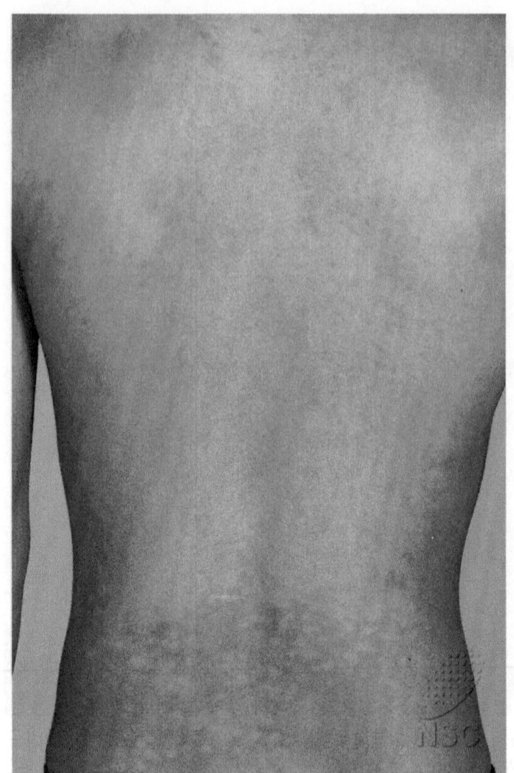

Fig. 15. Progressive macular hypomelanosis: confluent hypopigmented patch on the back, with small nummular macules radiating from the margins. (*Courtesy of* National Skin Centre, Singapore; with permission.)

In a patient with generalized depigmentation, congenital disorders such as oculocutaneous albinism should be differentiated from vitiligo universalis. In oculocutaneous albinism, the entire integument is involved, together with ocular abnormalities such as strabismus and nystagmus.

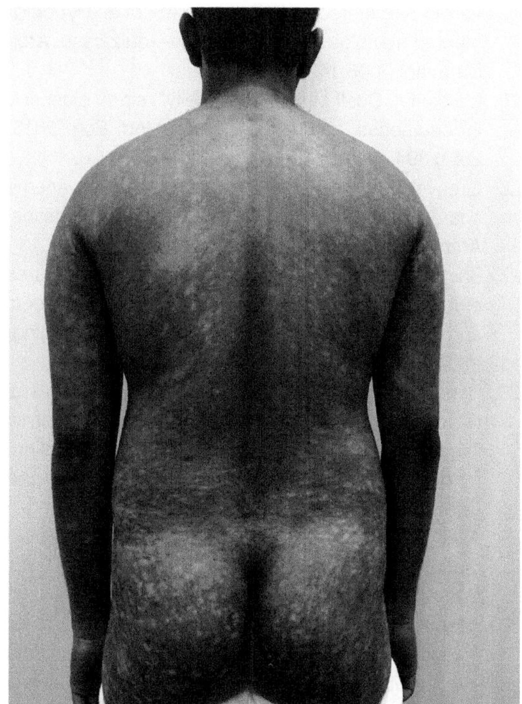

Fig. 16. Hypopigmented mycosis fungoides. Extensive hypopigmented and erythematous patches (of varied sizes and shapes) on the body, including buttocks.

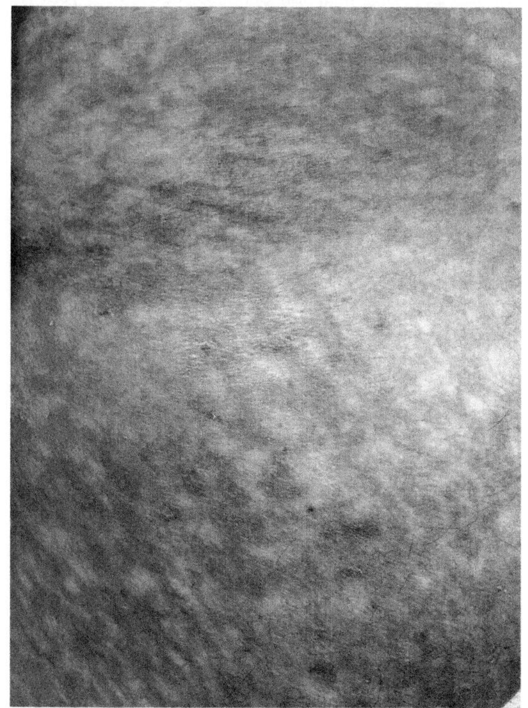

Fig. 17. Hypopigmented mycosis fungoides. Close up of the lesions on buttocks. Note the epidermal changes of atrophy (wrinkling) and scaling.

SUMMARY

Vitiligo presents with a variety of manifestations. Although generalized vitiligo is fairly straightforward to diagnose, early disease can be difficult to distinguish from other forms of hypopigmentation and depigmentation. In addition, signs of activity are important to recognize to select the correct therapy and determine prognosis. Knowledge of common and uncommon causes of pigment loss is essential when evaluating a patient with suspected vitiligo.

REFERENCES

1. Ezzedine K, Lim HW, Suzuki T, et al. Revised classification/nomenclature of vitiligo and related issues: the Vitiligo Global Issues Consensus Conference. Pigment Cell Melanoma Res 2012;25:E1–13.
2. Hann SK, Lee HJ. Segmental vitiligo: clinical findings in 208 patients. J Am Acad Dermatol 1996;35:671–4.
3. Ezzedine K, Gauthier Y, Leaute-Labreze C, et al. Segmental vitiligo associated with generalized vitiligo (mixed vitiligo): a retrospective case series of 19 patients. J Am Acad Dermatol 2011;65:965–71.
4. Sharma S, Sarkar R, Garg VK, et al. Coexistence of lip-tip vitiligo and disseminated discoid lupus erythematosus with hypothyroidism: need for careful therapeutic approach. Indian Dermatol Online J 2013;4:112–4.
5. Martis J, Bhat R, Nandakishore B, et al. A clinical study of vitiligo. Indian J Dermatol Venereol Leprol 2002;68:92–3.
6. van Geel N, Speeckaert R, De Wolf J, et al. Clinical significance of Koebner phenomenon in vitiligo. Br J Dermatol 2012;167:1017–24.
7. Hann S-K, Kim Y-S, Yoo JH, et al. Clinical and histopathologic characteristics of trichrome vitiligo. J Am Acad Dermatol 2000;42:589–96.
8. Le Poole IC, van den Wijngaard RM, Westerhof W, et al. Presence of T cells and macrophages in inflammatory vitiligo skin parallels melanocyte disappearance. Am J Pathol 1996;148:1219–28.
9. Sosa JJ, Currimbhoy SD, Ukoha U, et al. Confetti-like depigmentation: a potential sign of rapidly progressing vitiligo. J Am Acad Dermatol 2015;73(2):272–5.
10. Kanwar AJ, Mahajan R, Parsad D. Low-dose oral mini-pulse dexamethasone therapy in progressive unstable vitiligo. J Cutan Med Surg 2013;17:259–68.
11. Tey HL. Approach to hypopigmentation disorders in adults. Clin Exp Dermatol 2010;35:829–34.
12. Klatte JL, van der Beek N, Kemperman PMJH. 100 years of Wood's lamp revised. J Eur Acad Dermatol Venereol 2015;29:842–7.
13. Pandhi RK, Bedi TR, Bhutani K. Leucoderma in early syphilis. Br J Vener Dis 1977;53(1):19–22.

14. Uprety S, Vinay K, De D, et al. Hypopigmented patches on a young man. Clin Exp Dermatol 2016; 41(1):100–2.
15. Miranda MFR, Bettencourt MJS, Lopes IC, et al. Leucoderma syphiliticum - a rare expression of the secondary stage diagnosed by histopathology. An Bras Dermatol 2010;85(4):512–5.
16. Poulsen A, Secher L, Kobayasi T, et al. Treponema pallidum in leukoderma syphiliticum demonstrated by electron microscopy. Acta Derm Venereol 1988; 68:102–6.
17. Marquez F, Rein CR, Arias O. Mal del pinto in Mexico. Bull World Health Organ 1955;13(2):299–322.
18. Sánchez JL, Vázquez M, Sánchez NP. Vitiligolike macules in systemic scleroderma. Arch Dermatol 1983;119(2):129–33.
19. Teulings HE, Limpens J, Jansen SN, et al. Vitiligo-like depigmentation in patients with stage III–IV melanoma receiving immunotherapy and its association with survival: a systematic review and meta-analysis. J Clin Oncol 2015;33:773–81.
20. Bajaj AK, Gupta SC, Chatterjee AK. Contact depigmentation from free para-tertiary-butylphenol in bindi adhesive. Contact Dermatitis 1990;22: 99–102.
21. Liu WC, Tey HL, Lee JSS, et al. Exogenous ochronosis in a Chinese patient: use of dermoscopy aids early diagnosis and selection of biopsy site. Singapore Med J 2014;55(1):e1–3.
22. Jow T, Hantash BM. Hydroquinone-Induced depigmentation: case report and review of the literature. Dermatitis 2014;25(1):e1–5.
23. Nishigori C, Aoyama Y, Ito A, et al. Guide for medical professionals (i.e. dermatologists) for the management of Rhododenol-induced leukoderma. J Dermatol 2015;42:113–28.
24. Verma S, Patterson JW, Derdeyn AS, et al. Hypopigmented macules in an Indian man—quiz case. Arch Dermatol 2006;142(12):1643–8.
25. Matos D, Coelho R. "Apple jelly" sign: diascopy in cutaneous sarcoidosis. Acta Med Port 2015; 28(3):394.
26. Greaves MW, Birkett D, Johnson C. Nevus anemicus: a unique catecholamine-dependent nevus. Arch Dermatol 1970;102(2):172–6.
27. Shin M-K, Jeong K-H, Oh I-H, et al. Clinical features of idiopathic guttate hypomelanosis in 646 subjects and association with other aspects of photoaging. Int J Dermatol 2011;50:798–805.
28. Rerknimitr P, Disphanurat W, Achariyakul M. Topical tacrolimus significantly promotes repigmentation in idiopathic guttate hypomelanosis: a double-blind, randomized, placebo-controlled study. J Eur Acad Dermatol Venereol 2013;27:460–4.
29. Asawanonda P, Sutthipong T, Prejawai N. Pimecrolimus for idiopathic guttate hypomelanosis. J Drugs Dermatol 2010;9:238–9.
30. Relyveld GN, Westerhof W, Woudenberg J, et al. Progressive macular hypomelanosis is associated with a putative Propionibacterium species. J Invest Dermatol 2010;130:1182–4.
31. Westerhof W, Relyveld G, Kingswijk MM, et al. Propionibacterium acnes and the pathogenesis of progressive macular hypomelanosis. Arch Dermatol 2004;140:210–4.
32. Tan ES, Tang MB, Tan SH. Retrospective 5-year review of 131 patients with mycosis fungoides and Sézary syndrome seen at the National Skin Centre, Singapore. Australas J Dermatol 2006;47:248.
33. Heng YK, Koh MJA, Giam YC, et al. Pediatric mycosis fungoides in Singapore: a series of 46 children. Pediatr Dermatol 2014;31:477–82.

Segmental Vitiligo

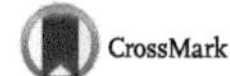

Nanja van Geel, MD, PhD*, Reinhart Speeckaert, MD, PhD

KEYWORDS

• Vitiligo • Segmental vitiligo • Halo nevi • Classification • Mosaicism • Segmental • Lines of blaschko • Surgical treatment

KEY POINTS

- Segmental vitiligo, a subtype of vitiligo, is characterized by its early onset, rapid stabilization, and unilateral distribution.
- It has been suggested that segmental and nonsegmental vitiligo are not 2 completely separate entities, but could represent variants of the same disease spectrum.
- Recent observational studies with respect to its distribution pattern point to a possible role of cutaneous mosaicism in segmental vitiligo.
- Good results are reported in stabilized forms of segmental vitiligo after a surgical treatment (pigment transplantation).

CLINICAL PRESENTATION

Clinical Signs

It is generally important to differentiate at least 2 types of vitiligo: the nonsegmental and segmental types. The nonsegmental type of vitiligo is characterized by its symmetric distribution, unpredictable course, and association with autoimmune diseases. In contrast, the segmental type has a typical unilateral distribution, is less strongly associated with autoimmune diseases, and shows a rapid stabilization. In an observational study from the authors' group, 41/141 patients (85.4%) observed disease stabilization within the first year after onset and 8 patients (16.7%) even mentioned a stabilization in only a few days after the initial appearance of the lesions.[1] Sometimes further progression is observed at later stages, although this is more exceptional. A study of Park and colleagues[2] found disease recurrence in 21.8% of segmental vitiligo patients 4 or more years after disease onset.

However, most studies with long-term follow-up after pigment cell transplantation for segmental vitiligo did not show high rates of unexpected disease activity.[3,4] Segmental vitiligo is associated more with an earlier age of onset compared with nonsegmental vitiligo.[1] The reported prevalence of segmental vitiligo within a total vitiligo population varies between studies (5% and 27.9%)[5,6] and was 11.6% (89/770) in the authors' department.[1]

Some variants of segmental vitiligo have also been described. The concomitant presence of segmental vitiligo and nonsegmental vitiligo has been termed mixed vitiligo, and if 2 segmental vitiligo lesions are present on opposite body sides, it is called a bilateral segmental vitiligo.[1] If 2 distinct segments on the same side are present, it could be called multisegmental vitiligo. Furthermore, segmental vitiligo lesions can be present with associated halo nevi. In this article describing the distribution patterns of segmental vitiligo, halo nevi were present in 26 of 179 segmental vitiligo patients (14.4%), whereas this was even remarkably higher (24.2%; 16/65) in the authors' study evaluating specifically segmental vitiligo lesions on the trunk. The latter might be due to the fact that the trunk is a predilection area for halo nevi.[7]

Disclosure Statement: The authors have nothing to disclose.

Department of Dermatology, Ghent University Hospital, De Pintelaan 185, Ghent 9000, Belgium
* Corresponding author.
E-mail address: Nanja.vangeel@ugent.be

Dermatol Clin 35 (2017) 145–150
http://dx.doi.org/10.1016/j.det.2016.11.005

Distribution Pattern

Segmental vitiligo has often been linked in the literature to a dermatomal distribution. However, several recent studies observed that most segmental vitiligo lesions did not fit exactly within the borders of the commonly mentioned "dermatomal" lines. It was therefore hypothesized that segmental vitiligo has probably been classified incorrectly in the past to a dermatomal distribution. However, a typical unique recurring pattern could be observed with a very clear midline demarcation. More recently, it was suggested that this recurring pattern could fit to the theory of cutaneous mosaicism.[8] This hypothesis was also supported by the authors' study describing convincing similarities between segmental vitiligo and other mosaic skin disorders, especially segmental lentiginosis and verrucous epidermal nevus.[8] These observations support the possible role of cutaneous mosaicism for at least a part of the segmental vitiligo lesions.

Classification

So far, a classification of segmental vitiligo on the face (see later discussion) and the trunk (see later discussion) has been proposed.[7,9] These classifications can help to predict the possible susceptible areas of future distribution of early developing segmental vitiligo lesions.

Face

The classification of segmental vitiligo on the face was determined by comparing the distribution patterns of 257 Korean patients with segmental vitiligo on the face.[9] Six subtypes were described by this Korean group: type Ia, Ib, II, III, IV, and V (**Figs. 1**A and **2**). *Type Ia* was most frequently observed (28.8%). It affects a large part of the left side of the face. Type Ia starts on the forehead at the right side of the midline and crosses the central part of the forehead, extending laterally and downwards. Overall, it resembles a reversed V-shaped pattern. Involvement of the right side of the face is rare in this subtype. *Type Ib* is located high on the forehead on the left or right side with frequently signs of poliosis. *Type II* lesions follow an archlike pattern starting from the auricular area until reaching the midline area at the philtrum. In *type III*, the depigmentation starts at one side of the lower lip spreading in a downwards and slightly lateral way toward the neck. *Type IV* closely resembles type I but does not cross the midline (unlike type 1a) and is exclusively located on the right side of the face. Finally, *type V* involves the right orbital area, and further spreading to the temporal area is possible. After type Ia, the most frequent subtypes were type II (16.0%), III (14.4%), IV (10.9%), Ib (10.5%), followed by type V (8.6%).[10]

Trunk

In the authors' retrospective observational study, the distribution pattern of 106 segmental vitiligo lesions on the trunk was analyzed and classified into 6 recurring subtypes.[7] Type 1, 2, and 3 involved the upper part of the trunk, type 4 and 5, the middle part of the trunk, and type 6, the lower part of the trunk (**Fig. 1**B). *Type 1* is a small linear band located at the central part of the upper trunk just lateral from the midline. It extends from the chin toward the sternal area. *Type 2* is a depigmentation on the upper part of the shoulder

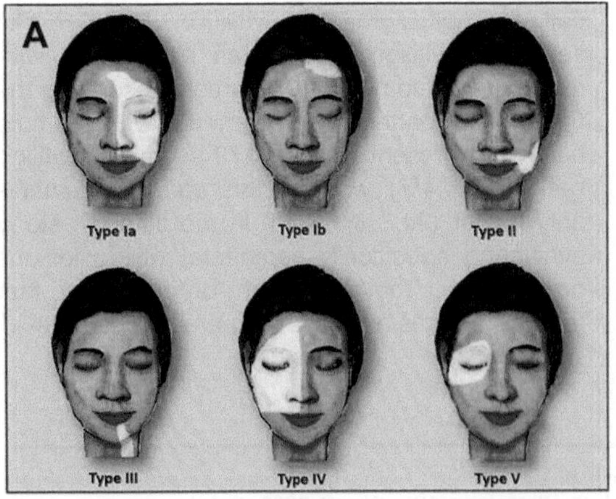

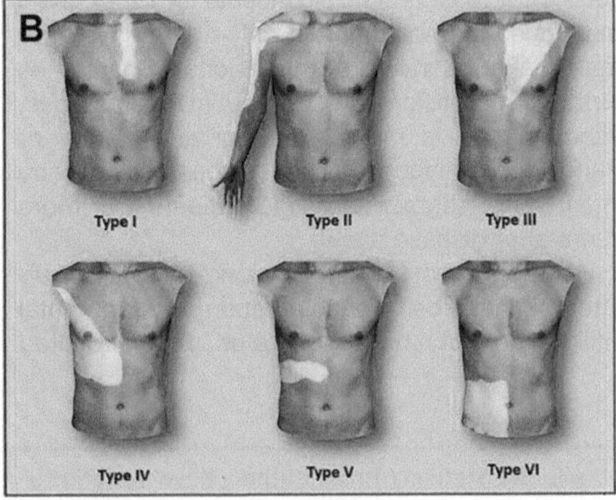

Fig. 1. (*A*) Distribution patterns of segmental vitiligo on the face. (*B*) Distribution patterns of segmental vitiligo on the trunk. (*Data from* [A] Kim D-Y, Oh SH, Hann S-K. Classification of segmental vitiligo on the face: clues for prognosis. Br J Dermatol 2011;164(5):1004–9; and [B] van Geel N, Bosma S, Boone B, Speeckaert R. Classification of segmental vitiligo on the trunk. Br J Dermatol 2014;170(2):322–7.)

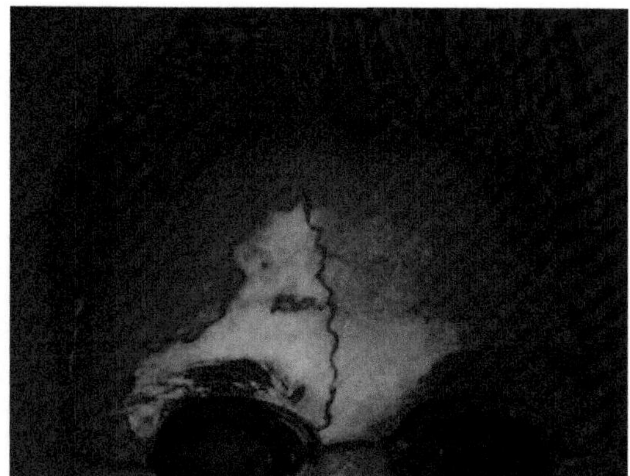

Fig. 2. Segmental vitiligo on the face corresponding to a partial involvement of type IV.

running from the neck to the lateral side of the arm. *Type 3* is a characteristic V-shaped pattern on the ventral side of the trunk. It starts on the lower edge of the shoulder and spreads down to the midline of the thorax. *Type 4* is located below the type 3 pattern. The lesions start at the axilla and spread lateral and down until the midline. *Type 5* is a horizontal bandlike lesion at the lower part of the trunk. It is located above the waist and expands to the lateral side of the trunk. *Type 6* presents as a rectangular depigmented area, which also develops on the lower part of the trunk, although it can extend below the waist. Type 6 can mostly be observed on the abdomen. It is similar to the checkerboard pattern as described by Happle.[11]

Type 3 was the most common observed segmental vitiligo pattern and can easily be recognized by its "triangle shape," which can be observed on the upper trunk against the midline of the upper thorax. This specific pattern (type 3) has also been reported in other mosaic disorders, such as segmental lentiginosis and epidermal nevus verrucosus.[8] Furthermore, the distribution of a triangle-shaped lesion on the upper part of the trunk resembled a combination of the type 1b (broadband Blaschko linear) and type 2 pattern of mosaicism as described by Happle.[11]

Segmental vitiligo was more frequently observed on the ventral side (85.9%) compared with the lateral part (52.8%) or back (36.8%) of the trunk; this may reflect the migration pattern of the melanoblasts during embryogenesis from their origin in the neural crest. Most melanocyte precursors migrate dorsolaterally and proliferate while they travel through the dermis until they reach the ventral midline. As such, melanocytes at the ventral side of the body could be at increased risk for acquiring somatic mosaicism due to their increased proliferation until they reside in their final destination at the epidermis or hair follicle.[12]

PATHOPHYSIOLOGY

Histologic and Immunohistochemical Data

Immunohistochemical data with respect to segmental vitiligo are rather scarce, and significant lymphocytic infiltrates have only occasionally been observed. The scarce observation of a lymphocytic infiltrate may be explained by the fact that the depigmented patches are clinically manifest a few weeks after the initial melanocyte damage and thus after the essential immunologic phenomena have occurred. Although the exact origin of melanocyte destruction is still unclear, increasing evidence has been published now on a possible autoimmune/inflammatory destruction of segmental vitiligo. Attili and Attili[13] found that segmental vitiligo corresponds histologically to nonsegmental vitiligo with an inflammatory infiltrate present in most patients with evolving or recently evolved lesions (87% for segmental vs 71% in nonsegmental vitiligo). Currently, it remains ambiguous whether the inflammatory process is based on a deregulated immune system or can be regarded as a secondary event to cellular abnormalities in the epidermis.

The authors described in 2010 the early dynamic clinical and immunologic sequence of segmental vitiligo appearing in a patient with halo nevi.[14] This study was the first that described the histopathological events and phenotypic characteristics, including antigen specificities of T cells isolated from lesional and nonlesional skin. This study provided evidence that a cell-mediated immune response is involved in the early phases of segmental vitiligo with associated halo nevi. Histopathological analysis revealed a lymphocytic infiltrate, mainly composed of $CD8^+$ T cells and some $CD4^+$ T cells around the dermoepidermal junction. Flow cytometry analysis of lesional T cells revealed a clear enrichment of proinflammatory interferon-γ-producing $CD8^+$ T cells compared with the nonlesional skin. Using HLA-peptide tetramers (MART-1, tyrosinase, gp100), increased numbers of T cells recognizing melanocyte antigens were found in segmental vitiligo lesional skin, as compared with the nonlesional skin and the blood. These findings indicated that a $CD8^+$ melanocyte-specific T-cell–mediated immune response, as observed in generalized vitiligo, could also play a role in segmental vitiligo.[14] This observation was also supported by another case report that described an exceptional combination of segmental vitiligo, alopecia areata, psoriasis, and a halo nevus.[15] As these disorders are supposed to be inflammation-driven conditions, this additional observation strengthened the likelihood of an immune-mediated pathophysiology in segmental vitiligo.

Hypotheses

So far, several theories for the pathogenesis of segmental vitiligo have been offered, including neuronal mechanisms, somatic mosaicism, and microvascular skin homing of immune cells, whether leading to an autoimmune destruction of melanocytes or not.

Neuronal mechanisms

The first hypothesis involves neural mechanisms (eg, sympathetic nerve function, neuropeptides), which is mainly based on the previous thought that segmental vitiligo is following the course of dermatomes. Some studies reported results in favor of this theory. Clinical observations have been reported in which a segmental vitiligo lesion appeared in areas corresponding to local neurologic damage (eg, subacute encephalitis, spinal cord tumor, or following trauma).[16] Furthermore, physiologic abnormalities associated with sympathetic nerve function (acetylcholine activity, neuropeptide distribution, and catecholamine metabolism) were demonstrated in lesional segmental vitiligo skin. Wu and colleagues[17] reported an increased cutaneous blood flow compared with the contralateral normal skin and a significantly increased α- and β-adrenoceptor response in segmental vitiligo lesions. Finally, experimental findings in animals could demonstrate that abnormalities in neuropeptides or other neurochemical mediators secreted by nerve endings could harm nearby melanocytes.[18] However, it might be assumed that this reaction can also be explained as a bystander effect of inflammation instead of a triggering factor.

Somatic mosaicism

As most segmental vitiligo lesions did not exactly fit within the borders of dermatomal lines, a second theory has been suggested.[8] According to this theory, segmental vitiligo lesions represent a vulnerable subpopulation of melanocytes as seen in cutaneous mosaicism.[8] Pigmentary mosaicism has been linked to migration pattern of skin cells during embryogenesis. When clinically visible, these pigmentary patterns (eg, Blaschko lines) are suggested to reflect an underlying mosaicism of different cell lines.[11]

In the authors' observational study, the pattern of segmental vitiligo resembled to a certain extent some patterns of cutaneous mosaicism.[8] Furthermore, convincing similarities were found with other mosaic skin disorders, in particular, segmental lentiginosis and verrucous epidermal nevi. In that observational study, a typical recurring "segmental vitiligo pattern" was observed that could not yet be clearly classified in the 6 subtypes of mosaicism as described by Happle,[11] although some overlap existed.

So far, convincing data at the molecular genetic level of lesional and nonlesional segmental vitiligo skin to prove the theory of mosaicism are not available yet. However, a clinical observation after surgical treatment of segmental vitiligo is supporting this theory. It is generally known that there is a superior long-term take of epidermal cellular grafting in segmental vitiligo lesions compared with the moderate to limited results in patients with generalized vitiligo. This better take assumes that the transplanted cells of autologous donor skin are genetically not affected in the isolated type of segmental vitiligo.[4]

Microvascular skin homing

It has also been suggested that the midline delineation in unilateral lesion could represent the migration pattern of cytotoxic T cells from specific lymph nodes along the microvascular system via homing receptors. According to the literature, it has been demonstrated that these homing receptors can have a unique unilateral homing code.[19]

The observation of associated halo nevi in segmental vitiligo patients may support this theory. Based on the authors' experience, the appearance of halo nevi occurs often before the development of the segmental vitiligo lesions, suggesting a clonal expansion of melanocyte-specific T lymphocytes in the regional lymph node. However, it seems reasonable that this theory of skin-homing receptors cannot entirely explain the specific disease pattern of segmental vitiligo.

Combination theory (3-step theory)

Whether different etiopathologic mechanisms as described above underlie the clinical phenotypes of segmental vitiligo remain to be elucidated. Furthermore, the theory of cutaneous mosaicism does not exclude the neuronal theory, as a neurogenic factor can still be one of the initial triggers to induce the whole process in its early stage. Furthermore, the possible existence of different or combined etiopathologic pathways (eg, neuronal, mosaicism, microvascular skin homing) underlying the same clinical presentation of segmental vitiligo cannot be ruled out. This possible combination was proposed as a 3-step theory, including the 3 etiopathogenic pathways, providing hereby a more integrated view into the current evidence on segmental vitiligo. It summarizes the different proposed etiopathogenic mechanisms for segmental vitiligo into one model. The first step includes the release of inflammatory factors, neuropeptides, and catecholamines, which can be considered as the triggering factor. This triggering factor leads to a small inflammatory response at a site where melanocytes are more vulnerable to immune-mediated destruction (possibly due to somatic mosaicism) (step 2). Subsequently, an antimelanocyte-specific response develops in the draining lymph node, and specific T cells migrate by binding to their vascular adhesion receptors toward the segmental vitiligo area, causing the characteristic skin depigmentations.[15]

TREATMENT

It is generally known that segmental vitiligo is less responsive to medical treatments like local steroids, topical calcineurin inhibitors, and phototherapy compared with nonsegmental vitiligo. This reduced response can be related to the absence of a melanocyte reservoir in the hair follicles (leukotrichia), which is typically present in segmental vitiligo. However, when treated early after onset, lesions seem to be more sensitive to response.[20] Furthermore, medical treatment may possibly be helpful to stop further progression. Topical treatment (corticosteroids, tacrolimus, pimecrolimus) and also targeted UVB therapy can therefore be recommended in progressive patients.[21] Combination treatments (eg, topical tacrolimus + excimer laser + systemic corticosteroids) have been tested with beneficial results.[22] However, it is generally accepted that surgical methods are an interesting therapeutic option in patients with segmental vitiligo. Different surgical techniques have been devised over the years and include tissue grafts (full-thickness punch grafts, split-thickness grafts, suction blister grafts) and cellular grafts (cultured melanocytes, cultured epithelial sheet grafts, and noncultured epidermal cellular grafts). According to many publications, best results after surgical treatment are obtained in segmental vitiligo, whereas results in generalized or mixed vitiligo are inferior. Furthermore, repigmentation seems to be maintained during follow-up in most segmental vitiligo patients.[4]

SUMMARY

Segmental vitiligo is a subtype of vitiligo with a specific unilateral distribution. It develops fast and remains stable in most cases over time. Based on the distribution pattern and other characteristics, most evidence supports the theory of somatic mosaicism combined with an autoimmune destruction of melanocytes, although confirmation on the genetic level is currently lacking. Based on these new insights, the authors suggest meanwhile to avoid using the term dermatomal distribution. Early developing vitiligo can be treated with topical anti-inflammatory treatments, and UVB treatment has been shown to induce possible repigmentation. Nonetheless, given the excellent results obtained with surgery, pigment cell transplantation can also be considered as a first-line option to repigment stabilised forms of segmental vitiligo.

REFERENCES

1. van Geel N, De Lille S, Vandenhaute S, et al. Different phenotypes of segmental vitiligo based on a clinical observational study. J Eur Acad Dermatol Venereol 2011;25(6):673–8.
2. Park J-H, Jung M-Y, Lee J-H, et al. Clinical course of segmental vitiligo: a retrospective study of eighty-seven patients. Ann Dermatol 2014;26(1):61–5.
3. Hann SK, Lee HJ. Segmental vitiligo: clinical findings in 208 patients. J Am Acad Dermatol 1996; 35(5 Pt 1):671–4.
4. van Geel N, Wallaeys E, Goh BK, et al. Long-term results of noncultured epidermal cellular grafting in vitiligo, halo naevi, piebaldism and naevus depigmentosus. Br J Dermatol 2010;163(6):1186–93.
5. el-Mofty AM, el-Mofty M. Vitiligo A symptom complex. Int J Dermatol 1980;19(5):237–44.
6. Koga M, Tango T. Clinical features and course of type A and type B vitiligo. Br J Dermatol 1988;118(2):223–8.
7. van Geel N, Bosma S, Boone B, et al. Classification of segmental vitiligo on the trunk. Br J Dermatol 2014;170(2):322–7.
8. van Geel N, Speeckaert R, Melsens E, et al. The distribution pattern of segmental vitiligo: clues for somatic mosaicism. Br J Dermatol 2013;168(1):56–64.
9. Kim D-Y, Oh SH, Hann S-K. Classification of segmental vitiligo on the face: clues for prognosis. Br J Dermatol 2011;164(5):1004–9.
10. Hann SK, Chang JH, Lee HS, et al. The classification of segmental vitiligo on the face. Yonsei Med J 2000; 41(2):209–12.
11. Happle R. Mosaicism in human skin. Understanding the patterns and mechanisms. Arch Dermatol 1993; 129(11):1460–70.
12. Gilbert SF. The neural crest. 2000. Available at: http://www.ncbi.nlm.nih.gov/books/NBK10065/. Accessed May 18, 2016.
13. Attili VR, Attili SK. Segmental and generalized vitiligo: both forms demonstrate inflammatory histopathological features and clinical mosaicism. Indian J Dermatol 2013;58(6):433–8.
14. van Geel NAC, Mollet IG, De Schepper S, et al. First histopathological and immunophenotypic analysis of early dynamic events in a patient with segmental

vitiligo associated with halo nevi. Pigment Cell Melanoma Res 2010;23(3):375–84.
15. van Geel N, Mollet I, Brochez L, et al. New insights in segmental vitiligo: case report and review of theories. Br J Dermatol 2012;166(2):240–6.
16. Singh A, Kornmehl H, Milgraum S. Segmental vitiligo following encephalitis. Pediatr Dermatol 2010;27(6):624–5.
17. Wu CS, Yu HS, Chang HR, et al. Cutaneous blood flow and adrenoceptor response increase in segmental-type vitiligo lesions. J Dermatol Sci 2000;23(1):53–62.
18. Miniati A, Weng Z, Zhang B, et al. Neuro-immuno-endocrine processes in vitiligo pathogenesis. Int J Immunopathol Pharmacol 2012;25(1):1–7.
19. Sackstein R. The lymphocyte homing receptors: gatekeepers of the multistep paradigm. Curr Opin Hematol 2005;12(6):444–50.
20. Park J-H, Park SW, Lee D-Y, et al. The effectiveness of early treatment in segmental vitiligo: retrospective study according to disease duration. Photodermatol Photoimmunol Photomed 2013;29(2):103–5.
21. Ezzedine K, Eleftheriadou V, Whitton M, et al. Vitiligo. Lancet 2015;386(9988):74–84.
22. Bae JM, Yoo HJ, Kim H, et al. Combination therapy with 308-nm excimer laser, topical tacrolimus, and short-term systemic corticosteroids for segmental vitiligo: a retrospective study of 159 patients. J Am Acad Dermatol 2015;73(1):76–82.

Chemical-Induced Vitiligo

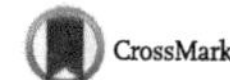

John E. Harris, MD, PhD

KEYWORDS

• Vitiligo • Leukoderma • Chemical • Phenol • Rhododendrol • Monobenzone • Cellular stress • Autoimmunity

KEY POINTS

- Chemical exposure may serve as an environmental risk factor for developing vitiligo.
- Chemical-induced depigmentation is indistinguishable from vitiligo, and should be considered "chemical-induced vitiligo."
- Chemical-induced vitiligo is typically found at to the site of application and may also spread to remote, unexposed locations.
- Monobenzyl ether of hydroquinone was the first chemical noted to induce depigmentation in the skin, and is now used therapeutically in patients with vitiligo to complete their depigmentation.
- Most chemicals that induce vitiligo are phenols that act as tyrosine analogs to disrupt melanocyte function, resulting in autoimmunity.

INTRODUCTION

Like many autoimmune diseases, vitiligo pathogenesis is influenced by genetic, stochastic, and environmental factors. This is clear from the fact that first-degree relatives of patients with vitiligo have a 5-fold to 6-fold increased risk of disease and identical twins have a 23-fold increased risk, clearly implicating genetics as an important risk factor for vitiligo. However, despite sharing almost all of their genes, identical twins are only 23% concordant for disease, meaning that if one has vitiligo the other will have it only 23% of the time.[1] This clearly implicates other, nonheritable risk factors for developing vitiligo as well. Stochastic mechanisms, or the influence of random chance, likely play a role, particularly during the development of the immune system, which occurs through random recombination of T-cell receptors and antibodies. This process is responsible for "building" the autoreactive cells that ultimately attack melanocytes in vitiligo. The role of stochastic factors in developing vitiligo and other autoimmune diseases is not likely to account for all of the nongenetic risk, and so many believe that factors from the environment strongly influence the likelihood of developing autoimmunity.

Vitiligo is one of the few autoimmune diseases in which environmental factors are well-known, including the depigmenting effect of the chemical monobenzyl ether of hydroquinone (MBEH) discovered by Oliver and colleagues[2] in a tanning factory, but includes many others as well. Some have been directly implicated via topical challenge through patch testing, others through large population studies, and still others more indirectly. This article summarizes the chemicals that have been clearly implicated as causing or exacerbating vitiligo, as well as the mechanism by which this occurs. Recognizing these chemicals and their implications for managing vitiligo is important during patient counseling and follow-up, both when thinking about disease prevention, as well as improving therapeutic responses.

Disclosures: Consultant for Combe, Inc. Funded by NIH grant number AR069114; NIHMS-ID: 829384.
Department of Dermatology, University of Massachusetts Medical School, 364 Plantation Street, LRB 225, Worcester, MA 01605, USA
E-mail address: John.Harris@umassmed.edu

Dermatol Clin 35 (2017) 151–161
http://dx.doi.org/10.1016/j.det.2016.11.006
0733-8635/17/

CHEMICALS DIRECTLY IMPLICATED IN INDUCING VITILIGO

Monobenzyl Ether of Hydroquinone

In 1939, Oliver and colleagues[2] reported a case series of workers in a leather manufacturing company who developed patchy depigmentation on their hands and arms. In fact, 50% of the workers in this factory and others who wore a particular brand of gloves developed depigmentation on skin that contacted the gloves, and several of them also had similar lesions on remote areas that did not contact the gloves. The ingredients used in manufacturing the gloves were obtained by the medical team, and each systematically applied to the workers through patch testing. Only patches containing the antioxidant MBEH induced an inflammatory response, which was then followed by depigmentation. This chemical ingredient was removed from the gloves, and workers subsequently repigmented.[2] Depigmentation was also reported following exposure to other products that contained MBEH, primarily by items made of rubber.[3] MBEH has been removed from manufacturing in the US rubber industry, although may still be in use in other countries.[4]

After this observation, others attempted to use MBEH as a treatment for hypermelanoses[5–7]; however, reports of complete and irreversible depigmentation at the site of application and in remote areas limited its use,[8–11] and resulted in its removal from commercial products. The ability of MBEH to permanently remove skin pigment prompted Mosher and colleagues[12] to test it as a topical treatment for patients with severe vitiligo. They recommended the use of MBEH in patients with vitiligo who failed to respond to therapy with psoralen ultraviolet A (PUVA) and with depigmentation of more than 50% of their body surface area. Their retrospective study of 18 patients who used topical MBEH revealed that 8 patients completely depigmented in 4 to 12 months.[12] Since then, dermatologists have used this as a therapy in severe patients who desired it, noting also depigmentation remote from the site of application, and sparing of hair and eye color.[3] It is currently the only treatment approved by the Food and Drug Administration for vitiligo, and details about its use are in the article by Pearl Grimes, "Depigmentation Therapy for Vitiligo," elsewhere in this issue. In addition, monomethyl ether of hydroquinone has been reported to induce depigmentation in 2 subjects,[13] and has been used therapeutically to depigment patients with vitiligo.[14,15]

Hydroquinone, a chemical structurally related to MBEH and frequently used in skin-lightening agents, has not been clearly implicated in inducing or exacerbating vitiligo when used for cosmetic purposes. Despite many cases attributed to MBEH, only 2 patients reportedly developed depigmentation after exposure to photographic developing solution containing hydroquinone, and in both patients the depigmentation was preceded by allergic dermatitis.[16,17] However, despite the use of hydroquinone creams for many years, including to "feather" the border of vitiligo lesions to make them less apparent, it results in only uniform lightening of the skin, and no cases of focal depigmentation have been reported following this method of treatment.[3] Thus, hydroquinone-containing topical treatments are probably safe to use in patients with vitiligo who request treatment for coexisting hyperpigmentation (ie, melasma, for example), although this should be considered on a case-by-case basis.

4-Tert-Butylcatechol

The application of a single chemical-soaked patch to the skin was also used to implicate other phenols in products that induced depigmentation in patients with vitiligo. In the 1970s, a smaller percentage (4/75, ~5%) of factory workers in a tappet (valve lifters) assembly plant developed acral depigmentation due to contact with 4-tert-butylcatechol (4-TBC) present in a lubricating oil. All patients had severe inflammation before depigmentation at the site of contact, and three-fourths had remote depigmentation as well.[18] Patch testing with 4-TBC induced an inflammatory response in 3 of the 4 affected, with clear depigmentation in 1, whereas none of 6 healthy volunteers developed depigmentation.[18] Studies in guinea pigs confirmed the ability of 4-TBC to depigment the skin, particularly in high concentrations and in strong solvents.[19]

4-Tert-Butylcatechol and 4-Tert-Amylphenol

Bajaj and colleagues[20] reported the characteristics of 100 consecutive patients who presented with depigmentation under their bindi, a decorative item worn on the forehead of many Indian women, often using an adhesive resin. Seventy-three exhibited dermatitis at the site before depigmentation, and 34 had depigmentation remote from the site of bindi application. On patch testing of 15 patients with the adhesive resin, 5 had irritant reactions and 3 of those depigmented 15 to 60 days later. The chemical 4-tert-butylphenol (4-TBP) was the suspected culprit based on its high content in the samples tested, as well as a number of other reports that implicated the chemical in other occupations. An additional report described perioral depigmentation in a patient after the use of lip liner that contained 4-TBP. Patch testing to the chemical was positive in this patient.[21] Other groups similarly implicated 4-TBP and 2,4-ditert-butylphenol (2,4-dTBP) in causing depigmentation after occupational exposures,[22–25] and 3 groups reported a variety of systemic abnormalities, including thyroid, liver, and/or splenic changes after exposure. Based on these observations, they suggested that the chemical may be capable of inducing inflammation in organs beyond the skin.[25–27]

Kahn[28] reported depigmentation in hospital workers at 2 separate locations: 5 in one hospital and 7 in another. Both groups worked directly with germicidal detergents, although the specific detergents were different brands: 5 were exposed to O-Syl (similar to Lysol) and 7 to Ves-Phene. Although the ingredients between these products varied, one contained 4-TBP and the other contained 4-tert-amylphenol (4-TAP). Both reproduced depigmentation with patch testing in all subjects, supporting the results discussed previously. Three of 5 and 4 of 7 subjects experienced pruritus and erythema before depigmentation of the patch testing sites. Sites of contact with the detergent were affected in all workers, and 2 had involvement of remote sites as well (1 in each group). One of the hospitals discontinued use of the detergent (O-Syl), and the other did not (Ves-Phene). Two of the 5 workers who discontinued using O-Syl regained their pigment.[28]

An additional study from Russia implicated 4-TBP in workers who manufactured synthetic condensation resins. Interestingly, of those who were in contact with the chemical for fewer than 2 years in total, 15% were affected, and of those who were exposed for more than 2 years, more than 40% were affected,[29] suggesting that length of exposure influenced the incidence of disease.

Dyes

Taylor and colleagues[30] first reported the ability of hair dyes and, specifically, para-phenylenediamine (PPD) to induce depigmentation. They described 4 subjects who developed depigmentation of the scalp and hair after using hair dyes, and found that 3 of the subjects exhibited depigmentation following patch testing (2 with PPD and 1 with the hair dye itself). Three of the subjects at least partially repigmented after discontinuing use of the dyes.[30] Other cases implicating PPD in hair dyes have been reported as well, although not all cases confirmed depigmentation through patch testing.[31–35] One group published a case series of 3 subjects who developed depigmentation of the scalp that abruptly stopped at the hair line, but was independent from hair dye use. They postulated that scalp depigmentation alone did not necessarily implicate the use of hair dyes as causative.[36] Patients may develop hair dye–induced depigmentation on the scalp or face, depending on the site of application (**Fig. 1**A, B).

Alta is a red dye solution used in India as a cosmetic coloring agent for the feet. The dye has been reported to induce vitiligo at the location of application, and patch testing in 1 subject implicated the dye components Crocein Scarlet MOO, or brilliant crocein, and rhodamine B, or tetraethyl rhodamine. Depigmentation was preceded by contact dermatitis in this subject, and she also developed remote depigmentation on the hands. Negative results were observed in more than 20 controls who were also patch tested with the dyes. The subject also developed a similar reaction to PPD, thought to be a well-known cross-reaction between the chemicals, as the alta contained no trace of PPD. All sites depigmented approximately 6 weeks after application of the patch tests, and repigmented after 6 months.[37] Some have reported that depigmentation occurred following direct exposure to dyes in leather products and other clothing when in close contact with the skin, such as shoes, wallets, and sandals[4,38,39] (**Fig. 1**C).

PRODUCTS INDIRECTLY IMPLICATED IN VITILIGO INDUCTION THROUGH POPULATION-BASED STUDIES

The critical importance of commercial products in the induction of vitiligo became evident in the summer of 2013 when Kanebo, a Japanese cosmetics company, was forced to recall a new skin-lightening cream after more than 16,000 users developed vitiligo (~2% of all users). The active ingredient was rhododendrol.[40,41] A large retrospective analysis of users revealed that most experienced depigmentation only at the site of exposure to the cream; however, a small percentage (5%) experienced depigmentation at remote sites as well.[42] Data acquired through questionnaires of affected individuals reported that following discontinuation of the cream, 7% of lesions had completely resolved, 27% had improved by more than half, 38% were improved by less than half, 25% were unchanged, and 2% had increased in size (1% could not be determined). Many patients (67%) improved even without therapy, whereas slightly more (77%) reported improvement when treated with standard

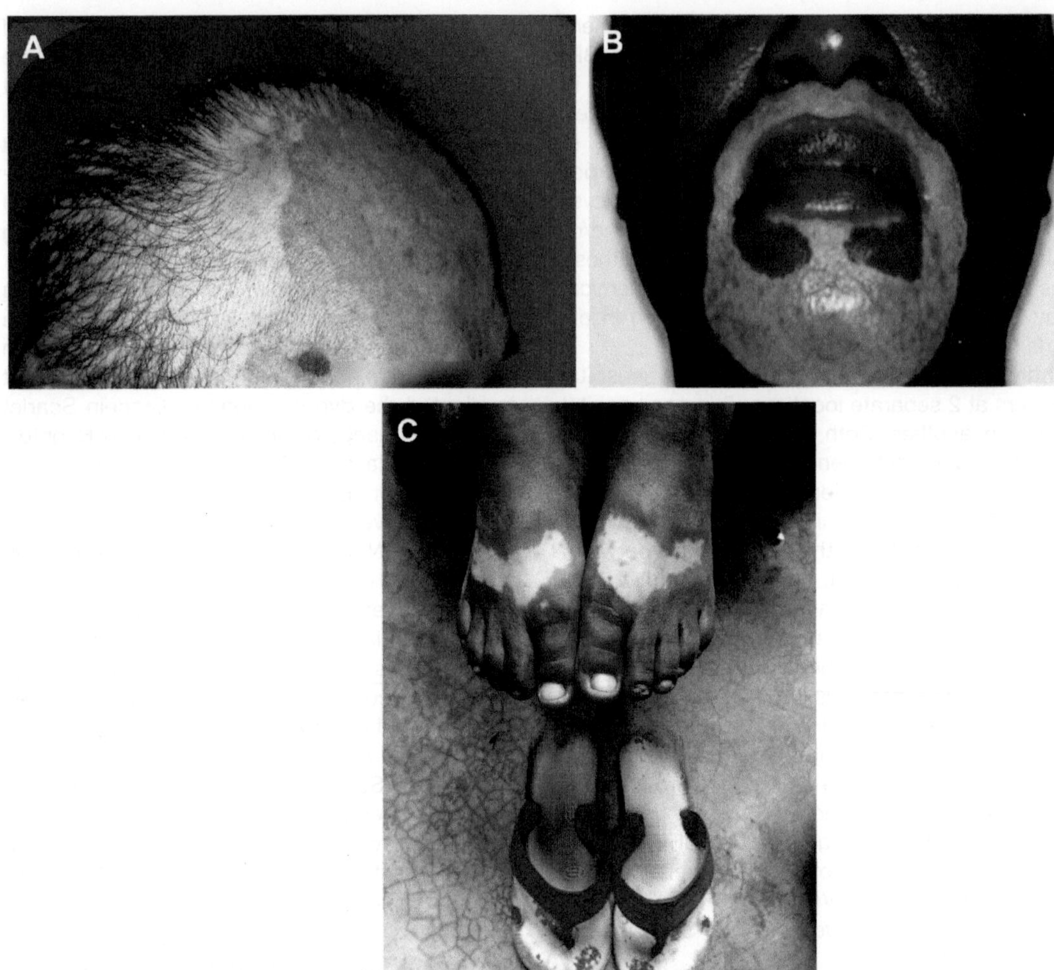

Fig. 1. (*A*) Man who used hair dyes and developed scalp depigmentation at the hairline. (*B*) Man with depigmentation on the face after treating his goatee with a comb-in dye. (*C*) Depigmentation of the feet in the distribution of sandal straps. (*Courtesy of* [*A*] William James, MD, Philadelphia, PA; [*B*] Pearl E. Grimes, MD, Los Angeles, CA; and [*C*] Inbal Braunstein, MD, Baltimore, MD.)

therapies for vitiligo.[41] Lesions induced by rhododendrol were mostly indistinguishable from vitiligo clinically and histologically,[41,42] although 1 report suggested that melanocytes were largely reduced in number but not always completely absent in chemical-induced lesions.[43] Some affected users developed eczematous reactions after using the cosmetic, and 14% reacted to rhododendrol patch testing with pruritus and erythema, although the number of those who depigmented at the location of the patch has not been reported.[41]

A large, prospective population-based study reported that the use of hair dyes increased the risk of developing vitiligo. This group queried a database from the Nurses Health Study, established in 1976, in which a cohort of more than 68,000 participants provided information on their health conditions and exposures on a yearly basis. The study had a more than 90% response rate to biennial questionnaires, and validated accurate reporting of the incidence of vitiligo. The investigators found that women who started using hair dyes before the age of 30 and those who used hair dyes for more than 5 years (regardless of the starting age) had a 50% higher risk of developing vitiligo.[44] This used an unbiased approach in a large cohort to support earlier case studies that implicated hair dyes in causing vitiligo. One caveat of the study was that it could not rule out an association between early hair graying and vitiligo, which has been reported previously,[3,45] as the causative factor in the use of hair dyes at a young age.

HOUSEHOLD PRODUCTS THOUGHT TO INDUCE VITILIGO

A variety of common household products have been reported to induce and/or worsen vitiligo in patients; however, the offending chemical ingredients have not necessarily been identified.[28,30,46,47] This has resulted in numerous lawsuits against the manufacturers, but no option for making safer products or educating patients about which ingredients to avoid. Phenol was used as the first surgical antiseptic by Joseph Lister in 1865.[48] Because it is inexpensive, water-soluble, mildly acidic, and highly reactive, phenol derivatives are used to produce a wide variety of common household products, including disinfectants, cosmetics, diaper creams, detergents, cosmetic dyes, adhesives, pharmaceutical drugs, and others. According to a search of the Household Products Database (US Department of Health and Human Services), 44 unique phenols are used as ingredients in more than 8400 household products sold by 81 distinct manufacturers.[49]

Outside of patch testing a specific suspected chemical, as described previously, it is difficult, if not impossible, to definitively implicate a product as a causative initiator of vitiligo, because there are currently no ways to distinguish this from spontaneous or idiopathic vitiligo. Thus, causation by a commercial product can be strongly inferred only based on patient history, physical examination, exposures, and knowledge about the chemical content of suspected products. Ghosh and Mukhopadhyay[46] reported the largest study of the role of exposures in patients with vitiligo. They extensively interviewed all patients with vitiligo over a 5-year period and identified 864 cases in which they strongly suspected chemically induced disease. They reported that of these cases, 66% were thought to be initiated by the exposure, whereas 34% had preexisting vitiligo that was thought to be exacerbated by use of the product. Depigmentation was limited to the site of exposure in 74%, whereas 26% developed lesions remote from the site of contact. Although pruritus was present in 22% of cases, only a minority (5%) had evidence of contact dermatitis through an eczematous eruption at the site of contact and depigmentation. Hair dye was the most commonly implicated product (27%), and this was presumably due to PPD. Other products contained 4-TBP, MBEH, and Azo dyes, previously implicated by patch testing in other studies (see earlier in this article). The investigators reported that a better response to therapy was observed in patients with depigmentation localized to the site of chemical contact (de novo vitiligo) than those with preexisting vitiligo, suggesting that identifying and eliminating the chemical improved treatment responses.[46]

Interestingly, the investigators noted the presence of "confetti macules" in most (89%) of their suspected patients with chemical-induced vitiligo, and suggested their presence as a distinct sign of chemical-induced vitiligo.[46] This had previously been described by Ortonne and colleagues[3] as well. However, the presence of confetti-like depigmentation was recently reported to be a clinical sign of highly active vitiligo.[50] I have personally observed these macules to be widely distributed in patients with rapidly progressing disease, in areas distinct from exposure to chemicals or products (Harris JE, personal observations, 2016). Thus, I suspect that confetti macules are not necessarily indicative of chemical-induced vitiligo, but rather that chemical-induced vitiligo is often rapidly progressing, which is why it may be marked by the presence of confetti macules.

Other products reported to have induced vitiligo through case reports and case studies are prevalent in the literature, and include condoms, colored strings, herbal oils, detergents, footwear, hair color, dental acrylics, nylon thread, Vick's Vaporub, compounded phenol-containing cream, a methylphenidate patch, electrocardiogram pads, synthetic leather wallets, ornamental Azo dyes, cinnamon toothpaste, eye drops, rubber, and "black henna" tattoos (although the reaction was likely due to PPD in the product, as black henna is not actual henna, which is orange or red).[4,24,30,37,38,51–62] All of these reported cases occurred through topical exposures, which theoretically deliver a high concentration of the chemical to melanoyctes in their epidermal niche. It is unknown whether systemic exposures to similar agents (through diet, medications, or supplements) could result in a similar effect. If so, it could have serious implications for individuals who use future "skin-whitening candy" or other supplements, which appear to contain phenols.[63,64] One study found that intramuscular injection of 4-TBP in black rabbits and dogs caused depigmentation,[29] whereas there are conflicting reports of depigmentation after feeding MBEH to guinea pigs.[5,65]

MECHANISM OF CHEMICAL-INDUCED VITILIGO

Depigmentation from chemicals may be associated with an initial reaction consistent with allergic contact dermatitis, and so some have dismissed chemical-induced depigmentation as a nonspecific postinflammatory change or Koebner response to inflammation. However, many cases occur in the absence of any apparent dermatitis, and most who experience contact dermatitis to these agents do not develop depigmentation. In fact, they typically develop postinflammatory hyperpigmentation.[3] Also, many subjects with chemical-induced depigmentation also develop lesions at sites that are remote from the site of contact with the chemical.[47,66] These observations are particularly apparent following the therapeutic administration of MBEH cream, which most often (>80% of patients) does not induce a contact dermatitis, and results in depigmentation of the entire body, including untreated sites. Thus, the evidence strongly supports a more complicated pathogenesis, one that involves either direct toxicity to melanocytes or subclinical inflammation that can be communicated to remote, unexposed melanocytes.

The common feature shared by offending chemicals in this category is their chemical structure, which typically includes a phenol group, composed of a benzene ring with a hydroxyl side chain. Phenols with a nonpolar side chain in the para (or 4-) position, and in particular an ether group at that position, appear to be the most potent depigmenting chemicals.[67] This chemical structure is shared with the amino acid tyrosine, which is the basic building block of melanin, on which tyrosinase and other melanogenic enzymes make key modifications[3] (**Table 1**). Thus, offending phenols appear to act as tyrosine analogs that interfere with melanogenesis. A small number of these chemicals are not phenols (ie, PPD), and whether these chemicals are "close enough" to phenols or are metabolized into phenols before becoming toxic is currently unknown. Early hypotheses suggested that depigmenting chemicals entering the melanogenesis pathway generated toxic metabolites that destroyed melanocytes from the inside out.[3,47]

Initial studies found that adding these chemicals to human melanocytes cultured in vitro resulted in toxicity at high concentrations, suggesting that they could be directly toxic to melanocytes. This required either tyrosinase or tyrosinase-related protein 1 (Tyrp1), depending on the chemical studied.[68,69] However, this seemed too simplistic, because the chemical concentrations required to induce melanocyte death in vitro are likely much higher than what is achievable in the basal epidermis following topical exposure, as typically only a fraction of chemicals penetrate the skin. According to previous studies with phenol, approximately 4% of the total topical dose was ultimately absorbed through the skin, at a rate of 0.25% per hour.[70] When hair dyes are used on the scalp, resorcinol is systemically absorbed at 0.076% of the total applied dose,[71] although the highest concentration reached in the epidermis is unknown. In addition, most individuals do not depigment after exposure, and a large subset of exposed subjects develop lesions remote from the site of exposure. This was particularly evident in the large population of Japanese exposed to rhododendrol: only 2% of users developed depigmentation, and approximately 5% of those had remote depigmentation.[41] Therefore, it is likely that chemicals induce depigmentation through an indirect mechanism that requires predisposition of the individual (likely genetic), and can spread to unexposed skin following an initial induction event.[47]

Kroll and colleagues[72] first demonstrated that a depigmenting phenol could act to induce melanocyte death indirectly, by activating an inflammatory cascade in dendritic cells co-cultured with exposed melanocytes. They added 4-TBP to melanocytes and found that this induced the cellular stress response, resulting in the secretion of HSP70, a proinflammatory heat shock protein. This secreted protein activated dendritic cells that were co-cultured with the melanocytes, which then killed the melanocytes.[72] A separate study found that 4-TBP and MBEH induced reactive oxygen species (ROS) in melanocytes and also activated the unfolded protein response (UPR), a cellular stress response that results in the production of chaperone proteins (including heat shock proteins like HSP70) to aid in protein folding. A key mediator of the UPR, a protein called XBP1, induced the production of interleukin (IL)-6 and IL-8, both inflammatory cytokines. These data also suggested that vitiligo-inducing phenols indirectly caused melanocyte death by stressing the cells and inducing the secretion of proinflammatory signals.

Van den Boorn and colleagues[73] found that in addition to these pathways, MBEH treatment of melanocytes initiated autophagy in the cells, a condition in which cells under significant stress begin to break down organelles and other cytoplasmic contents to recycle those contents and survive the assault. They observed that tyrosinase became modified by the chemical through quinone haptenation, a covalent linking of the enzyme and chemical that created a novel protein that could act as a foreign antigen to initiate an immune response. This was then secreted from the cells packaged into small nanoparticles called exosomes, which were absorbed by co-cultured dendritic cells and presented to autoreactive T cells.[68] More recent work in mice revealed that skin macrophages and natural killer cells activated by MBEH-stressed melanocytes through innate

Table 1
The amino acid tyrosine and its chemical structure along with patch test–proven vitiligo-inducing chemicals and the products in which they are used as ingredients

Chemical Name	Structure	Commercial Products	References
Tyrosine	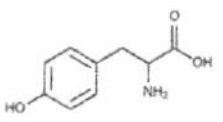		
Monobenzyl ether of hydroquinone (MBEH)	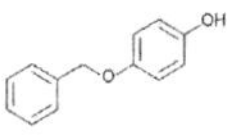	Benoquin cream, rubber	2,8–12
4-tert-butylcatechol (4-TBC)	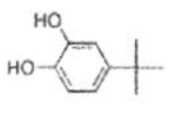	Lubricating oil	18
4-tert-butylphenol (4-TBP)	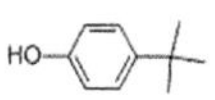	Detergents/disinfectants, sealant/adhesive	20–25,28,29
4-tert-amylphenol (4-TAP)	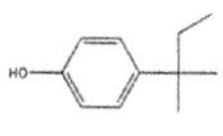	Detergents/disinfectants	28
Para-phenylenediamine (PPD)	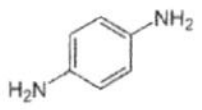	Hair dyes, "black henna"	30–35
Brilliant crocein	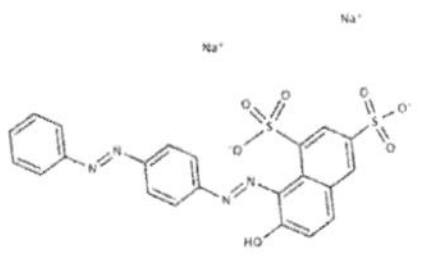	Alta dyes	4,37
Rhodamine B	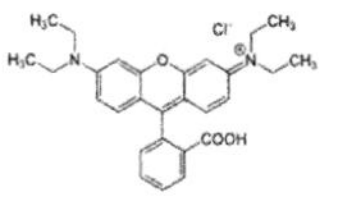	Alta dyes, air freshener dyes	4,37
Rhododendrol	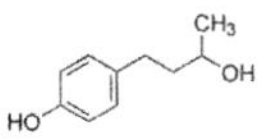	Skin-lightening cosmetic	40–43

pattern recognition receptors may participate in melanocyte destruction as well.[73]

Rhododendrol treatment of human melanocytes induced tyrosinase-dependent apoptosis, activation of endoplasmic reticulum (ER) stress through the UPR, IL-8 production, and autophagy, but not ROS.[40,74,75] Interestingly, rhododendrol toxicity correlated with tyrosinase activity in human melanocyte cell lines tested from a variety of donors from different racial backgrounds, suggesting that individual variability in tyrosinase activity could at least partially be responsible for the variable response to rhododendrol.[74] Histology of rhododendrol-induced lesions revealed a significant reduction of melanocytes, melanin incontinence, and an increased infiltration of T cells.[43,76] Patients also had more melanocyte-specific CD8+ T cells in their blood compared with controls,[77] suggesting that these chemically induced melanocyte changes activated an

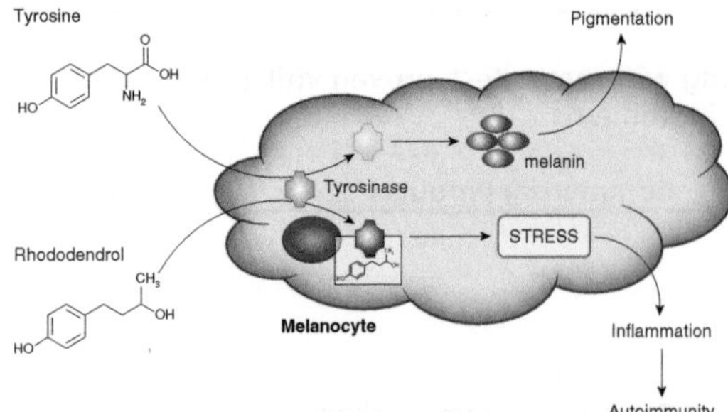

Fig. 2. Schematic of the pathogenesis of chemical-induced vitiligo. Tyrosine is processed into melanin by the enzyme tyrosinase. Chemicals that act as tyrosine analogs interact with tyrosinase (or other melanin-producing enzymes), disrupt melanin production, and induce the cellular stress response, which leads to inflammation and autoimmune destruction of melanocytes.

autoimmune response that has been observed in patients with conventional vitiligo as well.[78–80]

Thus, the pathogenicity of vitiligo-inducing phenols appears to be due to their structural similarity to the amino acid tyrosine, which is the basic building block of the pigment melanin. As a consequence, tyrosinase or other enzymes of melanogenesis engage the chemicals as they would tyrosine, but instead covalently bind to it, resulting in persistent ROS generation (in some cases), UPR activation, autophagy, and exosome production. Exosomes deliver new antigens to neighboring immune cells, which initiate inflammation and activate autoreactive T cells, so the chemical-induced stress in melanocytes initiates an autoimmune response that results in their destruction (**Fig. 2**, reviewed in Refs.[81]). This may explain why not all exposed individuals develop depigmentation, as genetic influences likely predispose affected subjects through more sensitive melanocytes, a predisposition toward autoimmunity, or both. It also may explain why exposed subjects can develop depigmentation remote from the site of chemical exposure, as an initiated immune response would likely target other melanocytes that are not directly stressed through chemical exposure. Sparing of the hair pigment following chemical exposure may be due to immune privilege of the follicle, meaning that it is protected from immune attack, a phenomenon observed in non–chemically induced vitiligo as well.

SUMMARY

Skin depigmentation after exposure to chemical phenols is indistinguishable from vitiligo,[3,30,41,66,82] and appears to be due to activation of melanocyte-specific autoimmunity, as is also seen in non–chemically induced vitiligo.[81,83] In fact, chemicals may simply accelerate stress pathways that are already present in healthy melanocytes, but push them above a tolerated threshold to exceed the capacity that can be appropriately managed by healthy cells, leading to autoimmune inflammation. This is likely a mechanism by which non–chemically induced vitiligo is initiated as well, but genetic influences may increase cellular stress in melanocytes or set a lower threshold for stress that can be tolerated by the immune system.[81]

Therefore, because chemically induced vitiligo and non–chemically induced vitiligo appear on the same spectrum clinically, histologically, and pathogenically, chemical-induced depigmentation should be called "chemical-induced vitiligo," rather than other names that have been used, such as chemical leukoderma, occupational vitiligo/leukoderma, and contact vitiligo/leukoderma/depigmentation. Admittedly, it is difficult to rule out a component of nonimmune direct melanocyte toxicity in subjects exposed to high concentrations of chemical, in whom the effect remains localized to the site of contact. However other terms are either less specific or do not apply in all cases, as "contact" implies only a local effect as well as allergic response, "leukoderma" is nonspecific and could apply to any form of hypopigmentation including postinflammatory changes, and "occupational" does not include the large number of subjects affected at home by commercial products. In addition, these chemicals should not be considered "bleaching chemicals" when used in vitiligo, because bleaching implies denaturing of pigment proteins, and the mechanism of chemical-induced vitiligo is much more complex. The prevalence of phenols in many common household products makes this topic of significant importance, particularly in light of potential future oral skin-lightening supplements that may soon become available.[63,64]

REFERENCES

1. Alkhateeb A, Fain PR, Thody A, et al. Epidemiology of vitiligo and associated autoimmune diseases in Caucasian probands and their families. Pigment Cell Res 2003;16(3):208–14.
2. Oliver EA, Shwartz L, Warren LH. Occupational leukoderma. JAMA 1939;113:927–8.
3. Ortonne J-P, Mosher DB, Fitzpatrick TB. Vitiligo and other hypomelanoses of hair and skin. New York: Plenum Medical Book Co; 1983.
4. Bajaj AK, Saraswat A, Srivastav PK. Chemical leucoderma: Indian scenario, prognosis, and treatment. Indian J Dermatol 2010;55:250–4.

5. Denton CR, Lerner AB, Fitzpatrick TB. Inhibition of melanin formation by chemical agents. J Invest Dermatol 1952;18:119–35.
6. Lerner AB, Fitzpatrick TB. Treatment of melanin hyperpigmentation. J Am Med Assoc 1953;152: 577–82.
7. Kelly EW Jr. Pigmented skin lesions; treatment with monobenzyl-ether of hydroquinone. J Mich State Med Soc 1956;55:303–4. passim.
8. Canizares O, Uribe Jaramillo F, Kerdel Vegas F. Leukomelanoderma subsequent to the application of monobenzyl ether of hydroquinone; a vitiligoid reaction observed in Colombia and Venezuela. AMA Arch Derm 1958;77:220–3.
9. Dorsey CS. Dermatitic and pigmentary reactions to monobenzyl ether of hydroquinone: report of two cases. Arch Dermatol 1960;81:245–8.
10. Ito M. Monobenzylether-hydroquinone leukomelanoderma. Tohoku J Exp Med 1957;65:64.
11. Sidi E, Bourgeois-Spinasse J. Depigmentation resulting from the application of hydroquinone-monobenzylether. Sem Hop 1958;34:417–20 [in French].
12. Mosher DB, Parrish JA, Fitzpatrick TB. Monobenzylether of hydroquinone. A retrospective study of treatment of 18 vitiligo patients and a review of the literature. Br J Dermatol 1977;97:669–79.
13. Chivers CP. Two cases of occupational leucoderma following contact with hydroquinone monomethyl ether. Br J Ind Med 1972;29:105–7.
14. Di Nuzzo S, Masotti A. Depigmentation therapy in vitiligo universalis with cryotherapy and 4-hydroxyanisole. Clin Exp Dermatol 2010;35:215–6.
15. Njoo MD, Vodegel RM, Westerhof W. Depigmentation therapy in vitiligo universalis with topical 4-methoxyphenol and the Q-switched ruby laser. J Am Acad Dermatol 2000;42:760–9.
16. Das M, Tandon A. Occupational vitiligo. Contact Dermatitis 1988;18:184–5.
17. Duffield JA. Depigmentation of skin by quinol and its monobenzyl ether. Lancet 1952;259:1164.
18. Gellin GA, Possick PA, Davis IH. Occupational depigmentation due to 4-tertiarybutyl catechol (TBC). J Occup Med 1970;12:386–9.
19. Gellin GA, Maibach HI, Misiaszek MH, et al. Detection of environmental depigmenting substances. Contact Dermatitis 1979;5:201–13.
20. Bajaj AK, Gupta SC, Chatterjee AK. Contact depigmentation from free para-tertiary-butylphenol in bindi adhesive. Contact Dermatitis 1990;22:99–102.
21. Angelini E, Marinaro C, Carrozzo AM, et al. Allergic contact dermatitis of the lip margins from para-tertiary-butylphenol in a lip liner. Contact Dermatitis 1993;28:146–8.
22. Malten KE, Seutter E, Hara I, et al. Occupational vitiligo due to paratertiary butylphenol and homologues. Trans St Johns Hosp Dermatol Soc 1971;57: 115–34.
23. Okmura Y, Shirai T. Vitiliginous lesions occurring among workers in a phenol derivative factory. Jpn J Dermatol 1962;7:617–9.
24. O'Malley MA, Mathias CG, Priddy M, et al. Occupational vitiligo due to unsuspected presence of phenolic antioxidant byproducts in commercial bulk rubber. J Occup Med 1988;30:512–6.
25. James O, Mayes RW, Stevenson CJ. Occupational vitiligo induced by p-tert-butylphenol, a systemic disease? Lancet 1977;2:1217–9.
26. Rodermund OE, Wieland H. Vitiliginous depigmentation, liver and splenic lesions and struma due to occupational contact with paratertiary butylphenol–a new systemic occupational disease. Berufsdermatosen 1975;23:193–5 [in German].
27. Goldmann PJ, Thiess AM. Occupational vitiligo caused by para-tertiary-butylphenol, a trias of vitiligo, hepatosis and struma. Hautarzt 1976;27:155–9 [in German].
28. Kahn G. Depigmentation caused by phenolic detergent germicides. Arch Dermatol 1970;102: 177–87.
29. Babanov GP, Chumakov NN. The etiology and pathogenesis of occupational vitiligo. Vestn Dermatol Venerol 1966;40:44–8 [in Russian].
30. Taylor JS, Maibach HI, Fisher AA, et al. Contact leukoderma associated with the use of hair colors. Cutis 1993;52:273–80.
31. Bajaj AK, Gupta SC, Chatterjee AK, et al. Hair dye depigmentation. Contact Dermatitis 1996;35:56–7.
32. Brancaccio R, Cohen DE. Contact leukoderma secondary to para-phenylenediamine. Contact Dermatitis 1995;32:313.
33. Saitta P, Cohen D, Brancaccio R. Contact leukoderma from para-phenylenediamine. Dermatitis 2009;20:56–7.
34. Farsani TT, Jalian HR, Young LC. Chemical leukoderma from hair dye containing para-phenylenediamine. Dermatitis 2012;23:181–2.
35. Trattner A, David M. Hair-dye-induced contact vitiligo treated by phototherapy. Contact Dermatitis 2007;56:115–6.
36. Verma S, Kumar B. Contact leukoderma of the scalp or an unusual variant of vitiligo? J Dermatol 2001;28: 554–6.
37. Bajaj AK, Pandey RK, Misra K, et al. Contact depigmentation caused by an azo dye in alta. Contact Dermatitis 1998;38:189–93.
38. Bajaj AK, Gupta SC, Chatterjee AK. Contact depigmentation of the breast. Contact Dermatitis 1991;24:58.
39. Bajaj AK, Gupta SC, Chatterjee AK. Footwear depigmentation. Contact Dermatitis 1996;35:117–8.
40. Sasaki M, Kondo M, Sato K, et al. Rhododendrol, a depigmentation-inducing phenolic compound, exerts melanocyte cytotoxicity via a tyrosinase-dependent mechanism. Pigment Cell Melanoma Res 2014;27:754–63.

41. Nishigori C, Aoyama Y, Ito A, et al. Guide for medical professionals (i.e., dermatologists) for the management of rhododenol-induced leukoderma. J Dermatol 2015;42:113–28.
42. Tokura Y, Fujiyama T, Ikeya S, et al. Biochemical, cytological, and immunological mechanisms of rhododendrol-induced leukoderma. J Dermatol Sci 2015;77:146–9.
43. Tanemura A, Yang L, Yang F, et al. An immune pathological and ultrastructural skin analysis for rhododenol-induced leukoderma patients. J Dermatol Sci 2015;77:185–8.
44. Wu S, Li WQ, Cho E, et al. Use of permanent hair dyes and risk of vitiligo in women. Pigment Cell Melanoma Res 2015;28(6):744–6.
45. Lerner AB. Vitiligo. J Invest Dermatol 1959;32:285–310.
46. Ghosh S, Mukhopadhyay S. Chemical leucoderma: a clinico-aetiological study of 864 cases in the perspective of a developing country. Br J Dermatol 2009;160:40–7.
47. Boissy RE, Manga P. On the etiology of contact/occupational vitiligo. Pigment Cell Res 2004;17:208–14.
48. Lister J. On the antiseptic principle in the practice of surgery. Br Med J 1867;2:246–8.
49. U.S. Department of Health and Human Services, Household Products Database: National Institutes of Health, National Library of Medicine, Specialized Information Services; 2013. Available at: https://householdproducts.nlm.nih.gov/index.htm.
50. Sosa JJ, Currimbhoy SD, Ukoha U, et al. Confetti-like depigmentation: a potential sign of rapidly progressing vitiligo. J Am Acad Dermatol 2015;73:272–5.
51. Ghosh SK, Bandyopadhyay D. Chemical leukoderma induced by colored strings. J Am Acad Dermatol 2009;61:909–10.
52. Ghosh SK, Bandyopadhyay D. Chemical leukoderma induced by herbal oils. J Cutan Med Surg 2010;14:310–3.
53. Pandhi RK, Kumar AS. Contact leukoderma due to 'bindi' and footwear. Dermatologica 1985;170:260–2.
54. Kanerva L, Estlander T. Contact leukoderma caused by patch testing with dental acrylics. Am J Contact Dermatitis 1998;9:196–8.
55. Boyse KE, Zirwas MJ. Chemical leukoderma associated with Vicks Vaporub. J Clin Aesthet Dermatol 2008;1:34–5.
56. Hernandez C, Reddy SG, Barfuss A, et al. Contact leukoderma after application of a compounded phenol cream and narrowband-UVB. Eur J Dermatol 2008;18:593–5.
57. Ghasri P, Gattu S, Saedi N, et al. Chemical leukoderma after the application of a transdermal methylphenidate patch. J Am Acad Dermatol 2012;66:e237–8.
58. Valsecchi R, Leghissa P, Di Landro A, et al. Persistent leukoderma after henna tattoo. Contact Dermatitis 2007;56:108–9.
59. Banerjee R, Banerjee K, Datta A. Condom leukoderma. Indian J Dermatol Venereol Leprol 2006;72:452–3.
60. Bajaj AK, Misra A, Misra K, et al. The azo dye solvent yellow 3 produces depigmentation. Contact Dermatitis 2000;42:237–8.
61. Mathias CG, Maibach HI, Conant MA. Perioral leukoderma simulating vitiligo from use of a toothpaste containing cinnamic aldehyde. Arch Dermatol 1980;116:1172–3.
62. Suchi ST, Gupta A, Srinivasan R. Contact allergic dermatitis and periocular depigmentation after using olapatidine eye drops. Indian J Ophthalmol 2008;56:439–40.
63. Oaklander M. Skin whitening candy is coming. Time 2014. Available at: http://www.time.com/3181942/skin-whitening-candy/.
64. Lighter skin from within: melagenol offers an effective natural solution for skin whitening applications. 2014. Available at: http://www.monteloeder.com/system/novedades/1/Brochure_ML0814-SC0648_en.pdf.
65. Peck SM, Sobotka H. Effect of monobenzyl hydroquinone on oxidase systems in vivo and in vitro. J Invest Dermatol 1941;4:325–9.
66. Ghosh S. Chemical leukoderma: what's new on etiopathological and clinical aspects? Indian J Dermatol 2010;55:255–8.
67. Riley P. Pathological disturbances of pigmentation. In: Jarrett A, editor. The physiology and pathophysiology of the skin. Vol 3. New York: Academic Press; 1974. p. 1167–97.
68. van den Boorn JG, Picavet DI, van Swieten PF, et al. Skin-depigmenting agent monobenzone induces potent T-cell autoimmunity toward pigmented cells by tyrosinase haptenation and melanosome autophagy. J Invest Dermatol 2011;131:1240–51.
69. Yang F, Sarangarajan R, Le Poole IC, et al. The cytotoxicity and apoptosis induced by 4-tertiary butylphenol in human melanocytes are independent of tyrosinase activity. J Invest Dermatol 2000;114:157–64.
70. Feldmann RJ, Maibach HI. Absorption of some organic compounds through the skin in man. J Invest Dermatol 1970;54:399–404.
71. Wolfram LJ, Maibach HI. Percutaneous penetration of hair dyes. Arch Dermatol Res 1985;277:235–41.
72. Kroll TM, Bommiasamy H, Boissy RE, et al. 4-Tertiary butyl phenol exposure sensitizes human melanocytes to dendritic cell-mediated killing: relevance to vitiligo. J Invest Dermatol 2005;124:798–806.
73. van den Boorn JG, Jakobs C, Hagen C, et al. Inflammasome-dependent induction of adaptive NK cell memory. Immunity 2016;44:1406–21.

74. Kasamatsu S, Hachiya A, Nakamura S, et al. Depigmentation caused by application of the active brightening material, rhododendrol, is related to tyrosinase activity at a certain threshold. J Dermatol Sci 2014;76: 16–24.
75. Yang L, Yang F, Wataya-Kaneda M, et al. 4-(4-hydroroxyphenyl)-2-butanol (rhododendrol) activates the autophagy-lysosome pathway in melanocytes: insights into the mechanisms of rhododendrol-induced leukoderma. J Dermatol Sci 2015;77: 182–5.
76. Nishioka M, Tanemura A, Yang L, et al. Possible involvement of CCR4(+)CD8(+) T cells and elevated plasma CCL22 and CCL17 in patients with rhododenol-induced leukoderma. J Dermatol Sci 2015;77:188–90.
77. Fujiyama T, Ikeya S, Ito T, et al. Melanocyte-specific cytotoxic T lymphocytes in patients with rhododendrol-induced leukoderma. J Dermatol Sci 2015;77:190–2.
78. Ogg GS, Rod Dunbar P, Romero P, et al. High frequency of skin-homing melanocyte-specific cytotoxic T lymphocytes in autoimmune vitiligo. J Exp Med 1998;188:1203–8.
79. van den Boorn JG, Konijnenberg D, Dellemijn TA, et al. Autoimmune destruction of skin melanocytes by perilesional T cells from vitiligo patients. J Invest Dermatol 2009;129:2220–32.
80. Rashighi M, Agarwal P, Richmond JM, et al. CXCL10 is critical for the progression and maintenance of depigmentation in a mouse model of vitiligo. Sci Transl Med 2014;6:223ra23.
81. Harris JE. Cellular stress and innate inflammation in organ-specific autoimmunity: lessons learned from vitiligo. Immunol Rev 2016;269:11–25.
82. Lommerts JE, Teulings HE, Ezzedine K, et al. Melanoma-associated leukoderma and vitiligo cannot be differentiated based on blinded assessment by experts in the field. J Am Acad Dermatol 2016;75(6): 1198–204.
83. Richmond JM, Frisoli ML, Harris JE. Innate immune mechanisms in vitiligo: danger from within. Curr Opin In Immunol 2013;25:676–82.

Medical and Maintenance Treatments for Vitiligo

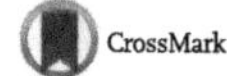

Thierry Passeron, MD, PhD

KEYWORDS

- Vitiligo • Medical treatments • Topical steroids • Calcineurin inhibitors • Sytemic steroids
- Methotrexate

KEY POINTS

- Medical treatments alone, or in combination with phototherapy, are key approaches for treating nonsegmental vitiligo and, to a lesser extent, for treating segmental vitiligo.
- The treatments can be useful for halting disease progression and have proved effective for inducing repigmentation and decreasing the risk of relapses.
- Although the treatments have some side effects and limitations, vitiligo often induces a marked decrease in the quality of life of affected individuals and in most cases the risk:benefit ratio is in favor of an active approach.
- Systemic and topical agents targeting the pathways involved in the loss of melanocytes and in the differentiation of melanocyte stem cells should provide even more effective approaches in the near future, thanks to the increased knowledge of the pathophysiology of vitiligo.

INTRODUCTION

There are 3 aims needed for the optimal care of vitiligo patients: first, halting the disease progression; then, allowing complete repigmentation of lesional areas; and, finally, preventing relapses. There is still no therapeutic panacea for vitiligo but current options can lead to significant improvement of vitiligo lesions. Some areas, such as the face, usually respond well to therapies whereas they remain mostly ineffective for others, such as hands and feet. Recent advances in the understanding of the pathophysiology of vitiligo foster new therapeutic opportunities. One of the most promising is the demonstration of the key role of the interferon gamma (INF-γ)/Janus kinase (JAK)/CXCL10 pathway in the depigmentation process of vitiligo.[1] Targeting this pathway might provide effective therapeutic approaches, as suggested by recent cases reports (discussed later).[2,3] The immune reaction is absent of complete depigmented lesions, however, and repigmentation may be difficult in lesions of some patients while their vitiligo remains inactive for years. Recent transcriptomic analysis showed an impaired Wnt signaling pathway in vitiligo lesions preventing the differentiation of melanocyte stem cells.[4] Fibroblasts of some areas, such as hands and feet, produce Wnt inhibitors.[5] This might contribute to a defect in melanocyte differentiation and could explain the difficulties for repigmenting those localizations. So far the best way to stimulate the differentiation of melanocytes is ultraviolet (UV) radiation. Recent data have shown that the action of UV on melanocyte stem cells is mediated by Wnt proteins.[6] Thus, stimulating the Wnt pathway by using topical agents might allow repigmenting even difficult-to-treat areas. Although phototherapy and surgery remain useful approaches for vitiligo, systemic or topical medical therapies are important alone or combined for optimal treatment of most vitiligo cases

Department of Dermatology and INSERM U1065, Team 12, C3M, Archet 2 Hospital, University Hospital of Nice, 150 Route de Ginestière, Nice 06200, France
E-mail address: passeron@unice.fr

Dermatol Clin 35 (2017) 163–170
http://dx.doi.org/10.1016/j.det.2016.11.007

and, in light of recent pathophysiologic advances, they offer encouraging options for the near future.

HALTING DISEASE PROGRESSION

The course of vitiligo is unpredictable. An active phase, however, can be clinically detected. Medical history of the vitiligo, reporting a rapid onset and ongoing extension of depigmented lesions, is highly suggestive of active disease. Wood lamp examination is of great importance because it can show blurred and hypochromic borders of lesions that are associated with ongoing depigmenting process.[7] The presence of a confetti sign was recently reported to be also associated with a marked spreading of vitiligo lesions within the following months.[8] Several medical approaches have been proposed for halting or decreasing the progression of active vitiligo.

Systemic Steroids

Systemic corticosteroids (high-dose pulsed therapy, minipulsed regimen, or daily oral low dose) have been reported to rapidly arrest spreading vitiligo and to induce repigmentation.[9] Low-dose oral prednisolone (0.3 mg/kg) taken daily for 2 months[10] and a high dose of intravenous methylprednisolone (8 mg/kg) administered on 3 consecutive days[11] were evaluated in open-label clinical studies. Both regimens were reported to halt disease progression in more than 85% of cases and to induce some repigmentation in more than 70% of cases. Most studies have evaluated oral minipulse (OMP) betamethasone or dexamethasone using 5 mg twice a week on 2 consecutive days usually for 3 months[12] to 6 months.[13] The progression of disease was stopped in more than 85% of cases but a marked repigmentation was observed in less than 7% of cases. Side effects included weight gain, insomnia, acne, agitation, menstrual disturbance, and hypertrichosis. The prevalence of side effects ranged from 12%[12] to 69%.[13] A large retrospective study confirmed these results, showing an arrest of disease activity in 91.8% of cases.[14] Adverse reactions, such as weight gain, lethargy, and acneiform eruptions, were observed in 9.2% of patients. Relapses after discontinuation of the treatment are not rare. In 138 children treated with OMP of methylprednisolone for 6 months, 34.8% had relapses over a period of 1 year. The rate of relapses was higher in children below 10 years of age (47.4%). Thus, systemic corticosteroids seem to halt disease progression in most cases. No prospective randomized trial against placebo, however, has been performed yet. Given the significant potential for side effects and the high rate of relapses, the use of such an approach remains controversial.

Methotrexate

The first case supporting the use of methotrexate in vitiligo was reported in a woman treated with 7.5 mg per week for rheumatoid arthritis. She had a 6-month history of rapidly progressing vitiligo. She stopped developing new lesions after 3 months of treatment.[15] More recently, the efficacy of methotrexate (10 mg per week) was compared with OMP dexamethasone (5 mg per week with 2.5 mg taken on 2 consecutive days) in a prospective randomized open-label study in 52 vitiligo patients.[16] After 6 months of treatment, 6 of 25 patients developed new lesions with methotrexate compared with 7 of 25 patients with OMP. Both groups had also a similar reduction in vitiligo disease activity score. The investigators concluded that both drugs are equally effective in controlling the disease activity of vitiligo. The data evaluating the use of methotrexate in vitiligo, however, remain limited.

Minocycline

Minocycline was proposed for treating vitiligo because of its anti-inflammatory, immunomodulatory, and free-radical scavenging properties. An initial open-label study reported an arrest in disease progression in 29 of 32 patients treated with 100 mg per day of minocycline.[17] The same group further reported a prospective randomized trial comparing OMP (5 mg per week) with minocycline (100 mg per day)[18]; 50 patients with active vitiligo were included. After 6 months of treatment, both groups showed a significant decrease in vitiligo disease activity score from 4.0 to 1.64 $\pm$ 0.86 ($P<.001$) and from 4.0 to 1.68 $\pm$ 0.69 ($P<.001$), for minocycline and OMP, respectively. The difference between the 2 groups was not statistically significant ($P = .60$). Minocycline (100 mg per day) was also compared with narrow-band (Nb)-UVB (twice weekly) in a prospective comparative trial performed in 42 patients with active vitiligo.[19] After 3 months of treatment, only 23.8% of patients still had active lesions with Nb-UVB compared with 66.1% with minocycline ($P<.05$). Patients in the Nb-UVB group also showed significantly higher repigmentation compared with those in minocycline group. Both studies lacked an untreated group to assess the evolution of vitiligo without treatment. These results need further evaluation, but Nb-UVB seems more important for halting disease progression and has the main advantage of also promoting more efficient repigmentation of vitiligo lesions.

REPIGMENTATION THERAPIES

Corticosteroids

Intralesional corticosteroids were first reported for use in vitiligo 30 years ago. The pain associated with injection and the risk of cutaneous atrophy (observed in approximately one-third of patients) was against further use of this approach.[20] Recently, a series of 9 patients with localized vitiligo were successfully treated with intralesional injections of triamcinolone acetonide, 3 mg/mL (0.05–0.1 mL for each site), every 4 to 6 weeks with an average duration of the treatment of 4 months (maximum 7 months).[21] Skin atrophy was seen in 1 patient and menstrual irregularity reported in 2 patients. A meta-analysis of nonsurgical approaches for treating vitiligo reported equal efficacy of intralesional and topical steroids.[22] Taking into account the side effects of intralesional steroids, the use of topical forms should thus be preferred. Systemic steroids can be beneficial for halting systemic progression of active vitiligo but they have limited efficacy in repigmenting the lesions.[13]

Topical corticosteroids are useful for small, localized areas and remain one of the gold standard treatments for vitiligo. Meta-analyses confirmed their effectiveness for localized vitiligo.[23] Steroid-induced repigmentation occurs within 1 to 4 months of treatment in a perifollicular pattern and from the margins of the lesions. Side effects include epidermal atrophy, steroid-induced acne, rosacea, telangiectasia, ecchymoses, and striae. Atrophy was observed in 14% and 21%, respectively (mean), of patients treated with potent versus very potent corticosteroids.[24] Corticosteroids of low potency, however, show no therapeutic effect at all. Furthermore, suppression of the hypothalamic-pituitary-adrenal axis may occur after prolonged applications on large areas. To minimize the incidence of these side effects, it is recommended to use topical steroids on limited skin areas; to avoid prolonged use on sensitive areas, such as face and body folds; and to use them once daily for only 6 to 8 weeks followed by a treatment-free interval of several weeks because mild steroid-induced skin atrophy is reversible. Other schedules of intermittent therapy (3 weeks on and 1 week off and 5 days a week) have also been proposed.[25] To minimize side effects, treatment should be discontinued if there is no visible improvement after 3 months.

Topical Calcineurin Inhibitors

Early observations suggested that tacrolimus and pimecrolimus may be effective treatments for both localized and generalized vitiligo.[26,27] A 2-month double-blind randomized trial compared 0.1% tacrolimus and 0.05% clobetasol propionate in children with vitiligo.[28] This study confirmed that tacrolimus stimulates vitiligo repigmentation; however, tacrolimus ointment was not superior to clobetasol in extent of repigmentation. These results were confirmed by a prospective randomized trial comparing tacrolimus 0.1%, clobetasol propionate, and placebo.[29] Tacrolimus and clobetasol propionate showed similar efficacy and both provided significantly better repigmentation compared with placebo. Facial lesions responded faster and better compared with nonfacial lesions. Twice-daily application of 0.1% tacrolimus provided better results compared with once-daily applications.[30] The same results were obtained in an open intraindividual study performed with 1% pimecrolimus cream.[31] Again, 0.05% clobetasol propionate induced a comparable rate of repigmentation to a topical calcineurin inhibitor. The best results were observed on sun-exposed areas. An intraindividual prospective comparative study has shown that tacrolimus monotherapy in the absence of UV has little or no repigmenting potential in vitiligo.[32] An open randomized study compared topical pimecrolimus and topical tacrolimus to Nb-UVB for treating vitiligo.[33] The investigators did not find statistically significant differences in repigmentation among the 3 groups. It is now demonstrated, however, that best results are achieved when phototherapy is combined with these topical treatments (**Fig. 1**) (See Samia Esmat and colleagues article, "Phototherapy and Combination Therapies for Vitiligo," in this issue).

Other Topical Medical Treatments

Topical vitamin D analogs have been proposed alone or combined with phototherapy for treating vitiligo. A prospective, right/left comparative, open-label study showed that calcipotriol in monotherapy is not effective for vitiligo.[34]

There are several conflicting results on the use of topical antioxidants for treating vitiligo. In most cases, however, topical antioxidants are used in combination with phototherapy. One prospective intraindividual study compared 0.05% betamethasone to topical catalase/dismutase superoxide.[35] After 10 months of treatment, there was no statistical differences between the 2 groups (P = .79), with mean repigmentation of 18.5% with betamethasone and 12.4% with topical catalase/dismutase superoxide. Although the rationale for using topical antioxidants in vitiligo is strong, the data remain limited and controversial. One possible explanation is the difficulty of delivering active antioxidants into the skin. Double-blind

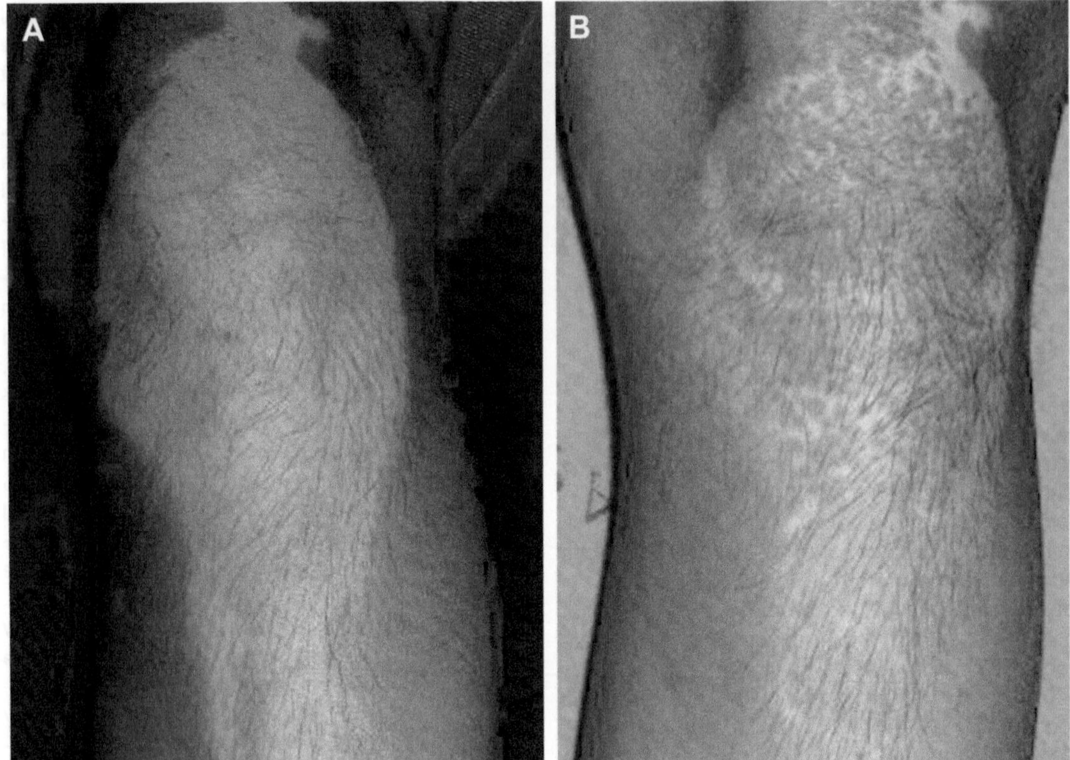

Fig. 1. Vitiligo of the leg and knee (*A*) before treatment and (*B*) after 30 sessions of 308-nm excimer laser combined with twice-daily applications of 0.1% of tacrolimus ointment.

placebo-controlled studies are mandatory to further investigate the real efficacy of such an approach for treating vitiligo.

INDICATIONS AND LIMITATIONS OF USING MEDICAL APPROACHES FOR TREATING VITILIGO

The use of systemic treatments, such as systemic corticosteroids or methotrexate, can induce potential serious side effects. The limited data actually available for their efficiency in treating vitiligo should prompt caution on their use in current practice. Their use remains controversial and should be limited to active vitiligo to halt the disease. Periodic monitoring of their efficacy and tolerance are important. Although comparative data are limited, the good safety profile of Nb-UVB, its ability to decrease disease progression, and its effectiveness for also inducing repigmentation should make Nb-UVB the first-line option for halting disease progression.

Vitiligo usually requires several months for repigmentation and patients have to be informed about the length of the treatment to avoid premature discontinuation of the treatment; many expect to observe rapid repigmentation. Potent topical steroids and calcineurin inhibitors have proved their efficacy and are the best options for repigmenting localized vitiligo.[36,37] Topical steroids or calcineurin inhibitors can also be proposed for segmental vitiligo, although they are less effective than in nonsegmental forms.[38] They can be useful before surgical approaches, however, because they can reduce the size of the area to graft and sometimes completely repigment the lesions (**Fig. 2**).

Due to the risk of atrophy when using potent or very potent topical steroids for a long period, their efficacy has to be assessed after 3 months. Although data remain limited, intermittent therapy with application 5 days a week can be proposed to decrease the risk of atrophy. On sensitive areas, such as folds, neck, and face (and mostly eyelids), twice-daily application of topical calcineurin inhibitors are preferred.[28] Calcineurin inhibitors are significantly more effective on sun-exposed areas or when combined with phototherapy (See Samia Esmat and colleagues article, "Phototherapy and Combination Therapies for Vitiligo," in this issue). Avoidance of UV light is suggested, however, by the package insert. This recommendation was

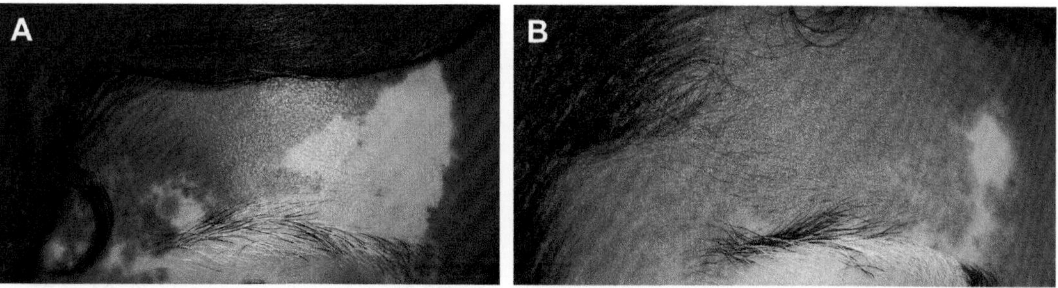

Fig. 2. (*A*) Segmental vitiligo affecting the V1 segment of the face before treatment and (*B*) partial repigmentation after 1 year of twice-daily applications of 0.1% of tacrolimus ointment and sun exposures. The repigmentation remains incomplete but allows decreasing the size of the surgical graft.

based on mouse models and on the immunosuppression that can be induced when a high quantity of calcineurin inhibitors penetrates through the skin and reaches systemic levels. The mouse models have strong limitations, however, when drawing definitive conclusions, and reassuring data on the use of topical calcineurin inhibitors have since been reported.[39,40] Moreover, penetration of high quantities of calcineurin inhibitors can mostly be observed when used over large surfaces in atopic dermatitis patients where the skin barrier is altered, which is not the case for vitiligo skin. Topical calcineurin inhibitors have been used for vitiligo alone or combined with phototherapy for more than 10 years without any indication of risk. Taken together, these data are reassuring concerning the use of topical calcineurin inhibitors combined with UV exposures in vitiligo patients; however, a total follow-up of 20 to 25 years may be required to be completely reassured concerning a potential increased risk of skin cancers. Thus, the risk:benefit ratio needs to be discussed with patients when topical calcineurin inhibitors are proposed. A treatment algorithm is proposed in **Fig. 3**.

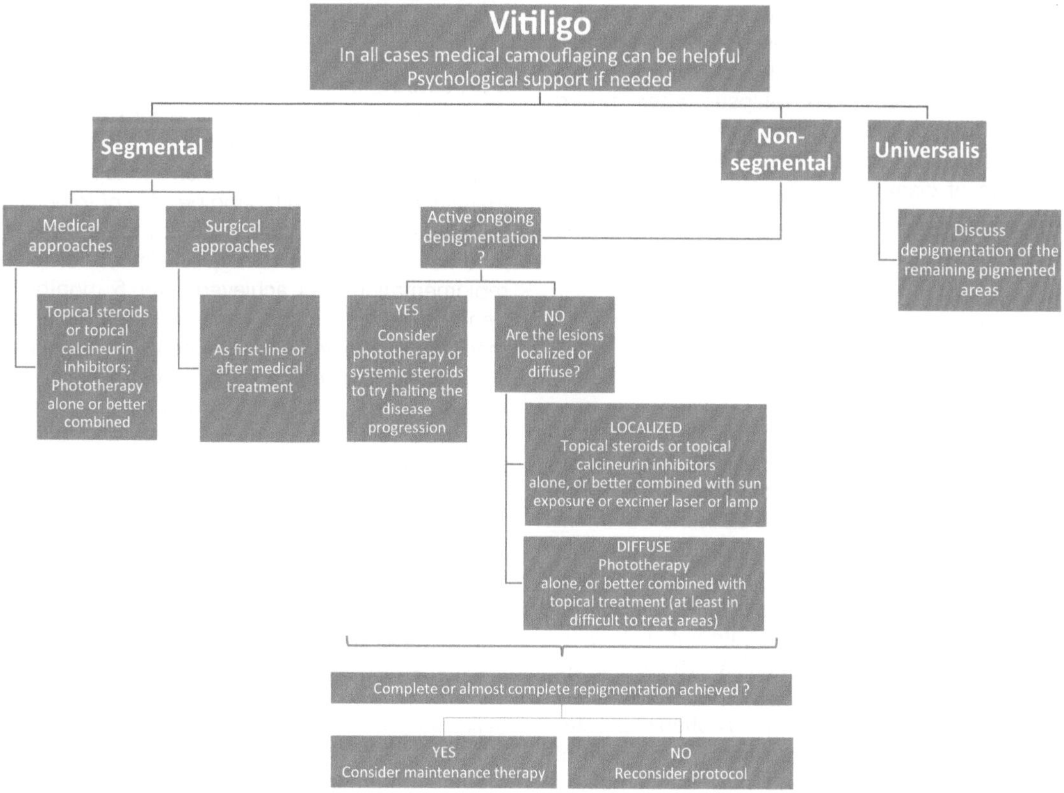

Vitiligo
In all cases medical camouflaging can be helpful
Psychological support if needed

Segmental
- Medical approaches
  - Topical steroids or topical calcineurin inhibitors; Phototherapy alone or better combined
- Surgical approaches
  - As first-line or after medical treatment

Non-segmental
- Active ongoing depigmentation ?
  - YES
    Consider phototherapy or systemic steroids to try halting the disease progression
  - NO
    Are the lesions localized or diffuse?
    - LOCALIZED
      Topical steroids or topical calcineurin inhibitors alone, or better combined with sun exposure or excimer laser or lamp
    - DIFFUSE
      Phototherapy alone, or better combined with topical treatment (at least in difficult to treat areas)

Complete or almost complete repigmentation achieved ?
- YES
  Consider maintenance therapy
- NO
  Reconsider protocol

Universalis
- Discuss depigmentation of the remaining pigmented areas

Fig. 3. Treatment algorithm.

PREVENTING VITILIGO RELAPSES

After successful repigmentation, the rate of relapse in vitiligo patches is approximately 40%.[41] In atopic dermatitis, proactive treatment with topical steroids or calcineurin inhibitors has demonstrated efficacy to decrease flares of the disease.[42] In a 2-center, prospective randomized study, the use of biweekly application of 0.1% tacrolimus ointment was compared with placebo[43]; 35 patients with 72 nonsegmental vitiligo lesions who achieved at least 75% of repigmentation after phototherapy, topical treatment, or a combination approach were included. After 6 months, 40% of lesions showed depigmentation in the placebo group compared with 9.7% with tacrolimus (P = .0075). The tolerance was good and the side effects limited to transient erythema and stinging or burning sensations. This study shows that twice-weekly applications of 0.1% of tacrolimus are effective for decreasing vitiligo relapses.

According to the data available in atopic dermatitis and the comparable efficacy of topical steroids and tacrolimus for treating vitiligo, it may be hypothesized that topical steroids could also be effective for preventing vitiligo relapse. Many questions remain. How long should this preventive treatment be continued? Are applications 3 times per week more effective than only 2 times per week and thus could they further reduce the risk of relapse? The author proposed this maintenance treatment only in patients with active vitiligo or patients who already had relapses after having achieved repigmentation and continues this proactive approach for at least 6 months without any sign of disease activity. Further studies are clearly required, however, to answer to these questions.

POTENTIAL EMERGING MEDICAL TREATMENTS

Topical Prostaglandins

Prostaglandin E2 can stimulate the proliferation of melanocytes and melanogenesis.[44] Two open-label prospective studies tested twice-daily application of topical prostaglandin E2 in the treatment of localized and stable vitiligo; 15 of the 24 patients in the first study[45] and 20 of the 56 patients in the second trial[46] achieved repigmentation of greater than 75% after 6 months of treatment. The tolerance was good in both studies. Those results need confirmation but they are potentially interesting because the mechanism of action of prostaglandins probably differs from the current therapeutic approaches and may be combined with them to enhance the repigmentation rate.

Afamelanotide

Afamelanotide is a melanocortin-1 receptor agonist. A prospective randomized trial provided encouraging results when afamelanotide, administrated monthly by subcutaneous implants, was combined with UVB (repigmentation rate of 48.64% at day 168) compared with UVB alone (repigmentation rate of 33.26%).[47] Only 17 of 28 patients completed the study in the combination arm (39.3% dropout) compared with 24 of 27 patients (11.1% dropout) in the UVB-only arm. The most frequent side effects were nausea (18%) and fatigue (11%). Better results were obtained, however, in dark-skinned patients. The potent tanning of the nonlesional skin is also a limitation in fair-skinned patients because it increases the contrast between healthy and lesional skin. Additional studies are clearly required to determine the indications and the limitations of this approach.[48]

Janus Kinase Inhibitors

The IFN-γ/JAK/CXCL10 pathway seems to play a key role in the depigmentation process of vitiligo.[1] Every component of this pathway represents a potential therapeutic target.[49] For now, clinical data are limited to 2 case reports using JAK inhibitors. IFN-γ signals through its receptor, which activates JAK1 and JAK2 to induce the transcription of CXCL10, which is important in vitiligo pathogenesis. The first clinical response was reported using a JAK1/JAK3 inhibitor, called tofacitinib, which is Food and Drug Administrant approved for the treatment of rheumatoid arthritis.[2] A 50-year-old woman with vitiligo nonresponsive to topical treatments was treated with 3 mg per day of tofacitinib for 3 weeks and then 5 mg per day (daily dose for rheumatoid arthritis is 10 mg). An almost-complete repigmentation was achieved after 5 months of treatment. The second case was a 35-year-old man with vitiligo and alopecia areata.[3] He received oral ruxolitinib during a phase 2 trial for alopecia areata. Ruxolitinib is a JAK1/JAK2 inhibitor approved for treating myelofibrosis and polycythemia vera. After 20 weeks of treatment, he repigmented from 0.8% to 51% on his face. Unfortunately, the repigmentation was completely gone 12 weeks after the discontinuation of the treatment. Prospective randomized trials are now required for assessing the long-term efficacy and the safety of such approaches but they seem of great interest, especially for active vitiligo.

SUMMARY

Medical treatments alone or in combination with phototherapy are key approaches for treating nonsegmental vitiligo and to a lesser extent for treating segmental vitiligo. They can be useful for halting disease progression and have proved effective for inducing repigmentation and more recently to decrease the risk of relapses. They have some side effects and limitations that have to be discussed with patients. Vitiligo often induces a marked decreased in the quality of life of affected individuals, however, and the risk:benefit ratio is in favor of an active approach in most cases. Thanks to increased knowledge of the pathophysiology of vitiligo, systemic and topical agents targeting more specifically the pathways involved in the loss of melanocytes and also in the differentiation of melanocyte stem cells should provide in the near future even more effective approaches.

REFERENCES

1. Rashighi M, Agarwal P, Richmond JM, et al. CXCL10 is critical for the progression and maintenance of depigmentation in a mouse model of vitiligo. Sci Transl Med 2014;6:223ra23.
2. Craiglow BG, King BA. Tofacitinib citrate for the treatment of vitiligo: a pathogenesis-directed therapy. JAMA Dermatol 2015;151:1110–2.
3. Harris JE, Rashighi M, Nguyen N, et al. Rapid skin repigmentation on oral ruxolitinib in a patient with coexistent vitiligo and alopecia areata (AA). J Am Acad Dermatol 2016;74:370–1.
4. Regazzetti C, Joly F, Marty C, et al. Transcriptional analysis of vitiligo skin reveals the alteration of WNT pathway: a promising target for repigmenting vitiligo patients. J Invest Dermatol 2015;135:3105–14.
5. Yamaguchi Y, Passeron T, Hoashi T, et al. Dickkopf 1 (DKK1) regulates skin pigmentation and thickness by affecting Wnt/beta-catenin signaling in keratinocytes. FASEB J 2008;22:1009–20.
6. Fukunaga-Kalabis M, Hristova DM, Wang JX, et al. UV-Induced Wnt7a in the Human Skin Microenvironment Specifies the Fate of Neural Crest-Like Cells via Suppression of Notch. J Invest Dermatol 2015;135:1521–32.
7. Benzekri L, Gauthier Y, Hamada S, et al. Clinical features and histological findings are potential indicators of activity in lesions of common vitiligo. Br J Dermatol 2013;168:265–71.
8. Sosa JJ, Currimbhoy SD, Ukoha U, et al. Confetti-like depigmentation: A potential sign of rapidly progressing vitiligo. J Am Acad Dermatol 2015;73:272–5.
9. Imamura S, Tagami H. Treatment of vitiligo with oral corticosteroids. Dermatologica 1976;153:179–85.
10. Kim SM, Lee HS, Hann SK. The efficacy of low-dose oral corticosteroids in the treatment of vitiligo patients. Int J Dermatol 1999;38:546–50.
11. Seiter S, Ugurel S, Tilgen W, et al. Use of high-dose methylprednisolone pulse therapy in patients with progressive and stable vitiligo. Int J Dermatol 2000;39:624–7.
12. Pasricha JS, Khaitan BK. Oral mini-pulse therapy with betamethasone in vitiligo patients having extensive or fast-spreading disease. Int J Dermatol 1993;32:753–7.
13. Radakovic-Fijan S, Furnsinn-Friedl AM, Honigsmann H, et al. Oral dexamethasone pulse treatment for vitiligo. J Am Acad Dermatol 2001;44:814–7.
14. Kanwar AJ, Mahajan R, Parsad D. Low-dose oral mini-pulse dexamethasone therapy in progressive unstable vitiligo. J Cutan Med Surg 2013;17:259–68.
15. Sandra A, Pai S, Shenoi SD. Unstable vitiligo responding to methotrexate. Indian J Dermatol Venereol Leprol 1998;64:309.
16. Alghamdi K, Khurrum H. Methotrexate for the treatment of generalized vitiligo. Saudi Pharm J 2013;21:423–4.
17. Parsad D, Kanwar A. Oral minocycline in the treatment of vitiligo–a preliminary study. Dermatol Ther 2010;23:305–7.
18. Singh A, Kanwar AJ, Parsad D, et al. Randomized controlled study to evaluate the effectiveness of dexamethasone oral minipulse therapy versus oral minocycline in patients with active vitiligo vulgaris. Indian J Dermatol Venereol Leprol 2014;80:29–35.
19. Siadat AH, Zeinali N, Iraji F, et al. Narrow-Band Ultraviolet B versus Oral Minocycline in Treatment of Unstable Vitiligo: A Prospective Comparative Trial. Dermatol Res Pract 2014;2014:240856.
20. Vasistha LK, Singh G. Vitiligo and intralesional steroids. Indian J Med Res 1979;69:308–11.
21. Wang E, Koo J, Levy E. Intralesional corticosteroid injections for vitiligo: a new therapeutic option. J Am Acad Dermatol 2014;71:391–3.
22. Njoo MD, Spuls PI, Bos JD, et al. Nonsurgical repigmentation therapies in vitiligo. Meta-analysis of the literature. Arch Dermatol 1998;134:1532–40.
23. Whitton M, Pinart M, Batchelor JM, et al. Evidence-Based Management of vitiligo: summary of a Cochrane systematic review. Br J Dermatol 2015;174(5):962–9.
24. Whitton ME, Ashcroft DM, Gonzalez U. Therapeutic interventions for vitiligo. J Am Acad Dermatol 2008;59:713–7.
25. Sassi F, Cazzaniga S, Tessari G, et al. Randomized controlled trial comparing the effectiveness of 308-nm excimer laser alone or in combination with topical hydrocortisone 17-butyrate cream in the treatment of vitiligo of the face and neck. Br J Dermatol 2008;159:1186–91.
26. Mayoral FA, Gonzalez C, Shah NS, et al. Repigmentation of vitiligo with pimecrolimus cream: a case report. Dermatology 2003;207:322–3.

27. Smith DA, Tofte SJ, Hanifin JM. Repigmentation of vitiligo with topical tacrolimus. Dermatology (Basel, Switzerland) 2002;205:301–3.
28. Lepe V, Moncada B, Castanedo-Cazares JP, et al. A double-blind randomized trial of 0.1% tacrolimus vs 0.05% clobetasol for the treatment of childhood vitiligo. Arch Dermatol 2003;139:581–5.
29. Ho N, Pope E, Weinstein M, et al. A double-blind, randomized, placebo-controlled trial of topical tacrolimus 0.1% vs. clobetasol propionate 0.05% in childhood vitiligo. Br J Dermatol 2011;165:626–32.
30. Radakovic S, Breier-Maly J, Konschitzky R, et al. Response of vitiligo to once- vs. twice-daily topical tacrolimus: a controlled prospective, randomized, observer-blinded trial. J Eur Acad Dermatol Venereol 2009;23:951–3.
31. Coskun B, Saral Y, Turgut D. Topical 0.05% clobetasol propionate versus 1% pimecrolimus ointment in vitiligo. Eur J Dermatol 2005;15:88–91.
32. Ostovari N, Passeron T, Lacour JP, et al. Lack of efficacy of tacrolimus in the treatment of vitiligo in the absence of UV-B exposure. Arch Dermatol 2006; 142:252–3.
33. Stinco G, Piccirillo F, Forcione M, et al. An open randomized study to compare narrow band UVB, topical pimecrolimus and topical tacrolimus in the treatment of vitiligo. Eur J Dermatol 2009;19:588–93.
34. Chiaverini C, Passeron T, Ortonne JP. Treatment of vitiligo by topical calcipotriol. J Eur Acad Dermatol Venereol 2002;16:137–8.
35. Sanclemente G, Garcia JJ, Zuleta JJ, et al. A double-blind, randomized trial of 0.05% betamethasone vs. topical catalase/dismutase superoxide in vitiligo. J Eur Acad Dermatol Venereol 2008;22: 1359–64.
36. Ezzedine K, Eleftheriadou V, Whitton M, et al. Vitiligo. Lancet 2015;386:74–84.
37. Taieb A, Alomar A, Bohm M, et al. Guidelines for the management of vitiligo: the European Dermatology Forum consensus. Br J Dermatol 2013;168:5–19.
38. Kathuria S, Khaitan BK, Ramam M, et al. Segmental vitiligo: a randomized controlled trial to evaluate efficacy and safety of 0.1% tacrolimus ointment vs 0.05% fluticasone propionate cream. Indian J Dermatol Venereol Leprol 2012;78:68–73.
39. Doelker L, Tran C, Gkomouzas A, et al. Production and clearance of cyclobutane dipyrimidine dimers in UV-irradiated skin pretreated with 1% pimecrolimus or 0.1% triamcinolone acetonide creams in normal and atopic patients. Exp Dermatol 2006;15: 342–6.
40. Tran C, Lübbe J, Sorg O, et al. Topical calcineurin inhibitors decrease the production of UVB-induced thymine dimers from airless mouse epidermis. Dermatology 2005;211(4):341–7.
41. Nicolaidou E, Antoniou C, Stratigos AJ, et al. Efficacy, predictors of response, and long-term follow-up in patients with vitiligo treated with narrowband UVB phototherapy. J Am Acad Dermatol 2007;56: 274–8.
42. Schmitt J, von Kobyletzki L, Svensson A, et al. Efficacy and tolerability of proactive treatment with topical corticosteroids and calcineurin inhibitors for atopic eczema: systematic review and meta-analysis of randomized controlled trials. Br J Dermatol 2011;164:415–28.
43. Cavalie M, Ezzedine K, Fontas E, et al. Maintenance therapy of adult vitiligo with 0.1% tacrolimus ointment: a randomized, double blind, placebo-controlled study. J Invest Dermatol 2015;135:970–4.
44. Tomita Y, Maeda K, Tagami H. Melanocyte-stimulating properties of arachidonic acid metabolites: possible role in postinflammatory pigmentation. Pigment Cell Res 1992;5:357–61.
45. Parsad D, Pandhi R, Dogra S, et al. Topical prostaglandin analog (PGE2) in vitiligo–a preliminary study. Int J Dermatol 2002;41:942–5.
46. Kapoor R, Phiske MM, Jerajani HR. Evaluation of safety and efficacy of topical prostaglandin E2 in treatment of vitiligo. Br J Dermatol 2009;160: 861–3.
47. Lim HW, Grimes PE, Agbai O, et al. Afamelanotide and Narrowband UV-B Phototherapy for the Treatment of Vitiligo: A Randomized Multicenter Trial. JAMA Dermatol 2014;151(1):42–50.
48. Passeron T. Indications and limitations of afamelanotide for treating vitiligo. JAMA Dermatol 2015;151: 349–50.
49. Rashighi M, Harris JE. Interfering with the IFN-gamma/CXCL10 pathway to develop new targeted treatments for vitiligo. Ann Transl Med 2015;3:343.

Phototherapy and Combination Therapies for Vitiligo

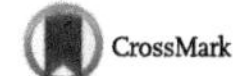

Samia Esmat, MD[a], Rehab A. Hegazy, MD[a], Suzan Shalaby, MD[a], Stephen Chu-Sung Hu, MBBS, MPhil[b], Cheng-Che E. Lan, MD, PhD[b,*]

KEYWORDS

• Vitiligo • Phototherapy • Narrowband ultraviolet B • Excimer

KEY POINTS

- Different forms of phototherapy for vitiligo include broadband UVB, narrowband UVB (NB-UVB), excimer light and excimer laser, and psoralen plus UVA.
- The main proposed mechanisms for induction of repigmentation in vitiligo by UV light include the induction of T-cell apoptosis, and stimulation of proliferation/migration of functional melanocytes in the perilesional skin and immature melanocytes in hair follicles.
- Optimizing NB-UVB requires consideration of different factors that affect the phototherapy protocol.
- Introducing the Vitiligo Working Group consensus to highlight possible answers to questions lacking evidence in phototherapy of vitiligo.
- Focusing on common obstacles met during phototherapy of vitiligo and how to overcome them.
- Different forms of combination therapies used with phototherapy in vitiligo and their various degrees of success.

INTRODUCTION

Vitiligo is a disease characterized by disappearance of melanocytes from the skin. It can negatively influence the physical appearance of affected individuals, and may profoundly affect a person's psychosocial function and quality of life.[1–4] Therefore, vitiligo should not be considered as merely a condition that affects a patient's appearance, but needs to be actively treated in patients who seek medical help. Phototherapy has been used as the main treatment modality for patients with vitiligo. Different forms of phototherapy for vitiligo include broadband UVB (BB-UVB), narrowband UVB (NB-UVB), excimer light and excimer laser, and psoralen plus UVA (PUVA).

PHOTOTHERAPY OF VITILIGO FROM EARLY AGES TO MODERN MEDICINE

Historically, phototherapy was first used to treat vitiligo more than 3500 years ago in ancient Egypt and India, when ancient healers used ingestion or topical application of plant extracts (*Ammi majus*

Conflicts of Interest: None declared.
Funding Sources: None.

[a] Phototherapy Unit, Dermatology Department, Faculty of Medicine, Cairo University, Egypt; [b] Department of Dermatology, College of Medicine, Kaohsiung Medical University Hospital, Kaohsiung Medical University, No 100, Tzyou 1st Road, Kaohsiung 807, Taiwan
* Corresponding author. Department of Dermatology, Kaohsiung Medical University Hospital, No 100, Tzyou 1st Road, Kaohsiung 807, Taiwan.
E-mail address: laneric@cc.kmu.edu.tw

Dermatol Clin 35 (2017) 171–192
http://dx.doi.org/10.1016/j.det.2016.11.008

Linnaeus in Egypt and *Psoralea corylifolia Linnaeus* in India) in combination with sunlight for the treatment of "leucoderma."[5]

Since the middle of the last century, PUVA or photochemotherapy had been the most popular form of phototherapy for patients with vitiligo.[6] However, in recent years, it has been gradually superseded by NB-UVB, which has been shown by various studies to have greater efficacy and fewer adverse effects than PUVA.

NARROW BAND ULTRAVIOLET B: THE WINNING HORSE

NB-UVB phototherapy is characterized by polychromatic light with a peak emission wavelength of 311 to 313 nm. In 1997, Westerhof and Nieuweboer-Krobotova[7] first reported the efficacy of NB-UVB phototherapy compared with topical PUVA for the treatment of vitiligo. They found that after 4 months of treatment, 67% of patients receiving NB-UVB phototherapy twice a week developed significant repigmentation, whereas only 46% of patients undergoing topical PUVA twice a week developed repigmentation. Since then, several other studies also have shown that NB-UVB is effective for the treatment of vitiligo both in adults and children.[8–18]

Various studies also have demonstrated that NB-UVB has superior efficacy compared with oral PUVA in the treatment of vitiligo.[19–22] In a double-blind randomized study, 25 patients with generalized vitiligo received twice-weekly NB-UVB phototherapy and 25 patients were treated with twice-weekly oral PUVA. It was found that 64% of patients in the NB-UVB group achieved more than 50% overall repigmentation, compared with 36% of patients in the oral PUVA group.[19] The efficacy of NB-UVB phototherapy in the treatment of vitiligo is summarized in (**Table 1**).

Because most studies have demonstrated that NB-UVB has superior efficacy compared with other forms of phototherapy, NB-UVB is now considered as the first-line treatment modality for generalized vitiligo.[36,55,56] Apart from its efficacy, NB-UVB has a better safety profile compared with PUVA, mainly due to absence of adverse effects related to psoralen.[57]

HOW DOES IT WORK?

The underlying mechanism for the repigmentation effects of NB-UVB phototherapy in vitiligo has not been completely defined, although several different mechanisms have been proposed.[58,59] Vitiligo is characterized by 2 stages: the active stage in which there is ongoing destruction of melanocytes by immune cells, and the stable stage in which the depigmented skin lesions remain constant over time.

In the active stage of vitiligo, the main mechanism of NB-UVB phototherapy may be explained by its immunomodulatory actions. NB-UVB may stimulate epidermal expression of interleukin-10, which induces differentiation of T-regulatory lymphocytes that can inhibit the activity of autoreactive T lymphocytes.[40] NB-UVB irradiation also has been shown to induce apoptosis of T cells in psoriatic skin lesions,[41] and a similar mechanism may occur in vitiligo.

In the stable stage of vitiligo, the major repigmentation effect of NB-UVB may be due to stimulation of functional melanocytes in the perilesional skin or immature melanocytes in hair follicles. This effect has been described as "biostimulation." In vitiligo lesional skin, there is a selective loss of active melanocytes in the epidermis, while the inactive/immature melanocytes in hair follicles are spared. UV radiation promotes the proliferation and migration of melanocytes located in the perilesional skin, and enhances activation and functional development of immature melanocytes in the outer root sheath of hair follicles.[60] The upward migration of melanocytes from the outer root sheath to the epidermis leads to the commonly observed formation of perifollicular pigmentation islands. Previously, we and others have shown that NB-UVB irradiation increased the expression of endothelin-1 and basic fibroblast growth factor by keratinocytes, which in turn may promote melanocyte proliferation.[42,61,62] Moreover, we demonstrated that NB-UVB irradiation may induce phosphorylated focal adhesion kinase (FAK) expression and matrix metalloproteinase (MMP)-2 activity in melanocytes, leading to increased melanocyte migration.[42] Therefore, NB-UVB phototherapy may promote vitiligo repigmentation directly by increasing melanocyte mobility and indirectly by inducing melanocyte-related growth factors from keratinocytes (**Fig. 1**). Furthermore, it is known that vitiligo lesions are characterized by increased oxidative stress, and treatment with NB-UVB had been found to reduce oxidative stress in patients with vitiligo.[63] Due to the differences in the mechanisms of action between active-stage and stable-stage vitiligo, we propose that higher fluence of NB-UVB may be required for stabilization of active disease and lower doses for repigmentation (biostimulation).

ADVERSE EFFECTS

Patients treated with NB-UVB phototherapy may experience various acute side effects, including

Table 1
Comparison of efficacy, side effects, and mechanisms of action of different forms of phototherapy for vitiligo

Phototherapy Modality	NB-UVB	Excimer Laser	Excimer Light	Oral PUVA	Topical PUVA
Efficacy (according to overall repigmentation)	>75% overall repigmentation: 63% of patients.[7] >75% overall repigmentation: 32% of patients.[19] >75% overall repigmentation: 53% of patients.[8] >75% overall repigmentation: 33% of patients.[10] >75% overall repigmentation: 48% of patients.[16] >75% overall repigmentation: 16% of patients.[22]	>75% overall repigmentation: 8% of patients.[23] >75% overall repigmentation: 16.6% of patients.[24] >75% overall repigmentation: 29% of patients.[25]	>75% overall repigmentation: 49% of patients.[26]	>75% overall repigmentation: 20% of patients.[19] >75% overall repigmentation: 18% of patients.[27] >75% overall repigmentation: 48% of patients.[28] >75% overall repigmentation: 8% of patients.[22]	>50% overall repigmentation: 36% of patients.[29]
Efficacy (according to lesional repigmentation)	>75% lesional repigmentation: 6% of lesions.[30]	>75% lesional repigmentation: 18% of lesions.[31] >75% lesional repigmentation: 26.9% of lesions.[32] >75% lesional repigmentation: 50.6% of lesions.[33] >75% lesional repigmentation: 61.4% of lesions.[34]	>75% lesional repigmentation: 37.5% of lesions.[30] >75% lesional repigmentation: 18.5% of lesions.[35]		

(*continued on next page*)

Table 1 (*continued*)

Phototherapy Modality	NB-UVB	Excimer Laser	Excimer Light	Oral PUVA	Topical PUVA
Side effects	Pruritus, erythema, burn, xerosis, eye injury, hyperpigmentation, photoaging, skin cancer.[5,13,36]	Erythema, blistering.[5,36]	Erythema, blistering.[5]	Erythema, skin and ocular phototoxicity, xerosis, nausea, headache, photoaging, skin cancer.[5,37–39]	Skin phototoxicity, perilesional tanning.[5]
Mechanism	Inhibit T-cell function,[40] induce T-cell apoptosis,[41] promote melanocyte proliferation (by increasing the expression of endothelin-1 and basic fibroblast growth factor from keratinocytes),[42] stimulate melanocyte migration (by inducing phosphorylated focal adhesion kinase expression and MMP-2 activity in melanocytes).[42]	Induce apoptosis of T lymphocytes,[43,44] promote melanocyte migration and proliferation (by inducing endothelin-1 secretion from keratinocytes).[45]	Induce T-lymphocyte apoptosis,[46] promote melanocyte migration and proliferation (by stimulating basic fibroblast growth factor and endothelin-1 release from keratinocytes),[45] promote differentiation of melanoblasts.[47]	Induce DNA cross-linking,[37,48] promote melanocyte proliferation (by stimulating the release of melanocyte growth factors by keratinocytes and fibroblasts),[49,50] promote melanocyte migration (by stimulating secretion of MMP-2 by melanoblasts),[51] stimulate melanogenesis,[52] induce T-cell suppression and apoptosis.[53,54]	Induce DNA cross-linking,[37,48] promote melanocyte proliferation and migration.[51]

Abbreviations: MMP, matrix metalloproteinase; NB-UVB, narrowband ultraviolet B; PUVA, psoralen plus ultraviolet A.

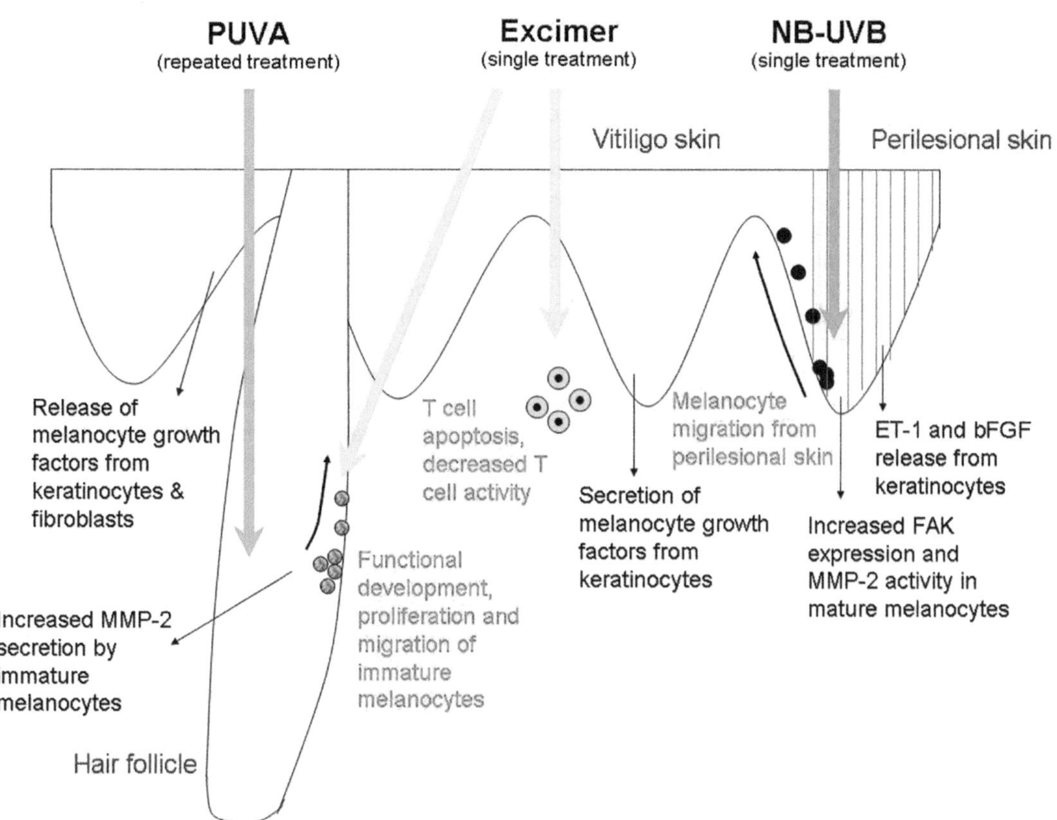

Fig. 1. Schematic diagram showing the proposed mechanisms of different forms of phototherapy (PUVA, excimer laser/excimer light, NB-UVB) in inducing vitiligo repigmentation. The main proposed mechanisms include the induction of T-cell apoptosis, release of melanocyte growth factors (such as endothelin-1 [ET-1] and basic fibroblast growth factor [bFGF]) from keratinocytes and fibroblasts, and increased MMP-2 secretion by melanocytes. This may lead to the proliferation and migration of functional melanocytes in the perilesional skin and immature melanocytes in hair follicles.

skin pruritus, erythema, burn injury, and xerosis. The adverse effects of UV radiation on the eyes should be considered in patients receiving treatment in periocular areas. Some phototherapy centers require patients to wear eye protection, whereas others allow patients to close their eyes during phototherapy, because theoretically NB-UVB does not penetrate the eyelids. The Vitiligo Working Group (VWG) consensus was to let patients with eyelid lesions close their eyes during the entire session and the possible the use of adhesive tape to keep the eye closed. Long-term adverse effects include darkening of normal skin and possible photoaging.

There is a possible long-term risk of skin cancer in patients undergoing UV light phototherapy. NB-UVB irradiation may induce DNA damage and cause carcinogenic changes.[64,65] However, a previous study found no increased risk of skin cancer in patients receiving BB-UVB or NB-UVB phototherapy for psoriasis.[66] Another study involving 3867 patients showed no significant increase in squamous cell carcinoma or melanoma in patients undergoing NB-UVB phototherapy for various diseases.[67] The carcinogenic risk of patients with vitiligo receiving NB-UVB treatment remains incompletely defined. Interestingly, despite the absence of melanin, the development of skin cancers in vitiligo lesions is rare.[68] Currently, NB-UVB is regarded to be less carcinogenic than PUVA.[69] Measuring 8-oxoguanine, a key parameter in the carcinogenic effect of ultraviolet radiation (UVR), it was found that cumulative doses of NB-UVB are safer than those of PUVA, with higher safety profile in higher skin phototypes.[70]

OTHER PHOTOTHERAPEUTIC MODALITIES

Excimer Laser

The excimer laser is characterized by a wavelength of 308 nm (also in the UVB region), and is generated using xenon and chlorine gases. It emits a monochromatic wavelength and is able to emit UVB radiation at high irradiance (defined as power output per unit area). The spot size may vary between 15 to 30 mm in diameter depending on the particular model that is used. Because of its smaller spot size, excimer laser allows the selective treatment of vitiligo lesional skin and is less likely to induce hyperpigmentation of perilesional skin. However, its small spot size means that this form of treatment is time-consuming and unsuitable for patients with vitiligo involving large body surface areas (>15%). Therefore, it is mainly used in the treatment of localized vitiligo. In addition, the cost of excimer laser is higher compared with other phototherapy devices.[5]

The excimer laser was first reported to be effective for treating vitiligo in 2001.[71,72] Since then, a number of reports have shown that this form of treatment is effective for inducing repigmentation of vitiligo lesions.[31–34,73–75] Treatments with excimer laser are usually undertaken twice or 3 times per week, and continue for 1 to 9 months. Although the rate of repigmentation is faster when treatments were administered 3 times a week, the ultimate degree of repigmentation appears to depend on the total number of treatments and not the frequency of treatments.[73] A summary of the clinical efficacy of excimer laser in vitiligo is presented in **Table 1**.

The mechanism of action for the therapeutic effect of excimer laser in vitiligo has not been well defined. Theoretically, it is possible the excimer laser may have a similar mechanism of action as NB-UVB, because both light sources contain similar wavelengths. However, excimer laser is characterized by monochromatic, coherent, and high-energy light, whereas NB-UVB consists of polychromatic, incoherent light with lower intensity. In fact, it has been shown that excimer laser is more effective in inducing apoptosis of T lymphocytes compared with NB-UVB.[43] Moreover, Novák and colleagues[44] compared the ability of different UVB light sources to induce T-lymphocyte apoptosis, and found that the 308-nm excimer laser is the greatest inducer of apoptosis. In addition, Noborio and Morita[45] compared the effectiveness of different wavelengths of UVB in inducing endothelin-1 secretion in a human epidermal tissue model, and found that the 308-nm excimer laser induced higher levels of endothelin-1 compared with broadband UVB and NB-UVB, implying that it may have more advantage in stimulating melanocytes. The proposed mechanism of excimer laser in inducing vitiligo repigmentation is presented in **Fig. 1**.

In general, excimer laser is a well-tolerated form of phototherapy. Possible side effects include skin erythema and occasionally blistering, which may be associated with higher treatment fluences. In addition, excimer laser is regarded as a safer form of treatment in pediatric patients due to its more localized field of irradiation.[5]

MONOCHROMATIC EXCIMER LIGHT/ EXCIMER LAMP

The monochromatic excimer light (excimer lamp) also emits light with 308-nm wavelength. It has also been shown to be effective in inducing repigmentation of vitiligo lesions.[26] The excimer lamp has a larger treatment field compared with excimer laser, which may enable irradiation of larger areas and shorter treatment times. Moreover, the cost of excimer lamp is cheaper compared with laser devices.

The mechanism of action of monochromatic excimer light in the treatment of vitiligo is not well defined. Similar to NB-UVB, excimer light may have immunomodulatory effects, by promoting T-lymphocyte apoptosis.[46] Moreover, excimer light may stimulate the release of endothelin-1 from keratinocytes, and thereby promote melanocyte proliferation.[45] We also have found that when administered at the same fluence, excimer light is more effective in stimulating basic fibroblast growth factor secretion from human keratinocytes compared with NB-UVB irradiation (Cheng-Che Lan, MD, PhD, unpublished data, 2016).

Regarding the differences in the mechanisms of action of excimer light and NB-UVB, it needs to be considered that excimer light is characterized by a higher irradiance compared with NB-UVB. Previously, we have shown that irradiance (the power delivered per unit area) has a more important role than fluence (amount of energy delivered per unit area) in UVB-induced melanoblast differentiation.[47] When administered at similar fluence, excimer light is effective in inducing melanoblast differentiation, whereas NB-UVB had no significant effect. Decreasing the irradiance of excimer light abolished its effects on melanoblasts, even though the same fluence was administered. This may provide an explanation for the superior efficacy of excimer light compared with NB-UVB for the treatment of localized vitiligo.

EXCIMER LASER AND EXCIMER LIGHT VERSUS NARROWBAND ULTRAVIOLET B FOR TREATMENT OF VITILIGO

Various studies have compared the therapeutic efficacy of excimer laser, excimer light, and NB-UVB in vitiligo.[30,76,77] Hong and colleagues[76] found that excimer laser had greater efficacy compared with NB-UVB in the treatment of vitiligo, and induced more rapid and greater degree of repigmentation. In Cairo University Hospital, a right-left comparison study between targeted NB-UVB and excimer light for 24 weeks showed similar repigmentation scores in both, but the onset was 2 weeks earlier on the excimer light side (unpublished data). In addition, several recent meta-analyses also have shown similar efficacy between excimer light, excimer laser, and NB-UVB for the treatment of vitiligo.[78–80]

EXCIMER LASER AND EXCIMER LIGHT FOR TREATMENT OF SEGMENTAL VITILIGO

Previously, several studies have shown that patients with segmental vitiligo respond poorly to NB-UVB phototherapy compared with patients with nonsegmental vitiligo. Anbar and colleagues[16] found that only 1 (7.7%) of 13 patients with segmental vitiligo achieved greater than 25% repigmentation following NB-UVB phototherapy for 6 months. The efficacy of excimer laser and excimer light in treating segmental vitiligo has not been clearly defined. In a study performed in Korea involving 80 patients with segmental vitiligo treated with excimer laser, Do and colleagues[81] found that 23.8% of patients achieved grade 4 (75%–99%) and 20% of patients achieved grade 3 (50%–74%) repigmentation. In addition, we have performed a retrospective review in our institution for patients with segmental vitiligo treated with excimer light for 3 months, and found that 9 (41%) of 22 patients achieved greater than 50% repigmentation, and 15 (68%) of 22 patients achieved greater than 25% repigmentation (unpublished data). These results indicate that excimer laser and excimer light may be effective forms of phototherapy for patients affected with segmental vitiligo.

BROADBAND ULTRAVIOLET B

BB-UVB is characterized by emission wavelengths ranging from 290 to 320 nm. Although it is widely used for the treatment of psoriasis and other skin diseases, there are few reports regarding its efficacy in vitiligo. A previous study involving 14 patients receiving BB-UVB showed that 8 patients (57.1%) obtained greater than 75% repigmentation after 12 months.[82] However, these results have not been confirmed by other studies. Therefore, BB-UVB is now rarely used for the treatment of vitiligo.

ORAL PSORALEN PLUS ULTRAVIOLET A

PUVA, otherwise known as photochemotherapy, has been the main form of treatment for generalized vitiligo since the 1950s until its replacement by NB-UVB. In this form of phototherapy, the patient first ingests a photosensitizer, and then is exposed to UVA (320–400 nm) irradiation. The most frequently used photosensitizer is 8-methoxypsoralen (methoxsalen, 8-MOP), which is ingested 2 hours before phototherapy, usually at a dose of 0.6 mg/kg. Other photosensitizers, including 5-methoxypsoralen (5-MOP) and trimethyl-psoralen (TMP), also have been used but have not been shown to be superior to 8-MOP.[5]

Oral PUVA is usually administered only to patients with generalized vitiligo.[83,84] Treatment is usually given twice weekly with an interval of at least 24 to 48 hours between treatment sessions. The starting irradiation dose depends on the skin phototype and can range between 0.5 and 1.0 J/cm^2. The irradiation dose is gradually increased until mild erythema develops in the vitiligo lesions.[5,37]

The underlying mechanism for the photosensitizing effect of methoxsalen has not been clearly defined. Following activation by light, methoxsalen forms covalent bonds with DNA, resulting in the generation of single-stranded and double-stranded DNA adducts.[37,48] PUVA phototherapy has also been found to stimulate the release of melanocyte growth factors by keratinocytes, induce proliferation of melanocytes, enhance melanocyte migration (by inducing MMP-2 secretion), stimulate melanogenesis, and decrease the expression of vitiligo-associated antigens on melanocyte cell membranes.[49,51,52] In addition, treatment with PUVA may induce lymphocyte apoptosis, and induces differentiation of T-regulatory lymphocytes with suppressor activity.[53,54]

Previously, we have investigated the effects of PUVA on melanocyte proliferation and migration.[50] Our findings showed that PUVA irradiation did not induce the secretion of melanocyte growth factors from keratinocytes, nor did it promote melanocyte migration on single treatment. On the other hand, we demonstrated that following oral PUVA treatment for vitiligo, patients who showed signs of repigmentation were characterized by higher serum levels of melanocyte growth factors (including basic fibroblast growth factor, stem cell factor, and hepatocyte growth factor). The difference in the in vitro and clinical findings may be possibly due to the longer duration of treatment in patients receiving oral PUVA compared with NB-UVB, or the presence of other cell types in vivo, such as fibroblasts that may contribute to the secretion of these melanocyte growth factors. Therefore, the repigmentation effect of oral PUVA may be partially explained by alterations in serum levels of melanocyte growth factors after long-term treatment.

Possible adverse effects of oral PUVA include erythema, skin and ocular phototoxicity, xerosis, and nausea and headache following psoralen intake.[37,38] In addition, long-term treatment with oral PUVA is associated with photoaging and an increased skin cancer risk (including squamous cell carcinoma, basal cell carcinoma, and melanoma).[39,85–88] In general, oral PUVA is considered to be more carcinogenic compared with BB-UVB and NB-UVB. Oral PUVA should not be administered to children or pregnant women. Due to the possibility of dangerous adverse effects, PUVA has been gradually replaced by NB-UVB in the treatment of vitiligo.

TOPICAL PSORALEN PLUS ULTRAVIOLET A

Topical PUVA may be a suitable treatment option for patients with localized vitiligo. It is safer than oral PUVA due to lower cumulative UVA dose and lack of systemic absorption of psoralen. It is also considered to be safe in children older than 2 years.[5] Topical PUVA treatment is performed using methoxsalen in solution or cream form, which is applied topically to the vitiligo lesions 20 to 30 minutes before UVA exposure.[29,89] Treatments are usually administered 1 to 3 times a week. The starting UVA dose is usually approximately 0.25 to 0.5 J/cm^2, which is gradually increased until mild erythema is observed in the vitiligo lesions.[29,89] Following phototherapy, the topical psoralen needs to be washed off with soap and water to avoid skin phototoxicity. In many patients with vitiligo receiving topical PUVA phototherapy, perilesional tanning develops and may be cosmetically unacceptable. This may prevent the continuation of topical PUVA treatment.

BROADBAND ULTRAVIOLET A

UVA alone (wavelength 320–400 nm), without the administration of photosensitizer before phototherapy, is usually ineffective for repigmenting vitiligo lesions.[90] Although this form of treatment has shown efficacy in a previous randomized trial involving 20 patients, with 50% of patients achieving greater than 60% repigmentation after 16 weeks,[91] this result has not been confirmed by other studies. Therefore, broadband UVA alone is now rarely used to treat vitiligo.

VISIBLE LIGHT

Previously, we also have shown that visible light, in the form of low energy helium-neon laser (wavelength 632.8 nm), is effective for segmental vitiligo, particularly in children with periorbital and perioral lesions. The therapeutic effects of helium-neon laser may be mediated via stimulation of melanocyte proliferation and migration, enhancement of primitive melanoblast differentiation, and improvement of lesional microcirculation.[92–94]

The clinical effects of different forms of phototherapy are summarized in **Table 1**, and the mechanisms involved in vitiligo repigmentation are presented in **Fig. 1**.

OPTIMIZING NARROWBAND ULTRAVIOLET B RESULTS

Among the numerous aforementioned phototherapeutic modalities, NB-UVB and excimer light/laser remain the most popular choice for dermatologists worldwide. Although a good response is not always observed in all lesions, every patient with vitiligo deserves a fair trial of this backbone treatment with an individualized protocol to reach optimum results.

FACTORS TO BE CONSIDERED IN TAILORING THE PHOTOTHERAPY PROTOCOL

Activity of Vitiligo

NB-UVB can be started regardless of disease activity, as it reportedly has both stabilizing[22,95,96] and repigmenting effects[10,95–99]; however, its repigmenting effects are less advantageous in active cases.[100] Most vitiligo specialists prefer combining phototherapy with other stabilizing medications.

Practical pearl: Activity should be monitored during the whole course of treatment, as stabilizing treatments could be re-administered whenever it becomes active.

Type of Vitiligo

Rapid progression[101] and early poliosis[102] are behind the poor response of segmental vitiligo to phototherapy compared with nonsegmental vitiligo. Early intervention in such cases could be beneficial,[102,103] where better responses were reported in cases of recent onset,[104,105] and normal pigmentation was achieved in 62.5% of cases with segmental vitiligo by Lotti and colleagues.[106] NB-UVB and targeted phototherapy were among the first-line therapies suggested by Lee and Choi[107] in their guidelines for treatment of segmental vitiligo.

Practical pearl: In patients, better responses are expected in cases with pigmented hairs and disease duration of 6 months or less.

Skin Phototype

A patient's skin phototype has recently been considered important for determination of the starting dose of NB-UVB dose.[108] Although a point of controversy,[99] it is suggested that patients with darker skin phototype ≥III are expected to achieve better prognosis with phototherapy.

Practical pearl: Applying efficient sunscreens to normal skin before the session can minimize increasing visibility of the lesions, especially in patients with lighter skin phototypes.

Disease Duration and Hair Color

Poliosis is a known unfavorable prognostic sign for repigmentation due to the total exhaustion of the melanocyte reservoir,[109,110] and is one of the poor prognostic signs in the recently proposed scoring system "Potential Repigmentation Index" of Benzekri and colleagues.[111]

Surprisingly, histopathological evidence failed to support the assumption that all black hairs should be dealt with as one category, denying its guarantee for favorable repigmentation.[112] In such lesions, disease duration was suggested to play an important role in the treatment response, in which patients with a recent onset show higher response rates, with no clear cutoff disease duration that bears a good prognosis.[9,16,112]

Practical pearl: Poor responses might be encountered in long-standing lesions even when pigmented hairs are present. In such cases, combination with surgical procedures could be considered.

Distribution of Lesions

In terms of location of lesions, several studies[7,12,15] have reported better response rates for facial lesions compared with lesions on other body areas, exposed or unexposed. Lesions on acral sites (hands and feet) consistently show minimal response rates.[7,12,15,17,21,97] In addition, resistant areas on the face include preauricular and postauricular areas, the lips, and mouth angles.[20] The reason for this anatomic variation in the response to treatment is still unclear, but may be attributed to the regional variation in the density of hair follicles, "the melanocytes reservoir."[60]

Lower melanocyte count and lower stem cell factor expression in acral compared with nonacral lesions both before and after PUVA therapy, as well as failure of elevation of MMPs 1, 2, and 9 in acral sites after PUVA, may be other factors behind the resistance of those areas to treatment.[113,114]

Furthermore, observations at the Phototherapy Unit Kasr Al Ainy showed that lesions in different sites of acral areas do not behave the same way, with periungual areas bearing the worst prognosis compared with more proximal areas.[115]

Practical pearl: Although not always successful, early intervention as well as combining phototherapy with other modalities is highly recommended in acral lesions.

Patient's Response to Light

Any history or sign of photosensitivity may preclude the decision of receiving phototherapy. Caution should be taken in patients bearing signs of photo koebnerization,[116] including those with lesions concentrated only on sun-exposed areas (dorsa of the hands, V-shaped area of the neck, forehead, nose), and those with history of exacerbation on previous exposure to natural sunlight.

Practical pearl: In such cases, investigations to exclude systemic lupus erythematosus[117] and hepatitis C virus infection[118] are recommended, as they may be the predisposing factors to photosensitivity; checking for a history of using photosensitizing medications is also important.[117]

Special Sites (Genitals)

It has long been recommended to cover male genitals during the session; this was also the VWG consensus. However, the consensus did not mention how to manage lesions in the genital areas. Apart from an old report of malignancy developing at exposed genitals, no studies have further supported or ruled out the hazard of phototherapy to these sites. Thus, excimer light might be a useful suggested line if topicals are not effective.[119]

PROTOCOL FOR PHOTOTHERAPY

Although NB-UVB has been in practice for more than 2 decades, no universally accepted protocol has been set. Reviewing the literature, many recommendations were lacking evidence as regards phototherapy protocols.[120] The phototherapy committee of VWG has put together a consensus to answer those inquiries through the collaboration of 6 institutions from different parts of the world[119]; the data are outlined as follows, and summarized in **Box 1**.[119]

Two Versus 3 Weekly Exposures

Although both frequencies proved to be effective in the treatment of vitiligo,[16,20,21,121,122] no controlled trials compared them. In a 1-year trial, the phototherapy unit in Cairo University Hospital accomplished better patient compliance and low load on the equipment with a twice-weekly regimen, but with a significantly slower repigmentation. The VWG consensus considered the thrice-weekly

Box 1
The Vitiligo Working Group phototherapy consensus recommendations

Frequency of administration

- Optimal: 3 times per week
- Acceptable: 2 times per week

Dosing protocol

- Initiate dose at 200 mJ/cm^2 irrespective of skin type
- Increase by 10% to 20% per treatment
- Fixed dosing based on skin type is another acceptable dosing strategy that takes inherent differences in the minimal erythema dose (MED) of various skin types into account

Maximum acceptable dose

- Face: 1500 mJ/cm^2
- Body: 3000 mJ/cm^2

Maximum number of exposures

- SKIN PHOTOTYPE IV–VI: No limit
- SKIN PHOTOTYPE I–III: More data on the risk of cutaneous malignancy is needed before a recommendation can be made

Course of narrowband ultraviolet B (NB-UVB)

- Assess treatment response after 18 to 36 exposures
- Minimum number of doses needed to determine lack of response: 48 exposures
- Due to the existence of slow responders, up to 72 exposures may be needed to determine lack of response to phototherapy

*Dose adjustment based on degree of erythema (see **Fig. 2**)*

- No erythema: Increase next dose by 10% to 20%
- Pink asymptomatic erythema: Hold at current dose until erythema disappears then increase by 10% to 20%
- Bright red asymptomatic erythema: Stop phototherapy until affected areas become light pink, then resume at last tolerated dose
- Symptomatic erythema (includes pain and blistering): Stop phototherapy until the skin heals and erythema fades to a light pink, then resume at last tolerated dose

Dose adjustment following missed doses

- 4 to 7 days between treatments: Hold dose constant
- 8 to 14 days between treatments: Decrease dose by 25%
- 15 to 21 days between treatments: Decrease dose by 50%
- More than 3 weeks between treatments: Re-start at initial dose

Device calibration or bulb replacement

- Decrease dose by 10% to 20%

Outcome measures to evaluate response

- Serial photography to establish baseline severity, disease stability, and response to treatment
- Validated scoring systems, such as the Vitiligo Area Scoring Index or Vitiligo European Task Force, to quantify degree of response

Posttreatment recommendations

- Application of sunscreen
- Avoidance of sunlight

Topical products before phototherapy

- Avoid all topical products for 4 hours EXCEPT mineral oil
- Mineral oil can be used to enhance light penetration in areas of dry, thickened skin, such as the elbows and knees

Tapering NB-UVB after complete repigmentation achieved

- First month: Phototherapy twice weekly
- Second month: Phototherapy once weekly
- Third and fourth months: Phototherapy every other week
- After 4 months, discontinue phototherapy

Follow-up

- SKIN PHOTOTYPE I–III: Yearly follow-up for total body skin examination to monitor for adverse effects of phototherapy, including cutaneous malignancy
- SKIN PHOTOTYPE IV–VI: No need to return for safety monitoring, as no reports of malignancy exist with this group
- All patients: Return on relapse for treatment

Minimum age for NB-UVB in children

- Minimum age is when children are able to reliably stand in the booth with either their eyes closed or wearing goggles
- Typically approximately 7 to 10 years of age depending on the child

Treatment of eyelid lesions

- Keep eyes closed during treatment, using adhesive tape if necessary

Special sites

- Cover face during phototherapy if uninvolved
- Shield male genitalia
- Protect female areola with sunscreen before treatment, especially in SKIN PHOTOTYPE I–III

Combination treatment for stabilization

- Oral antioxidants
- Topical treatments
- Oral-pulse corticosteroids

Treatment of NB-UVB induced skin changes

- Xerosis: Emollient or mineral oil
- Skin thickening: Topical corticosteroids or keratolytics

regimen the optimum because of the more accelerated response.[119]

Practical pearl: As a fast response is often desired by the patient of this slowly responding disease, you may counsel patients about the importance of adhering to a 3-times-weekly regimen.

Starting Dose

Measuring the minimal erythema dose is the most accurate means of determining the suitable starting dose; however, it is time-consuming and is not applied in most centers.[119] A fixed starting dose considering vitiligo as skin phototype I is often used.[123] Recent observation was raised that darker skin types have additional photoprotective mechanisms other than melanin, namely epidermal layer thickness, optical properties, and chromophores.[124] These findings mean that applying the starting dose for all skin phototypes as if it is type I may not be optimal. While fixing the starting dose according to the skin phototype increases the risk of phototoxicity,[119] it may be considered the most time-saving and practical method in planning the dosing schedule, especially for darker skin phototypes.

Erythema or Suberythema

In most of the studies,[16,21] a 10% to 20% increase of any given dose is used for patients with vitiligo per session. The target erythema is a point of debate, in which some protocols aim at rapid achievement of erythema,[7,16,19,22,96] and others stop at suberythema (70% of the MED).[121] Randomized controlled trials (RCTs) comparing both protocols are lacking; however, the VWG consensus described the target point (**Fig. 2**) as pink asymptomatic erythema, which was described by a member of the committee (Prof Amit Pandya) as carnation pink erythema.[119]

After reaching the target erythema, either the phototherapy dose is maintained constant or continuously increased until reaching first signs of repigmentation. On the basis of the assumption that a better response to treatment could be achieved on using a more aggressive treatment

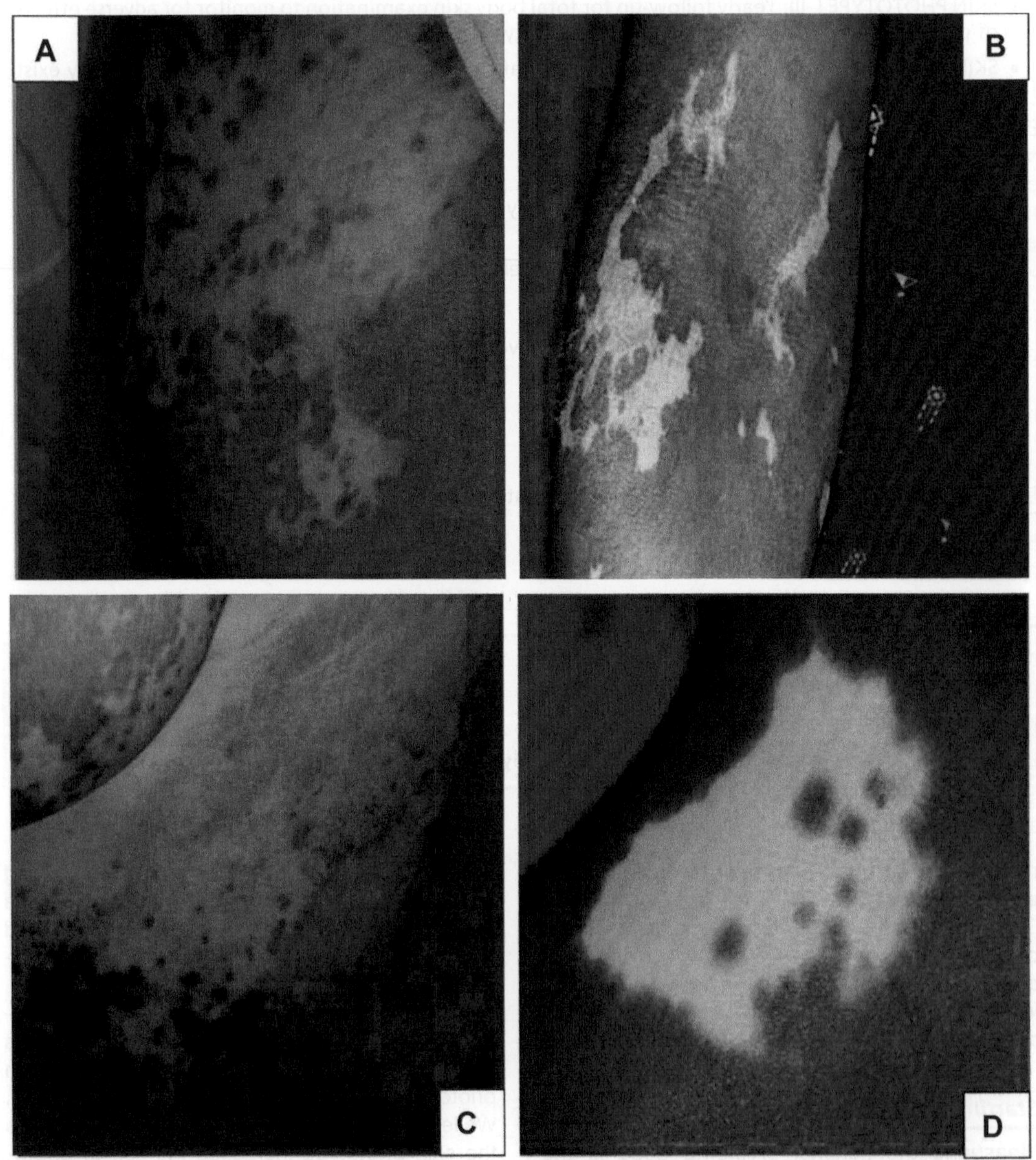

Fig. 2. Different grades of erythema encountered during NB-UVB phototherapy. (*A*) Optimal erythema. (*B*) Bright red asymptomatic erythema. (*C*) Symptomatic erythema. (*D*) No erythema.

protocol, a group of investigators carried out a continuous increase in the NB-UVB dose for as long as the patient could tolerate.[17] The protocol can be adjusted for darker skin phototypes. Anbar and colleagues[16] suggested calculating the dose according to each patient's daily sun exposure, differential dosimetry per body area, and individualization of increments. It is noteworthy that the optimal dose may differ at different sites; areas responsive to lower doses can be shielded until the optimal dose has been reached for areas requiring higher doses.[104]

Practical pearl: Patients with darker skin phototypes usually tolerate a high starting dose and larger incremental increases.

Combination with Other Therapies

Even though NB-UVB is the cornerstone treatment of vitiligo, combinations with medical and/or surgical therapies improve patients' odds in their battle against this disease.[13] Over the years, several combination plans were suggested, some with proven efficacy, others with controversial results, and the rest were of denied value (**Table 2**). Combination therapies serve multiple purposes.

INDUCTION OF STABILIZATION

Immunomodulation

Systemic steroids help with stabilization.[143] The evolution of oral-pulse and mini-pulse regimens provide the advantage of achieving stabilization with minimal or no side effects.[13] The use of other immunosuppressants such as cyclosporine[144] or methotrexate[145] to induce stabilization in vitiligo has been the subject of few recent studies but without similar efficacy.

Topical corticosteroids and calcineurin inhibitors with their immune-modulatory effects are commonly used in combination during the early stage of disease. The use of topical Vitamin D3 analogs also have been reported.[146]

Overcoming Oxidative Stress

Excessive oxidative stress is associated with vitiligo activity.[63] Systemic and to a less extent topical antioxidants (pseudocatalase, vitamin E, vitamin C, ubiquinone, lipoic acid, *Polypodium leucotomos*, catalase/superoxide dismutase combination, and *Ginkgo biloba*) represent newly emerging combination therapies, with the benefit of a high safety profile and a unique mechanism of action compacting the increased oxidative stress in vitiliginous lesions or even that induced by phototherapy itself.[133–139]

ENHANCEMENT OF REPIGMENTATION

Stimulation of Melanogenesis

Different topical therapies can be used simultaneously with phototherapy to achieve better response, including calcineurin inhibitors and vitamin D analogs which, in addition to immune modulation, may stimulate melanocyte proliferation/migration through increased MMP2 and enhanced topical drug absorption.[13] A recent meta-analysis advised that the combination of calcineurin inhibitors with NB-UVB should be used cautiously, as both are associated with theoretic risk of malignancy.[147] Although sparing psoralen intake was the main factor encouraging the use of NB-UVB, Bansal and colleagues[148] suggested that addition of psoralen might increase the extent of repigmentation induced by NB-UVB. Afamelanotide, a synthetic analog of the naturally occurring alpha-melanocyte–stimulating hormone (α-MSH), stimulates melanogenesis and protects against UV-induced damage.[141]

A recent study suggested that the combination of NB-UVB with excimer laser enhanced the treatment response for cases previously resistant to NB-UVB therapy. To avoid side effects, the NB-UVB dose was fixed while the excimer laser increments were gradually increased.[149]

Improving the Melanocyte Environment

Although phototherapy alone effectively stimulates the outer root sheath melanocytes, their journey afterward may be hindered by unsuitable unfavorable environment, such as decreased cadherins[150] and MMPs.[13] Phototherapy itself has a role in improving such defects; however, different techniques (dermabrasion, fractional lasers, 5-fluorouracil, and chemical peels) were introduced to improve the melanocyte chances for better migration that may hasten regimentation, through elimination of hyperkeratosis as well as the controlled wounding that stimulates melanocyte proliferation, migration through increased MMP2, and enhanced topical drug absorption.[141–151] Topical therapies also can improve the cytokine milieu through decreasing inflammatory cytokines, such as tumor necrosis factor-α and interferon-Υ.[13]

SUPPLYING THE MISSING RESERVOIR

The introduction of different surgical techniques that allow melanocyte transplantation in areas of low melanocyte reservoir was a breakthrough in the treatment of vitiligo. These techniques include suction blister grafts, punch grafts, needling, minigrafts, and split-thickness skin grafts, cultured

Table 2
Combination therapies with NB-UVB

Drug	Efficacy on Combination with NB-UVB	Study		Combination, %	NB-UVB, %	Combination Advised or Not
Topical steroids	• Stabilization • Significant increase in mean repigmentation	Clobetasol	Lim-Ong et al,[125] 2005	55	40	+
Topical calcineurin inhibitors	• Results inferior to steroids • Faster regimentation when combined with NB-UVB • Treatment efficacy is dose dependent	Tacrolimus	Nordal et al,[126] 2011	42	29	+
			Mehrabi and Pandya,[127] 2006	49	41	–
			Satyanarayan et al,[128] 2013	33	28	–
			Klahan and Asawanonda,[129] 2009	33	15	+
		Pimecrolimus	Esfandiarpour et al,[130] 2009	64	25	+
Topical vitamin D analogs	• Contradictory results, no significant value vs rapid initiation of pigmentation on combination with NB-UVB	Calciptriol	Arca et al,[131] 2006	46	42	+
		Tacalcitol	Leone et al,[132] 2006	50	40	–
Antioxidants	• Systemic antioxidants showed significant increase in mean pigmentation area • Topical antioxidants showed no significant value in RCTs	Vitamin E	Elgoweini and Nour El Din,[133] 2009	73	56	+
			Dell Anna et al,[134] 2007	47	18	+
		CSOD gel	Doghim et al,[135] 2011	40	45	–
			Yuskel et al,[136] 2009	5	0	+/–
			Kostovic et al,[137] 2007	16	—	+
		PCAT	Bakis-Petsoglou et al,[138] 2009	6	5.5	–
			Patel et al,[139] 2002	0	—	–
Dermabrasion	• Pain and scarring on treated area with significant improvement	Erbium laser	Bayoumi et al,[140] 2012	46	4.2	+
Fractional lasers	• Significant improvement in repigmentation in resistant areas	CO_2 Laser	Shin et al,[141] 2012	10	0	+
Afamelanotide	• Analog of alpha-melanocyte–stimulating hormone	Grimes 50%: SC implant once/month[142]				+

Abbreviations: CSOD, catalase superoxide dismutase; NB-UVB, narrowband ultraviolet B; PCAT, pseudo catalase; RCT, randomized controlled trial; SC, subcutaneous.

and noncultured melanocyte transplants, and epidermal suspensions.[152–154] Studies suggest that best results were observed when NB-UVB was used before and after surgery to improve the viability, migration, and proliferation of the newly resident melanocytes.[154]

Common Obstacles

Obstacles encountered during phototherapy in patients with vitiligo are described in the following sections.

Arrest of repigmentation

In some cases, a plateau is reached with arrest in further repigmentation. Reasons behind this arrest may include epidermal thickening of the lesional skin, observed clinically as lichenification and slight roughness. It is a sign of photo adaptation defined as the skin's ability to withstand an increased dose of UV radiation with repeated exposure during a course of phototherapy.[155] This is an indication for letting the patient stop the sessions and use topical or intralesional steroids until this sign resolves, as assessed through palpation of the skin for pliability.

Failure of repigmentation

In some situations, lesions with a typically good prognosis fail to repigment. Checking the phototherapy equipment calibration, patient's positioning, and proper exposure of his or her lesions to the phototherapy source should be one of the primary steps to ensure the accurate delivery of the desired dose. Combination therapy is always advised as a secondary tool.[13]

New lesions developing while on treatment

Reconsideration of the stabilization plan[156] and trying to control precipitating factors, such as psychogenic stress, trauma, and sunburns, are important steps.

Persistent loss of pigment despite adoption of the previously mentioned measures should raise the suspicion of photo koebnerization, deeming this line of therapy an improper one.

Failure of compliance

Successful treatment is directly related to patient compliance. The anticipated long duration of treatment should be clarified to patients from the beginning to set their expectations, considering their schedule, lifestyle, and individual needs. If they cannot maintain a consistent schedule in phototherapy, other options should be considered. A recent study[157] concluded that younger patients and those with widespread disease and facial lesions were more compliant. Educational status and sex had no impact on default status.

Darkening of normal skin

Many patients are concerned when their normal perilesional skin becomes darker with phototherapy, making the lesions more obvious. In localized lesions, adoption of targeted therapy might overcome such a drawback, but may not be available in many centers. In such cases, coverage of unaffected areas, as well as application of sunscreens to normal skin surrounding the lesions, could aid in solving this dilemma.

Frequent development of marked erythema

This might occur in centers with a high, fixed starting dose. If this occurs, minimal erythema dosing may help. It is of extreme importance to make note of this sensitivity in the patient's file for future therapy. Sometimes patients might suffer from repeated development of marked erythema in certain locations rather than others. This usually occurs with uneven exposure in the phototherapy device; for example, an obese patient with abdomen and breasts at a closer distance to the light source, or a patient leaning on the device. In such cases, it is important to closely monitor their positioning.

Another cause of frequent development of marked erythema is the intake of photosensitizing drugs while receiving the sessions. These drugs include tetracycline antibiotics, nonsteroidal anti-inflammatory drugs, some diuretics, retinoids, and some antifungals, such as voriconazol.[13]

MACHINE CALIBRATION

Regular maintenance and calibration of the equipment is one step that could help ensure the delivery of the required dose and avoidance of side effects related to underdosing or overdosing.

WHEN TO STOP TREATMENT

Stopping treatment is a rather complex decision, with many controversies involved. The value of maintenance therapy in patients showing complete response should be considered. Another consideration is how long to continue therapy in patients showing an incomplete or minimal response. The European task force[55] suggested that a 3-month trial is a reasonable duration after which phototherapy should be stopped if no repigmentation is achieved, and 6 months in others with unsatisfactory ($\leq$25%) repigmentation. In their consensus, the phototherapy committee of the VWG considered 48 sessions over 4 months to be the minimum number of sessions to determine a lack of response. This decision could be delayed up to the 72nd session because of the existence of slow responders.

In cases showing ongoing repigmentation, phototherapy should be continued for as long as improvement is observed for a maximum of 2 years' duration; however, this point needs more elaborative detailed guidelines. These durations could be considered too short in sites that are slower to respond.[111] In addition, the different skin phototypes are expected to respond at different durations.[17,99] Gradual tapering of the frequency of exposures before stopping has been suggested in the VWG consensus regarding maintenance phototherapy over a 4-month schedule and regular follow-up examinations are important.[55]

NEW HORIZONS IN THE TREATMENT OF VITILIGO

Developments in the phototherapy field are never ending, with newer machines, protocols, combinations, and evaluation techniques emerging to improve results and safety profiles, and expand the sector of patients with vitiligo who benefit from this line of treatment.

Low-level laser therapy (LLLT) was found to improve the proliferation of melanocytes without causing any cytotoxic effects. The effects vary according to the applied energy density and wavelengths to which the target cells are subjected. An energy density value of 0.5 to 4.0 J/cm^2 and a visible spectrum ranging from 600 to 700 nm of LLLT are very helpful in enhancing the proliferation rate of various cell lines. With the appropriate use of LLLT, the proliferation rate of cultured cells, including stem cells, can be increased, which would be very useful in tissue engineering and regenerative medicine.[158] A recent study[159] shed light on the potential benefits of low-level lasers on the melanocyte viability, proliferation, and migration in vitro, with the blue light (457 nm) showing an upper hand in comparison with the red (635 nm), and UV (355 nm) lasers. These findings might have potential application in vitiligo treatment in the future.

Home-based phototherapy is another territory that is showing great advancements.[160–162] A randomized controlled study including 44 cases of focal vitiligo demonstrated that with careful selection of patients, home-based phototherapy can be as effective as institution-based treatment options.[161] This approach would offer better treatment adherence and compliance. Development of comprehensive training packages would help in improving the results and reducing complications.[162]

Several new medications based on our increasing understanding of the pathogenesis of vitiligo are still in the pipeline. The most interesting being those that inhibit the janus kinases or others interfering with the action of recently known to be involved chemokines, such as CXCL9 and 10.[163] Those drugs in the near future might be used in combination with phototherapy of vitiligo to achieve optimal management.

SUMMARY

There is no doubt that the therapeutic armamentarium for vitiligo will be witnessing a huge expansion in the coming years. Nevertheless, we believe that phototherapy will hold its ground and remain a cornerstone in the management of this enigmatic disease. Developments in the phototherapeutic field are never ending, with newer machines, protocols, combinations, and evaluation techniques emerging to improve results and safety profiles, and expand the sector of patients with vitiligo who benefit from this line of treatment.

REFERENCES

1. Ongenae K, Beelaert L, van Geel N, et al. Psychosocial effects of vitiligo. J Eur Acad Dermatol Venereol 2006;20(1):1–8.
2. Ongenae K, Van Geel N, De Schepper S, et al. Effect of vitiligo on self-reported health-related quality of life. Br J Dermatol 2005;152(6):1165–72.
3. Amer AA, Gao XH. Quality of life in patients with vitiligo: an analysis of the dermatology life quality index outcome over the past two decades. Int J Dermatol 2016;55(6):608–14.
4. Krüger C, Schallreuter KU. Stigmatisation, avoidance behaviour and difficulties in coping are common among adult patients with vitiligo. Acta Derm Venereol 2015;95(5):553–8.
5. Pacifico A, Leone G. Photo(chemo)therapy for vitiligo. Photodermatol Photoimmunol Photomed 2011;27(5):261–77.
6. Grimes PE. Psoralen photochemotherapy for vitiligo. Clin Dermatol 1997;15(6):921–6.
7. Westerhof W, Nieuweboer-Krobotova L. Treatment of vitiligo with UV-B radiation vs topical psoralen plus UV-A. Arch Dermatol 1997;133(12):1525–8.
8. Njoo MD, Bos JD, Westerhof W. Treatment of generalized vitiligo in children with narrow-band (TL-01) UVB radiation therapy. J Am Acad Dermatol 2000;42(2 Pt 1):245–53.
9. Scherschun L, Kim JJ, Lim HW. Narrow-band ultraviolet B is a useful and well-tolerated treatment for vitiligo. J Am Acad Dermatol 2001;44(6):999–1003.
10. Natta R, Somsak T, Wisuttida T, et al. Narrowband ultraviolet B radiation therapy for recalcitrant vitiligo in Asians. J Am Acad Dermatol 2003;49(3):473–6.
11. Samson Yashar S, Gielczyk R, Scherschun L, et al. Narrow-band ultraviolet B treatment for vitiligo,

pruritus, and inflammatory dermatoses. Photodermatol Photoimmunol Photomed 2003;19(4):164–8.
12. Kanwar AJ, Dogra S. Narrow-band UVB for the treatment of generalized vitiligo in children. Clin Exp Dermatol 2005;30(4):332–6.
13. Yazdani Abyaneh M, Griffith RD, Falto-Aizpurua L, et al. Narrowband ultraviolet B phototherapy in combination with other therapies for vitiligo: mechanisms and efficacies. J Eur Acad Dermatol Venereol 2014;28(12):1610–22.
14. Chen GY, Hsu MM, Tai HK, et al. Narrow-band UVB treatment of vitiligo in Chinese. J Dermatol 2005; 32(10):793–800.
15. Brazzelli V, Prestinari F, Castello M, et al. Useful treatment of vitiligo in 10 children with UV-B narrowband (311 nm). Pediatr Dermatol 2005;22(3): 257–61.
16. Anbar TS, Westerhof W, Abdel-Rahman AT, et al. Evaluation of the effects of NB-UVB in both segmental and non-segmental vitiligo affecting different body sites. Photodermatol Photoimmunol Photomed 2006;22(3):157–63.
17. Nicolaidou E, Antoniou C, Stratigos AJ, et al. Efficacy, predictors of response, and long-term follow-up in patients with vitiligo treated with narrowband UVB phototherapy. J Am Acad Dermatol 2007; 56(2):274–8.
18. Brazzelli V, Antoninetti M, Palazzini S, et al. Critical evaluation of the variants influencing the clinical response of vitiligo: study of 60 cases treated with ultraviolet B narrow-band phototherapy. J Eur Acad Dermatol Venereol 2007;21(10):1369–74.
19. Yones SS, Palmer RA, Garibaldinos TM, et al. Randomized double-blind trial of treatment of vitiligo: efficacy of psoralen-UV-A therapy vs Narrowband-UV-B therapy. Arch Dermatol 2007;143(5):578–84.
20. Parsad D, Kanwar AJ, Kumar B. Psoralen-ultraviolet A vs. narrow-band ultraviolet B phototherapy for the treatment of vitiligo. J Eur Acad Dermatol Venereol 2006;20(2):175–7.
21. El Mofty M, Mostafa W, Esmat S, et al. Narrow band ultraviolet B 311 nm in the treatment of vitiligo: two right-left comparison studies. Photodermatol Photoimmunol Photomed 2006;22(1):6–11.
22. Bhatnagar A, Kanwar AJ, Parsad D, et al. Comparison of systemic PUVA and NB-UVB in the treatment of vitiligo: an open prospective study. J Eur Acad Dermatol Venereol 2007;21(5):638–42.
23. Matin M, Latifi S, Zoufan N, et al. The effectiveness of excimer laser on vitiligo treatment in comparison with a combination therapy of Excimer laser and tacrolimus in an Iranian population. J Cosmet Laser Ther 2014;16(5):241–5.
24. Sassi F, Cazzaniga S, Tessari G, et al. Randomized controlled trial comparing the effectiveness of 308-nm excimer laser alone or in combination with topical hydrocortisone 17-butyrate cream in the treatment of vitiligo of the face and neck. Br J Dermatol 2008;159(5):1186–91.
25. Esposito M, Soda R, Costanzo A, et al. Treatment of vitiligo with the 308 nm excimer laser. Clin Exp Dermatol 2004;29(2):133–7.
26. Leone G, Iacovelli P, Paro Vidolin A, et al. Monochromatic excimer light 308 nm in the treatment of vitiligo: a pilot study. J Eur Acad Dermatol Venereol 2003;17(5):531–7.
27. Sahin S, Hindioğlu U, Karaduman A. PUVA treatment of vitiligo: a retrospective study of Turkish patients. Int J Dermatol 1999;38(7):542–5.
28. Chuan MT, Tsai YJ, Wu MC. Effectiveness of psoralen photochemotherapy for vitiligo. J Formos Med Assoc 1999;98(5):335–40.
29. Grimes PE, Minus HR, Chakrabarti SG, et al. Determination of optimal topical photochemotherapy for vitiligo. J Am Acad Dermatol 1982;7(6):771–8.
30. Casacci M, Thomas P, Pacifico A, et al. Comparison between 308-nm monochromatic excimer light and narrowband UVB phototherapy (311-313 nm) in the treatment of vitiligo–a multicentre controlled study. J Eur Acad Dermatol Venereol 2007;21(7): 956–63.
31. Spencer JM, Nossa R, Ajmeri J. Treatment of vitiligo with the 308-nm excimer laser: a pilot study. J Am Acad Dermatol 2002;46(5):727–31.
32. Ostovari N, Passeron T, Zakaria W, et al. Treatment of vitiligo by 308-nm excimer laser: an evaluation of variables affecting treatment response. Lasers Surg Med 2004;35(2):152–6.
33. Hadi S, Tinio P, Al-Ghaithi K, et al. Treatment of vitiligo using the 308-nm excimer laser. Photomed Laser Surg 2006;24(3):354–7.
34. Zhang XY, He YL, Dong J, et al. Clinical efficacy of a 308 nm excimer laser in the treatment of vitiligo. Photodermatol Photoimmunol Photomed 2010; 26(3):138–42.
35. Cheng YP, Chiu HY, Jee SH, et al. Excimer light photototherapy of segmental and non-segmental vitiligo: experience in Taiwan. Photodermatol Photoimmunol Photomed 2012;28(1):6–11.
36. Nicolaidou E, Antoniou C, Stratigos A, et al. Narrowband ultraviolet B phototherapy and 308-nm excimer laser in the treatment of vitiligo: a review. J Am Acad Dermatol 2009;60(3):470–7.
37. Gupta AK, Anderson TF. Psoralen photochemotherapy. J Am Acad Dermatol 1987;17(5 Pt 1):703–34.
38. Morison WL, Marwaha S, Beck L. PUVA-induced phototoxicity: incidence and causes. J Am Acad Dermatol 1997;36(2 Pt 1):183–5.
39. Hannuksela-Svahn A, Pukkala E, Koulu L, et al. Cancer incidence among Finnish psoriasis patients treated with 8-methoxypsoralen bath PUVA. J Am Acad Dermatol 1999;40(5 Pt 1):694–6.
40. Ponsonby AL, Lucas RM, van der Mei IA. UVR, vitamin D and three autoimmune diseases–multiple

sclerosis, type 1 diabetes, rheumatoid arthritis. Photochem Photobiol 2005;81(6):1267–75.
41. Ozawa M, Ferenczi K, Kikuchi T, et al. 312-nanometer ultraviolet B light (narrow-band UVB) induces apoptosis of T cells within psoriatic lesions. J Exp Med 1999;189(4):711–8.
42. Wu CS, Yu CL, Wu CS, et al. Narrow-band ultraviolet-B stimulates proliferation and migration of cultured melanocytes. Exp Dermatol 2004; 13(12):755–63.
43. Novák Z, Bónis B, Baltás E, et al. Xenon chloride ultraviolet B laser is more effective in treating psoriasis and in inducing T cell apoptosis than narrowband ultraviolet B. J Photochem Photobiol B 2002; 67(1):32–8.
44. Novák Z, Bérces A, Rontó G, et al. Efficacy of different UV-emitting light sources in the induction of T-cell apoptosis. Photochem Photobiol 2004; 79(5):434–9.
45. Noborio R, Morita A. Preferential induction of endothelin-1 in a human epidermal equivalent model by narrow-band ultraviolet B light sources. Photodermatol Photoimmunol Photomed 2010; 26(3):159–61.
46. Bianchi B, Campolmi P, Mavilia L, et al. Monochromatic excimer light (308 nm): an immunohistochemical study of cutaneous T cells and apoptosis-related molecules in psoriasis. J Eur Acad Dermatol Venereol 2003;17(4):408–13.
47. Lan CC, Yu HS, Lu JH, et al. Irradiance, but not fluence, plays a crucial role in UVB-induced immature pigment cell development: new insights for efficient UVB phototherapy. Pigment Cell Melanoma Res 2013;26(3):367–76.
48. Averbeck D. Recent advances in psoralen phototoxicity mechanism. Photochem Photobiol 1989; 50(6):859–82.
49. Abdel-Naser MB, Hann SK, Bystryn JC. Oral psoralen with UV-A therapy releases circulating growth factor(s) that stimulates cell proliferation. Arch Dermatol 1997;133(12):1530–3.
50. Wu CS, Lan CC, Wang LF, et al. Effects of psoralen plus ultraviolet A irradiation on cultured epidermal cells in vitro and patients with vitiligo in vivo. Br J Dermatol 2007;156(1):122–9.
51. Lei TC, Vieira WD, Hearing VJ. In vitro migration of melanoblasts requires matrix metalloproteinase-2: implications to vitiligo therapy by photochemotherapy. Pigment Cell Res 2002;15(6):426–32.
52. Kao CH, Yu HS. Comparison of the effect of 8-methoxypsoralen (8-MOP) plus UVA (PUVA) on human melanocytes in vitiligo vulgaris and in vitro. J Invest Dermatol 1992;98(5):734–40.
53. Bulat V, Situm M, Dediol I, et al. The mechanisms of action of phototherapy in the treatment of the most common dermatoses. Coll Antropol 2011;35(Suppl 2):147–51.
54. El-Domyati M, Moftah NH, Nasif GA, et al. Evaluation of apoptosis regulatory proteins in response to PUVA therapy for psoriasis. Photodermatol Photoimmunol Photomed 2013;29(1):18–26.
55. Taieb A, Alomar A, Böhm M, et al, Vitiligo European Task Force (VETF), European Academy of Dermatology and Venereology (EADV), Union Européenne des Médecins Spécialistes (UEMS). Guidelines for the management of vitiligo: the European Dermatology Forum consensus. Br J Dermatol 2013; 168(1):5–19.
56. Ling TC, Clayton TH, Crawley J, et al. British Association of Dermatologists and British Photodermatology Group guidelines for the safe and effective use of psoralen-ultraviolet A therapy 2015. Br J Dermatol 2016;174(1):24–55.
57. Felsten LM, Alikhan A, Petronic-Rosic V. Vitiligo: a comprehensive overview. Part II: treatment options and approach to treatment. J Am Acad Dermatol 2011;65(3):493–514.
58. Alikhan A, Felsten LM, Daly M, et al. Vitiligo: a comprehensive overview. Part I. Introduction, epidemiology, quality of life, diagnosis, differential diagnosis, associations, histopathology, etiology, and work-up. J Am Acad Dermatol 2011;65(3): 473–91.
59. Westerhof W, d'Ischia M. Vitiligo puzzle: the pieces fall in place. Pigment Cell Res 2007;20(5):345–59.
60. Cui J, Shen LY, Wang GC. Role of hair follicles in the repigmentation of vitiligo. J Invest Dermatol 1991;97(3):410–6.
61. Hirobe T. Role of keratinocyte-derived factors involved in regulating the proliferation and differentiation of mammalian epidermal melanocytes. Pigment Cell Res 2005;18(1):2–12.
62. Imokawa G. Autocrine and paracrine regulation of melanocytes in human skin and in pigmentary disorders. Pigment Cell Res 2004;17(2):96–110.
63. Karsli N, Akcali C, Ozgoztasi O, et al. Role of oxidative stress in the pathogenesis of vitiligo with special emphasis on the antioxidant action of narrowband ultraviolet B phototherapy. J Int Med Res 2014;42(3):799–805.
64. Tzung TY, Rünger TM. Assessment of DNA damage induced by broadband and narrowband UVB in cultured lymphoblasts and keratinocytes using the comet assay. Photochem Photobiol 1998; 67(6):647–50.
65. Budiyanto A, Ueda M, Ueda T, et al. Formation of cyclobutane pyrimidine dimers and 8-oxo-7,8-dihydro-2'-deoxyguanosine in mouse and organ-cultured human skin by irradiation with broadband or with narrowband UVB. Photochem Photobiol 2002;76(4):397–400.
66. Weischer M, Blum A, Eberhard F, et al. No evidence for increased skin cancer risk in psoriasis patients treated with broadband or narrowband

UVB phototherapy: a first retrospective study. Acta Derm Venereol 2004;84(5):370–4.
67. Hearn RM, Kerr AC, Rahim KF, et al. Incidence of skin cancers in 3867 patients treated with narrowband ultraviolet B phototherapy. Br J Dermatol 2008;159(4):931–5.
68. Teulings HE, Overkamp M, Ceylan E, et al. Decreased risk of melanoma and nonmelanoma skin cancer in patients with vitiligo: a survey among 1307 patients and their partners. Br J Dermatol 2013;168(1):162–71.
69. Ibbotson SH, Bilsland D, Cox NH, et al. British Association of Dermatologists. An update and guidance on narrowband ultraviolet B phototherapy: a British Photodermatology Group Workshop Report. Br J Dermatol 2004;151(2):283–97.
70. Youssef R, Mashaly H, Safwat M, et al. Lack of oxidative damage potential to DNA of different phototherapeutic modalities in dark-skinned individuals. Indian J Dermatol Venereol Leprol 2016;82(6):666–72.
71. Baltás E, Nagy P, Bónis B, et al. Repigmentation of localized vitiligo with the xenon chloride laser. Br J Dermatol 2001;144(6):1266–7.
72. Baltás E, Csoma Z, Ignácz F, et al. Treatment of vitiligo with the 308-nm xenon chloride excimer laser. Arch Dermatol 2002;138(12):1619–20.
73. Hofer A, Hassan AS, Legat FJ, et al. Optimal weekly frequency of 308-nm excimer laser treatment in vitiligo patients. Br J Dermatol 2005;152(5):981–5.
74. Passeron T, Ortonne JP. Use of the 308-nm excimer laser for psoriasis and vitiligo. Clin Dermatol 2006; 24(1):33–42.
75. Hofer A, Hassan AS, Legat FJ, et al. The efficacy of excimer laser (308 nm) for vitiligo at different body sites. J Eur Acad Dermatol Venereol 2006;20(5):558–64.
76. Hong SB, Park HH, Lee MH. Short-term effects of 308-nm xenon-chloride excimer laser and narrowband ultraviolet B in the treatment of vitiligo: a comparative study. J Korean Med Sci 2005;20(2): 273–8.
77. Le Duff F, Fontas E, Giacchero D, et al. 308-nm excimer lamp vs. 308-nm excimer laser for treating vitiligo: a randomized study. Br J Dermatol 2010; 163(1):188–92.
78. Lopes C, Trevisani VF, Melnik T. Efficacy and safety of 308-nm monochromatic excimer lamp versus other phototherapy devices for vitiligo: a systematic review with meta-analysis. Am J Clin Dermatol 2016;17(1):23–32.
79. Sun Y, Wu Y, Xiao B, et al. Treatment of 308-nm excimer laser on vitiligo: a systemic review of randomized controlled trials. J Dermatolog Treat 2015;26(4):347–53.
80. Xiao BH, Wu Y, Sun Y, et al. Treatment of vitiligo with NB-UVB: a systematic review. J Dermatolog Treat 2015;26(4):340–6.
81. Do JE, Shin JY, Kim DY, et al. The effect of 308 nm excimer laser on segmental vitiligo: a retrospective study of 80 patients with segmental vitiligo. Photodermatol Photoimmunol Photomed 2011;27(3): 147–51.
82. Köster W, Wiskemann A. Phototherapy with UV-B in vitiligo. Z Hautkr 1990;65(11):1022–4 [in German].
83. Kwok YK, Anstey AV, Hawk JL. Psoralen photochemotherapy (PUVA) is only moderately effective in widespread vitiligo: a 10-year retrospective study. Clin Exp Dermatol 2002;27(2):104–10.
84. Kovacs SO. Vitiligo. J Am Acad Dermatol 1998; 38(5 Pt 1):647–66 [quiz: 667–8].
85. Stern RS, Laird N. The carcinogenic risk of treatments for severe psoriasis. Photochemotherapy follow-up study. Cancer 1994;73(11):2759–64.
86. Stern RS. Malignant melanoma in patients treated for psoriasis with PUVA. Photodermatol Photoimmunol Photomed 1999;15(1):37–8.
87. Stern RS, PUVA Follow-Up Study. The risk of squamous cell and basal cell cancer associated with psoralen and ultraviolet A therapy: a 30-year prospective study. J Am Acad Dermatol 2012;66(4): 553–62.
88. Stern RS, Nichols KT, Väkevä LH. Malignant melanoma in patients treated for psoriasis with methoxsalen (psoralen) and ultraviolet A radiation (PUVA). The PUVA Follow-Up Study. N Engl J Med 1997; 336(15):1041–5.
89. Halpern SM, Anstey AV, Dawe RS, et al. Guidelines for topical PUVA: a report of a workshop of the British Photodermatology Group. Br J Dermatol 2000;142(1):22–31.
90. Westerhof W, Nieuweboer-Krobotova L, Mulder PG, et al. Left-right comparison study of the combination of fluticasone propionate and UV-A vs. either fluticasone propionate or UV-A alone for the long-term treatment of vitiligo. Arch Dermatol 1999; 135(9):1061–6.
91. El-Mofty M, Mostafa W, Youssef R, et al. Ultraviolet A in vitiligo. Photodermatol Photoimmunol Photomed 2006;22(4):214–6.
92. Lan CC, Wu CS, Chiou MH, et al. Low-energy helium-neon laser induces melanocyte proliferation via interaction with type IV collagen: visible light as a therapeutic option for vitiligo. Br J Dermatol 2009; 161(2):273–80.
93. Yu WT, Yu HS, Wu CS, et al. Noninvasive cutaneous blood flow as a response predictor for visible light therapy on segmental vitiligo: a prospective pilot study. Br J Dermatol 2011;164(4):759–64.
94. Lan CC, Wu CS, Chiou MH, et al. Low-energy helium-neon laser induces locomotion of the immature melanoblasts and promotes melanogenesis of the more differentiated melanoblasts: recapitulation of vitiligo repigmentation in vitro. J Invest Dermatol 2006;126(9):2119–26.

95. Dawe RS, Cameron H, Yule S, et al. A randomized controlled trial of narrowband ultraviolet B vs. bath-psoralen plus ultraviolet A photochemotherapy for psoriasis. Br J Dermatol 2003;148:1194–204.
96. Kishan Kumar YH, Rao GR, Gopal KV, et al. Evaluation of narrow-band UVB phototherapy in 150 patients with vitiligo. Indian J Dermatol Venereol Leprol 2009;75(2):162–6.
97. Sapam R, Agrawal S, Dhali TK. Systemic PUVA vs. narrowband UVB in the treatment of vitiligo: a randomized controlled study. Int J Dermatol 2012; 51(9):1107–15.
98. Percivalle S, Piccino R, Caccialanza M, et al. Narrowband UVB phototherapy in vitiligo: evaluation of results in 53 patients. G Ital Dermatol Venereol 2008;143(1):9–14.
99. Kanwar AJ, Dogra S, Parsad D, et al. Narrow-band UVB for the treatment of vitiligo: an emerging effective and well-tolerated therapy. Int J Dermatol 2005; 44(1):57–60.
100. Bhatnagar A, Kanwar AJ, Parsad D, et al. Psoralen and ultraviolet A and narrow-band ultraviolet B in inducing stability in vitiligo, assessed by vitiligo disease activity score: an open prospective comparative study. J Eur Acad Dermatol Venereol 2007;21(10):1381–5.
101. Park JH, Jung MY, Lee JH, et al. Clinical course of segmental vitiligo: a retrospective study of eighty-seven patients. Ann Dermatol 2014;26(1):61–5.
102. Koga M, Tango T. Clinical features and course of type A and type B vitiligo. Br J Dermatol 1988; 118:223–8.
103. Taïeb A, Picardo M. Clinical practice. Vitiligo. N Engl J Med 2009;360:160–9.
104. Park JH, Park SW, Lee DY, et al. The effectiveness of early treatment in segmental vitiligo: retrospective study according to disease duration. Photodermatol Photoimmunol Photomed 2013;29(2):103–5.
105. Lee DY, Park JH, Lee JH, et al. Poor response of phototherapy in segmental vitiligo with leukotrichia: role of digital microscopy. Int J Dermatol 2012; 51(7):873–5.
106. Lotti TM, Menchini G, Andreassi L. UV-B radiation microphototherapy. An elective treatment for segmental vitiligo. J Eur Acad Dermatol Venereol 1999;13:102–8.
107. Lee D-Y, Choi S-C. A proposal for the treatment guideline in segmental vitiligo. Int J Dermatol 2012;51(10):1274–5.
108. Sekar CS, Srinivas CR. Minimal erythema dose to targeted phototherapy in vitiligo patients in Indian skin. Indian J Dermatol Venereol Leprol 2013; 79(2):268.
109. Lee DY, Kim CR, Park JH, et al. The incidence of leukotrichia in segmental vitiligo: implication of poor response to medical treatment. Int J Dermatol 2011;50(8):925–7.
110. Gupta S, Narang T, Olsson MJ, et al. Surgical management of vitiligo and other leukodermas: evidence-based practice guidelines. In: Gupta S, Olsson MJ, Kanwar A, et al, editors. Surgical management of vitiligo. Malden (MA): Blackwell Publishing; 2007. p. 69–79.
111. Benzekri L, Ezzedine K, Gauthier Y. Vitiligo Potential Repigmentation Index: a simple clinical score that might predict the ability of vitiligo lesions to repigment under therapy. Br J Dermatol 2013;168(5): 1143–6.
112. Anbar TS, Abdel-Raouf H, Awad SS, et al. The hair follicle melanocytes in vitiligo in relation to disease duration. J Eur Acad Dermatol Venereol 2009; 23(8):934–9.
113. Kumar R, Parsad D, Kanwar AJ, et al. Altered levels of Ets-1 transcription factor and matrix metalloproteinases in melanocytes from patients with vitiligo. Br J Dermatol 2011;165(2):285–91.
114. Lee D, Kim C, Lee J. Recent onset vitiligo on acral areas treated with phototherapy: need of early treatment. Photodermatol Photoimmunol Photomed 2010;26(5):266–8.
115. El-Zawahry B, Esmat S, Bassiouny D, et al. Effect of procedural-related variables on melanocyte-keratinocye suspension transplantation in stable vitiligo: a clinical and immunohistochemical study. Pigment Cell Melanoma Res 2014;27(5):903.
116. Ezzedine K, Lim HW, Suzuki T, et al. Revised classification/nomenclature of vitiligo and related issues: the Vitiligo Global Issues Consensus Conference. Pigment Cell Melanoma Res 2012;25(3):E1–13.
117. Chen YT, Chen YJ, Hwang CY, et al. Comorbidity profiles in association with vitiligo: a nationwide population-based study in Taiwan. J Eur Acad Dermatol Venereol 2015;29(7):1362–9.
118. Esmat S, Elgendy D, Ali M, et al. Prevalence of photosensitivity in chronic hepatitis C virus patients and its relation to serum and urinary porphyrins. Liver Int 2014;34(7):1033–9.
119. Consensus. 2016. Available at: http://www.vitiligoworkinggroup.com. Accessed February, 2016.
120. Madigan LM, Al-Jamal M, Hamzavi I. Exploring the gaps in the evidence-based application of narrowband UVB for the treatment of vitiligo. Photodermatol Photoimmunol Photomed 2016;32(2):66–80.
121. Hamzavi I, Jain H, McLean D, et al. Parametric modeling of narrowband UV-B phototherapy for vitiligo, using a novel quantitative tool: the vitiligo area scoring index. Arch Dermatol 2004;140:677–83.
122. Honigsmann H, Krutmann J. Practical guidelines for broad-band UVB, UVA-1 phototherapy and PUVA photochemotherapy. Chapter 19. In: Krutmann J, Honigsmann H, Elements CA, et al, editors. Textbook of dermatology, dermatological phototherapy and photodiagnostic methods. Berlin: Springer; 2000. p. 371–80.

123. Jeon SY, Lee CY, Song KH, et al. Spectrophotometric measurement of minimal erythema dose sites after narrowband ultraviolet B phototesting: clinical implication of spetrophotometric values in phototherapy. Ann Dermatol 2014;26(1):17–25.
124. El-Khateeb EA, Ragab NF, Mohamed SA. Epidermal photoprotection: comparative study of narrowband ultraviolet B minimal erythema doses with and without stratum corneum stripping in normal and vitiligo skin. Clin Exp Dermatol 2011; 36(4):393–8.
125. Lim-Ong M, Leveriza RM, Ong BE, et al. Comparison between narrow-band UVB with topical corticosteroid and narrow-band UVB with placebo in the treatment of vitiligo: a randomized controlled trial. J Philipp Dermatol Soc 2005;14:17–22.
126. Nordal EJ, Guleng GE, Rönnevig JR. Treatment of vitiligo with narrowband- UVB (TL01) combined with tacrolimus ointment (0.1%) vs. placebo ointment, a randomized right/left double-blind comparative study. J Eur Acad Dermatol Venereol 2011;25: 1440–3.
127. Mehrabi D, Pandya AG. A randomized, placebo-controlled, doubleblind trial comparing narrowband UV-B plus 0.1% tacrolimus ointment with narrowband UV-B plus placebo in the treatment of generalized vitiligo. Arch Dermatol 2006;142: 927–9.
128. Satyanarayan HS, Kanwar AJ, Parsad D, et al. Efficacy and tolerability of combined treatment with NB-UVB and topical tacrolimus versus NBUVB alone in patients with vitiligo vulgaris: a randomized intra-individual open comparative trial. Indian J Dermatol Venereol Leprol 2013;79:525–7.
129. Klahan S, Asawanonda P. Topical tacrolimus may enhance repigmentation with targeted narrowband ultraviolet B to treat vitiligo: a randomized, controlled study. Clin Exp Dermatol 2009;34:e1029–30.
130. Esfandiarpour I, Ekhlasi A, Farajzadeh S, et al. The efficacy of pimecrolimus 1% cream plus narrowband ultraviolet B in the treatment of vitiligo: a double-blind, placebo-controlled clinical trial. J Dermatolog Treat 2009;20:14–8.
131. Arca E, Tastan HB, Erbil AH, et al. Narrow-band ultraviolet B as monotherapy and in combination with topical calcipotriol in the treatment of vitiligo. J Dermatol 2006;33:338–43.
132. Leone G, Pacifico A, Iacovelli P, et al. Tacalcitol and narrow-band phototherapy in patients with vitiligo. Clin Exp Dermatol 2006;31:200–5.
133. Elgoweini M, Nour El Din N. Response of vitiligo to narrowband ultraviolet B and oral antioxidants. J Clin Pharmacol 2009;49:852–5.
134. Dell'Anna ML, Mastrofrancesco A, Sala R, et al. Antioxidants and narrow band-UVB in the treatment of vitiligo: a double-blind placebo controlled trial. Clin Exp Dermatol 2007;32:631–6.
135. Doghim NN, Hassan AM, El-Ashmawy AA, et al. Topical antioxidant and narrowband versus topical combination of calcipotriol plus betamethathone dipropionate and narrowband in the treatment of vitiligo. Life Sci J 2011;8:186–97.
136. Yuksel EP, Aydin F, Senturk N, et al. Comparison of the efficacy of narrow band ultraviolet B and narrow band ultraviolet B plus topical catalase-superoxide dismutase treatment in vitiligo patients. Eur J Dermatol 2009;19:341–4.
137. Kostovic K, Pastar Z, Pasic A, et al. Treatment of vitiligo with narrow-band UVB and topical gel containing catalase and superoxide dismutase. Acta Dermatovenerol Croat 2007;15:10–4.
138. Bakis-Petsoglou S, Le Guay JL, Wittal R. A randomized, double blinded, placebo-controlled trial of pseudocatalase cream and narrowband ultraviolet B in the treatment of vitiligo. Br J Dermatol 2009;161:910–7.
139. Patel DC, Evans AV, Hawk JL. Topical pseudocatalase mousse and narrowband UVB phototherapy is not effective for vitiligo: an open, single centre study. Clin Exp Dermatol 2002; 27:641–4.
140. Bayoumi W, Fontas E, Sillard L, et al. Effect of a preceding laser dermabrasion on the outcome of combined therapy with narrowband ultraviolet B and potent topical steroids for treating nonsegmental vitiligo in resistant localizations. Br J Dermatol 2012;166:208–11.
141. Shin J, Lee JS, Hann SK, et al. Combination treatment by 10 600 nm ablative fractional carbon dioxide laser and narrowband ultraviolet B in refractory nonsegmental vitiligo: a prospective, randomized half-body comparative study. Br J Dermatol 2012; 166:658–61.
142. Grimes PE, Hamzavi I, Lebwohl M, et al. The efficacy of afamelanotide and narrowband UV-B phototherapy for repigmentation of vitiligo. JAMA Dermatol 2013;149:68–73.
143. Radakovic-Fijan S, Furnsinn-Fridl AM, Honigsmann H, et al. Oral dexamethasone pulse treatment for vitiligo. J Am Acad Dermatol 2001;44:814–7.
144. Gupta AK, Ellis CN, Nickoloff BJ, et al. Oral cyclosporine in the treatment of inflammatory and non inflammatory dermatoses. A clinical and immunopathologic analysis. Arch Dermatol 1990;126: 339–50.
145. Singh H, Kumaran MS, Bains A, et al. A randomized comparative study of oral corticosteroid minipulse and low-dose oral methotrexate in the treatment of unstable vitiligo. Dermatology 2015;231(3):286–90.
146. Speeckaert R, Speeckaert M, Van Geel N. Why treatments do(n't) work in vitiligo: an autoinflammatory perspective. Autoimmun Rev 2015;14(4):332–40.
147. Dang YP, Li Q, Shi F, et al. Effect of topical calcineurin inhibitors as monotherapy or combined

with phototherapy for vitiligo treatment: a meta-analysis. Dermatol Ther 2016;29:126–33.

148. Bansal S, Sahoo B, Garg V. Psoralen-narrowband UVB phototherapy for the treatment of vitiligo in comparison to narrowband UVB alone. Photodermatol Photoimmunol Photomed 2013;29(6):311–7.
149. Shin S, Hann SK, Oh SH. Combination treatment with excimer laser and narrowband UVB light in vitiligo patients. Photodermatol Photoimmunol Photomed 2016;32:28–33.
150. Wagner RY, Luciani F, Cario-André M, et al. Altered E-cadherin levels and distribution in melanocytes precede clinical manifestations of vitiligo. J Invest Dermatol 2015;135:1810–9.
151. Anbar TS, Westerhof W, Abdel-Rahman AT, et al. Effect of one session of ER:YAG laser ablation plus topical 5fluorouracil on the outcome of short term NB-UVB phototherapy in the treatment of non-segmental vitiligo: a left-right comparative study. Photodermatol Photoimmunol Photomed 2008;24:322–9.
152. Falabella R, Barona MI. Update on skin repigmentation therapies in vitiligo. Pigment Cell Melanoma Res 2009;22:42–65.
153. Khunger N, Kathuria SD, Ramesh V. Tissue grafts in vitiligo surgery - past, present, and future. Indian J Dermatol 2009;54:150–8.
154. Zhang DM, Hong WS, Fu LF, et al. A randomized controlled study of the effects of different modalities of narrow-band ultraviolet B therapy on the outcome of cultured autologous melanocytes transplantation in treating vitiligo. Dermatol Surg 2014;40:420–6.
155. Darné S, Stewart LC, Farr PM, et al. Investigation of cutaneous photoadaptation to narrowband ultraviolet B. Br J Dermatol 2014;170(2):392–7.
156. Anbar TS, Hegazy RA, Picardo M, et al. Beyond vitiligo guidelines: combined stratified/personalized approaches for the vitiligo patient. Exp Dermatol 2014;23(4):219–23.
157. Kandaswamy S, Akhtar N, Ravindran S, et al. Phototherapy in vitiligo: assessing the compliance, response and patient's perception about disease and treatment. Indian J Dermatol 2013;58(4):325.
158. AlGhamdi KM, Kumar A, Moussa NA. Low-level laser therapy: a useful technique for enhancing the proliferation of various cultured cells. Lasers Med Sci 2012;27(1):237–49.
159. AlGhamdi KM, Kumar A, Ashour AE, et al. A comparative study of the effects of different low-level lasers on the proliferation, viability, and migration of human melanocytes in vitro. Lasers Med Sci 2015;30(5):1541–51.
160. Shan X, Wang C, Tian H, et al. Narrow-band ultraviolet B home phototherapy in vitiligo. Indian J Dermatol Venereol Leprol 2014;80(4):336–8.
161. Tien Guan ST, Theng C, Chang A. Randomized, parallel group trial comparing home-based phototherapy with institution-based 308 excimer lamp for the treatment of focal vitiligo vulgaris. J Am Acad Dermatol 2015;72(4):733–5.
162. Eleftheriadou V, Thomas K, Ravenscroft J, et al. Feasibility, double-blind, randomised, placebo-controlled, multi-centre trial of hand-held NB-UVB phototherapyfor the treatment of vitiligo at home (HI-Light trial: Home Intervention of Light therapy). Trials 2014;15:51. Available at: http://www.medgadget.com/2015/06/2015-vitiligo-treatment-market-pipeline-review-size-demands-and-opportunities.html.
163. Harris JE, Rashighi M, Nguyen N, et al. Rapid skin repigmentation on oral ruxolitinib in a patient with coexistent vitiligo and alopecia areata (AA). J Am Acad Dermatol 2016;74(2):370–1.

Surgical Therapies for Vitiligo

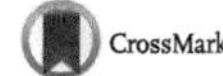

Tasneem F. Mohammad, MD, Iltefat H. Hamzavi, MD*

KEYWORDS

• Vitiligo • Surgery • Repigmentation • Graft • Recipient site • Donor site

KEY POINTS

- Vitiligo is a disorder characterized by the development of depigmented macules and patches that can be treated with surgical intervention.
- Surgery is a safe and effective treatment option in select candidates with vitiligo.
- Preoperative evaluation, choosing an appropriate surgical technique, and postoperative management are important components in ensuring optimal results.

INTRODUCTION

Vitiligo is a disorder of dyspigmentation characterized by the development of depigmented macules and patches over the body. Treatment is essential in patients who have a significantly diminished quality of life as the psychosocial impact of this condition is greater than many other diseases. Topical, oral, light-based, and surgical therapies are often used in combination to achieve optimal results. Vitiligo surgery is an important, but underperformed, treatment of vitiligo that was first reported in 1947 by Haxthausen and colleagues.[1] Since then, surgical techniques have become more sophisticated and varied, with each method having unique advantages and disadvantages. With this article, the authors hope to provide a comprehensive overview of vitiligo surgery, including preoperative, perioperative, and postoperative considerations.

Preoperative Evaluation

Patient selection

The selection of suitable candidates for surgical intervention is key, as not all patients will benefit from a surgical approach (**Table 1**). Usually, surgery is performed after failure of medical management for several different types of leukoderma, including vitiligo, piebaldism, halo nevi, physical and chemical leukodermas, and nevus depigmentosus. The difference among the variable responses to therapy seems to be based on the immunology of patients. Patients with stable disease or a nonimmune basis to their depigmentation usually have a better response to surgical intervention.

When evaluating patients with vitiligo for surgery, a detailed history needs to be obtained. First, the clinical subtype of vitiligo should be determined. Vitiligo is described as segmental and nonsegmental, with generalized vitiligo being the most common variant of nonsegmental vitiligo. Segmental vitiligo is unilateral, stable, and poorly responsive to medical management, whereas generalized vitiligo is bilateral and symmetric, with a waxing and waning course.[2] Patients with segmental or focal vitiligo have an extremely favorable response to vitiligo surgery, and it is a first-line option in this population.[3] In contrast, treatment of other subtypes with surgery

Disclosures: Dr I.H. Hamzavi is an investigator for Estee Lauder, Ferndale, and Allergan and has received equipment from Johnson and Johnson. Dr T.F. Mohammad is a subinvestigator for Estee Lauder, Ferndale, and Allergan.

Department of Dermatology, Henry Ford Hospital, 3031 West Grand Boulevard, Suite 800, Detroit, MI 48202, USA

* Corresponding author. Department of Dermatology, Henry Ford Hospital, 3031 West Grand Boulevard, Suite 800, Detroit, MI 48202.

E-mail address: ihamzav1@hfhs.org

Dermatol Clin 35 (2017) 193–203

http://dx.doi.org/10.1016/j.det.2016.11.009

0733-8635/17/

Table 1
Criteria for patient selection in vitiligo surgery

Positive prognostic indicators	Negative prognostic indicators
Leukoderma treatable with surgery	Koebnerization
Segmental/focal vitiligo > generalized vitiligo	New or growing lesions within the past 6 mo
Stable disease	Distal fingertip or perioral involvement
Lesions on face/neck > trunk > extremities	Lesions over bony prominences and distal extremities
	Keloidal tendencies
Additional screening questions	
• Previous treatments to ensure failure of medical management except in focal/segmental vitiligo where surgery is first-line option	
• Significant bleeding issues or comorbidities interfering with surgery	
• Medications, allergies, and past medical history	

is often less successful and should only be used when medical management has failed and patients have stable disease.

Disease stability is another parameter that must be evaluated before surgery and is defined by the lack of new or growing lesions within a given time frame, usually between 6 months to 2 years. Several methods can be used to assess stability, such as patient report, serial photography, and validated scoring systems. These methods of evaluation include a lack of change in the Vitiligo Area Scoring Index (VASI), Vitiligo European Task Force Assessment (VETF), and a low Vitiligo Disease Activity Score (VIDA). The VIDA is a scoring method that assesses disease stability in patients who have discontinued treatment of vitiligo for at least 6 months.[4] In cases whereby stability or treatment outcome is uncertain, performing a test spot with a single punch graft in the center of a stable, depigmented lesion to assess the degree of repigmentation is useful.[5,6] Koebnerization, which involves depigmentation at sites of previous trauma, is an indicator of unstable disease. Future methods for assessing disease stability include reflectance confocal microscopy,[7] total antioxidant status,[8] antimelanocyte antibody levels, and measurement of serum catecholamines and their metabolites.[9] Measurement of other cellular markers, such as interleukin 17,[10] chemokine (C-X-C motif) ligand (CXCL) 9 and 10,[11] and mircoRNA,[12] may also play a role in determining disease stability.

Recipient site location, which refers to the site of the lesion being treated, should be taken into account, as areas with a greater vascular supply and follicular density, such as the head and neck, have a better response to surgery than the extremities.[13,14] Presentations associated with poor outcomes include the acrofacial variant, which is characterized by perioral and distal fingertip involvement around the nail bed. Areas over joints also respond poorly, possibly because of repeated friction and injury at these locations.[14] Patients must also be screened for keloidal tendencies, significant bleeding issues, blood-borne infections, and additional contraindications to surgery.

Consultation

Preoperative discussion is focused on educating patients about the procedure, screening for candidacy, and obtaining informed consent. General information about vitiligo as well as perioperative and postoperative expectations are discussed. To ensure that no contraindications to surgery or potential allergies to anesthesia exist, past medical history, medications, and drug allergies are reviewed. Risks of the procedure and the measures taken to minimize their occurrence are also explained. These risks include bleeding, infection, scarring, pain, contact dermatitis from dressings, and anesthesia-related arrhythmias or allergy. To ensure that patients have realistic expectations, providers must emphasize that repigmentation and color matching takes several months to years and that surgery is a treatment, not a cure. Although patients may achieve long-term remission, even with focal or segmental vitiligo, there is always the possibility of reactivation of disease that patients should be aware of. Adjuvant treatments, including additional surgeries, may be necessary to achieve maximal repigmentation, especially if the treatment area was too large to complete in a single session or the degree of repigmentation after surgery is unacceptable.

Preoperative Work-up

Preoperative laboratory work includes screening for blood-borne diseases, such as human immunodeficiency virus, hepatitis B, and hepatitis C. This screening is especially important if dermabrasion is being used to prepare the recipient site, as infectious particles can aerosolize. Patients undergoing general anesthesia should have a preoperative evaluation for surgical fitness based on comorbidities and the extent of surgery. This evaluation should be done before any decisions to pursue surgery because of the significant additional cost general anesthesia adds to this procedure. General anesthesia is not commonly performed but is useful in patients who are extremely anxious or have large surface areas being treated. Photographs under appropriate lighting and measurements of the donor and recipient site are obtained before surgery and are critical in tracking progress. Woods lamp photographs are often valuable in patients in whom depigmented areas are not easily visualized, especially in lighter-skinned individuals. This high quality and woods lamp photographs enables a more accurate comparison of preoperative and postoperative photographs in evaluating treatment response.

PERIOPERATIVE CONSIDERATIONS

Once preoperative evaluation is completed, surgical techniques should be considered. There are several methods for preparing the donor and recipient site as well as a multitude of surgical techniques. Typically, skin is removed from normally pigmented skin at the donor site, which is then either directly transferred or manipulated and transferred to the recipient site. Lesion location, size, and clinic resources should all be taken into account when deciding on a specific method (**Table 2**).

Table 2
Consideration of surgical techniques

Surgical Method Preferred According to Area of Involvement and Site of Vitiligo			
		Preferred Technique	Alternative Technique
Area	Small	SBG, STSG, FTG	SG, PG
	Moderate	NCES, STSG, FTG	SG, PG
	Large	NCES, CM, CE	SG
Site	Fingers and toes	NCES, PG	SG, PG
	Palms and soles	PG	
	Lips	NCES, SBG	SG, PG
	Eyelids	NCES, SBG, STG	SG
	Nipple & areola	NCES, SBG	SG, PG
	Genitals	NCES, SBG	SG
	Eyebrows, scalp	HFG, NCFRS	

Abbreviations: CE, cultured epidermal cell grafting; CM, cultured melanocyte grafting; FTG, flip-top grafting; HFG, hair follicle grafting; NCES, noncultured epidermal cell suspension; NCFRS, noncultured follicular root sheath suspension; PG, punch grafting; SBG, suction blister grafting; SG, smash grafting; STSG, split-thickness skin grafting.

From Ghia D, Mulekar S. Surgical management of vitiligo. In: Hamzavi I, Mahmoud B, Isedeh P, editors. Handbook of vitiligo: basic science and clinical management. London: JP Medical Publishers; 2015. p. 133; with permission.

Site Preparation

Before preparation of the donor or recipient site, these areas must be cleaned and anesthetized. Alcohol, povidone iodine, and chlorhexidine are all options for disinfection and can be used in combination. If lasers are used for recipient site preparation, alcohol cannot be used because of its flammable nature.

Topical, local, and general anesthesias are all options for pain control depending on lesion size and location, patient preference, and resources of the performing facility. Topical formulations, which usually feature different concentrations of lidocaine in combination with prilocaine or tetracaine, can be used under occlusion for the donor site and for select small recipient sites. Injection of 1% to 2% lidocaine using a field block technique to prevent uneven surfaces or a nerve block can be used for more extensive and sensitive areas. If dermabrasion is being used, lidocaine without epinephrine is used to enable visualization of pinpoint bleeding. Weight-based calculation of maximal dose is also important because of the risk of cardiotoxicity with overdose.

Donor Site

Before obtaining a skin graft, hair from the donor site may be removed by shaving, depilation creams, or plucking in order to prevent hairs from interfering with graft manipulation.[14] The main methods of harvesting skin from the donor site include the shave, blister, and punch biopsy approaches. With the shave method, a thin (0.125 mm–0.250 mm) to ultrathin (less than 0.125 mm) skin graft is obtained using either a sterile razor blade held by hemostats, a silver skin grafting knife (E. Murray & Company, Cork, United Kingdom), a Goulian-Weck knife (Edward Weck & Co Inc, Research Triangle Park, NC), or a motorized dermatome (**Fig. 1**).[13,15,16]

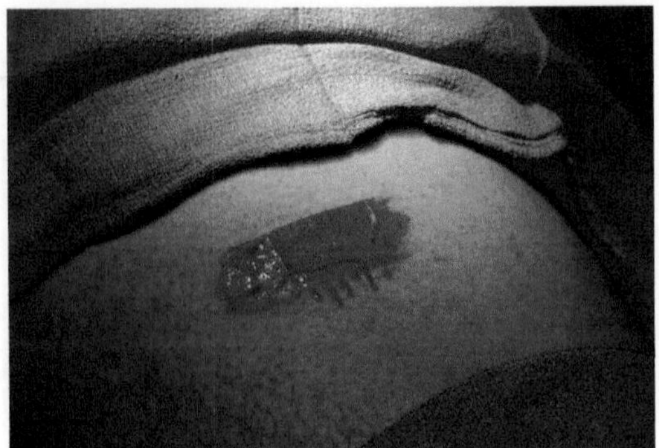

Fig. 1. Harvesting of an ultrathin skin graft.

Appropriate grafts are transparent and float when placed in sterile saline for rinsing.[17] If curling of the graft edges is noted, then the graft is too thick and another sample should be obtained. The straight razor allows maximal operator control of size and depth, but it takes considerable skill to obtain uniform grafts of appropriate thickness. A Goulion blade allows for uniform thickness but does not allow for adjustment of depth like the Silver's grafting knife. Motorized dermatomes provide uniform grafts quickly without the level of operator skill required for manual blades, but are more costly. A 1.0- to 1.5-mm punch biopsy can be used to harvest tissue but is typically only used for mini-grafting or test spots.[6,18] Suction blisters are also used to obtain grafts by using suction pressure to create mechanical disruption at the dermoepidermal junction (DEJ), resulting in a purely epidermal blister roof. The easiest method for blister induction is by using a Luer lock disposable syringe with a 3-way stopcock and pulling plunger (**Fig. 2**). The degree of negative pressure necessary for blister formation varies by age, with younger patients requiring higher pressure.[19] Depending on site and age, blister formation can take between 15 minutes to 3 hours. In order to facilitate more rapid blister formation, heat or injection of sterile normal saline can be used.[20,21] Scarring and dyspigmentation at the site of blister formation are uncommon.

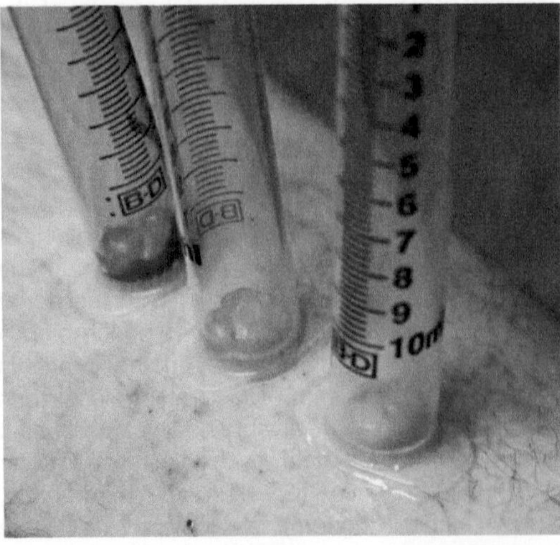

Fig. 2. Suction blister induction using a syringe, 3-way stopcock, and pulling plunger.

Recipient Site

The aim of recipient site preparation is to remove the epidermis to the level of the DEJ, allowing transplanted melanocytes to access structures necessary for adherence and nutrition. Depending on the type of surgery performed, hair removal may be performed to prevent hairs at the recipient site from pushing the transplanted graft away as they grow.[14] The first method for recipient site preparation is by using liquid nitrogen to create a cryoblister. Subsequent deroofing of the blister exposes the recipient site. Complications include peripheral hyperpigmentation or hypopigmentation and hypertrophic scarring.[22] Suction blisters can also be used, with lower incidence of these sequelae. These methods are feasible for small recipient sites, especially suction blisters, because harvesting blisters for large sites is time consuming.

Chemical means of recipient site preparation include psoralen with ultraviolet A (PUVA), phenol, and trichloroacetic acid (TCA). PUVA can be used to treat large sites through the formation of phototoxic blisters; 0.075% 8-methoxypsoralen is applied to the recipient site with subsequent exposure to 10 J/cm^2 of UVA for 2 consecutive days before surgery. Blister formation is present 24 hours later and the blister roof can be removed by rubbing with saline-soaked gauze and a wire brush if necessary. This method allows rapid preparation of the recipient site with lack of scarring because the reticular dermis is uninvolved. However, there may be some risk for carcinogenesis.[23] Eighty-eight percent phenol or 100% TCA can also be used to cause coagulation of epidermal proteins, which are rubbed off to expose the recipient site. However, it is difficult to control depth using this method.[14]

Dermabrasion is one of the most common methods for recipient site preparation, with pinpoint bleeding being the clinical end point. Although it is cost-effective and provides complete control over depth, manual dermabrasion is time consuming with rapid user fatigue. Motorized dermabrasion is more rapid but requires skill, as the depth is more difficult to control. This skill is especially important in areas with an uneven landscape or around the eyelids, as avulsion is possible if an eyelash gets caught. Compared with other options for recipient site preparation, dermabrasion is relatively inexpensive and can be used to prepare larger areas. There is aerosolization of blood and often splatter when using this method, so protective covering, including masks with a good seal, are important. Lasers, most commonly the carbon dioxide (CO_2) and erbium glass, can also be used for recipient site preparation. The wavelengths emitted by both lasers are absorbed by water causing tissue heating and subsequent destruction by vaporization (**Fig. 3**). The benefits of this method include speed, low user fatigue, and a bloodless field with uniform depth of ablation. The uniform depth of ablation is especially important for tendinous or concave areas, where there may be increased risk of scarring with other methods. However, this is the most costly method.[14]

Dressing

Choice of dressing is another important facet of vitiligo surgery that serves to promote adherence and maximize melanocyte survival. In addition, it decreases dyspigmentation and scarring while stimulating more rapid wound healing. Dressings also reduce the risk of infection postoperatively by preventing contamination and overhydration of the wound, which can lead to tissue maceration. However, direct application of antibacterial ointments or cotton gauze is not recommended because of the risk of contact dermatitis or trauma on removal. Providing an environment where the graft is able to readily obtain nutrition is another function of dressings. During the first 48 to 72 hours, graft nutrition is obtained by plasmatic imbibition, which involves passive absorption of serous drainage from the wound bed. Therefore, it is important to ensure that the graft has adequate moisture without overhydration. This plasmatic imbibition is followed by inosculation where vessels from the graft form connections with those of the wound bed. Angiogenesis occurs approximately 5 days postoperatively, which involves new vessels growing into the vascularized graft. Dressings prevent trauma to the wound during these processes. At least 72 hours should pass before dressing removal so that melanocytes are not inadvertently torn off. However, it is preferred to keep the dressing in place for a longer duration for all types of vitiligo surgery to prevent disruption of vessel in-growth that will lead to permanent graft viability. The dressing should also be kept dry to prevent nonadherent cells from being washed away. After reepithelialization, gauze and nonocclusive dressings can be applied to prevent traumatic removal of the graft.[22]

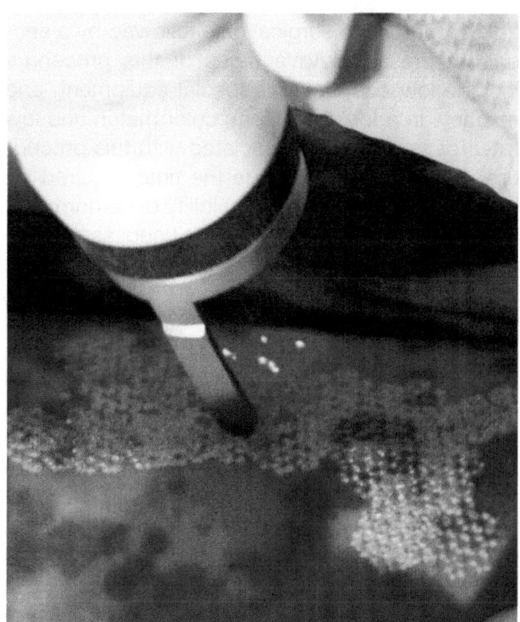

Fig. 3. Recipient site preparation using fractional CO_2 laser.

Typically, dressings used for vitiligo surgery are composed of multiple components. Low absorptive capacity dressings form the first layer as they prevent dehydration of the wound and increase adherence. Nonadherent dressings include paraffin gauze, which can directly contact wounds. It has pores to allow the passage of drainage while maintaining a moist environment.[24] Collagen can also be used as a primary dressing to maintain the microenvironment as it is impermeable to bacteria and can be applied directly over the recipient site. In addition, it helps direct fibroblast production and cellular migration as well as inhibits excessive production of matrix metalloproteinases.[25] Films and membranes, such as Tegaderm, come as adhesive sheets that are impermeable to liquids. As such, they should not be used alone, especially over areas that have copious quantities of exudates. However, they are useful in securing dressings.

Hydrocolloids, such as DuoDERM, are an example of moderately absorptive dressings. These hydrocolloids have a greater absorptive capacity and can stay in place over the wound for several days. The occlusive polyurethane within DuoDERM also prevents bacterial contamination, and this dressing can be directly applied to the wound. This dressing is ideal for use on the donor site. Highly absorptive dressings, such as cotton gauze, are primarily used as a secondary dressing. Cotton gauze is a cost-effective and widely available option that is optimal for wicking away excess drainage from wounds.[24] This gauze is especially useful for sites such as the face or neck, which tend to have greater production of exudates. Tails made from cotton gauze can be inserted between the primary and secondary dressing to prevent dressing saturation and detachment (**Fig. 4**).

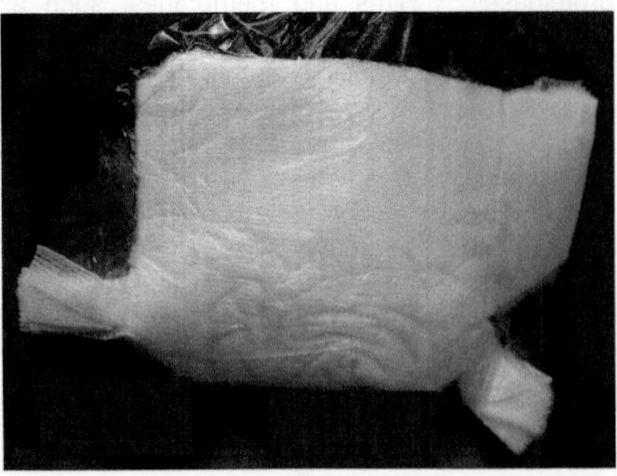

Fig. 4. Dressing with tails to allow drainage of exudates.

SURGICAL TECHNIQUES

Methods of vitiligo surgery can be classified as tissue grafts and cellular grafts.

Tissue Graft

Tissue grafts involve the transfer of tissue to the recipient site without processing and are ideal for treating smaller areas.

Mini-punch graft

Mini-punch grafts are performed by harvesting tissue from the donor site, which is typically on the upper thigh or gluteal region, with 1- to 2-mm punch biopsies. The recipient site is prepared using a punch biopsy tool to create chambers that are spaced approximately 5 mm apart. The size of punch tool used for the donor and recipient site can vary. In the author's experience, using a larger punch size at the donor site than the recipient site accounts for graft contracture, but using an equal or smaller punch tool at the donor site than at the recipient site to decrease the risk of textural abnormalities has also been reported. The harvested tissue is inserted into the chambers at the recipient site and dressed using paraffin gauze, followed by absorbent cotton gauze, and then a bio-occlusive dressing, such as Tegaderm. Alternatively, Steri-Strips can be applied over the punch graft and secured with mastisol with cotton gauze as a secondary dressing. Treated areas should be immobilized to prevent movement of the graft. Dressing changes are performed at 48 hours and again at 7 days postoperatively. Repigmentation is observed approximately 2 to 3 weeks postoperatively, and individual spots should coalesce between 4 to 6 months. This technique is easy to perform, inexpensive, and does not require any specialized equipment. However, it cannot be used to treat large areas and can lead to textural and pigmentary variations, such as cobblestoning. There is also a possibility of scarring and keloid formation.[13,14,18,26]

Blister graft

With blister grafting, chemical depilation is performed at the recipient site to prevent hair growth from pushing away the graft. Shaving is avoided as it can cause trauma and has a faster rate of hair growth. Once the blister has formed at the donor site using a suction apparatus, the roof is detached with curved scissors. The recipient site is prepared using dermabrasion, laser ablation, or blister formation, after which the blister roof is transferred dermal side down to the recipient site. To prevent confusion about which side of the blister is epidermal, a slide is placed underneath the blister as it is being cut to maintain its orientation. An alternative method is to mark the epidermal face with a surgical pen. Other ways to identify the dermal face include the presence of fibrin clots and a tendency to curl toward the dermal side. Increased creases on the epidermal side can also be visualized by digital microscopy. The recipient site is dressed using paraffin gauze and secured with surgical glue followed by a secondary dressing. Advantages of this procedure include low cost, lack of special equipment, and efficacy. In addition, uniform color match and low rates of scarring are associated with this procedure. Disadvantages include the time required for blister induction and the possibility of hemorrhagic blisters forming, which cannot be used, as they are too thick. Handling and placing the graft on the recipient site can also be difficult.[13,14,27–29]

Split-thickness skin graft

Split-thickness skin grafts (STSGs) are performed by harvesting a thin or ultrathin layer of epidermis from the donor site, which is then placed on the prepared recipient site. The graft is typically taken from a flat surface on the thigh, lower back, or gluteal region to allow for a graft of even thickness. Graft size is typically 10% to 20% larger than the recipient site, as graft contracture occurs during the healing process. This size ensures that the entire lesion will have coverage once healing is complete. To harvest the graft, lubricant is applied to the donor site. Traction is held to ensure that a thin and even graft is harvested. This graft is placed in a petri dish with lactated ringers or sterile saline to prevent the tissue from drying out. Then the recipient site is prepared, with dermabrasion or laser ablation, on which the graft is placed dermal side down. Fenestrations are made in grafts over large surface areas to allow for flexibility and release of exudates. Octyl cyanoacrylate can be used to fix the graft followed by paraffin gauze as a primary dressing and absorbent gauze as a secondary dressing. A wound check is performed 24 hours postoperatively followed by a dressing change 7 days postoperatively. This surgical technique is extremely effective and results in rapid, uniform repigmentation. Larger areas can be treated if meshing is performed, and it is possible for leukotrichia to achieve repigmentation with STSGs. This technique is difficult to use over areas such as the eyelids, areolae, and genitals; the size of the graft is often larger than the recipient site to account for graft contracture. Possible complications include hyperpigmentation of the graft or donor site, peripheral halo secondary to graft contracture, graft rejection, and scarring of the donor site if the graft is too thick. A thick graft can also lead to a stuck-on or tire-patch appearance at the recipient site. Beading, which is an inward curling of the graft rim during healing, can occur in addition to the formation of milia or inclusion cysts.[13,14,30,31]

Smash graft

Smash grafting is a modification of the STSG, which involves smashing the graft into tiny pieces before application over the recipient site. The graft is obtained in a similar fashion to an STSG but is cut into small pieces and then placed into a bowl of normal saline. The saline is poured off, leaving just enough to wet the tissue. A pair of curved scissors is used to cut or smash the tissue into miniscule pieces that have the consistency of a paste. This process takes approximately 15 to 20 minutes. The donor site is only one-tenth the size of the recipient site as the paste can be spread over larger surface areas of the prepared recipient site. The paste is left on the recipient site for 15 to 30 minutes for the exudates to dry and then dressed with a nonadherent material followed by gauze and dressing pads. The area is immobilized with dressing removal 7 days postoperatively. Patients should be warned that the graft will look like exfoliated skin and will peel. Repigmentation is typically seen within 2 weeks and is more prominent by 4 to 6 weeks. This technique is simple, cost-effective, and does not require special equipment. However, phototherapy is needed postoperatively to ensure pigment spread; further studies are necessary to determine the efficacy of this newer technique.[32]

Flip-top graft

Flip-top grafts are performed by placing minigrafts under a hinged epidermal flap at the recipient site. These mini-grafts act as a biological dressing and hold the graft in place. With this procedure, epidermal mini-grafts are obtained from the medial arm or axilla using a razor blade. These mini-grafts are further sectioned into strips that are approximately 1 to 2 mm in diameter and placed on saline-soaked gauze. After anesthetizing the recipient site, a 4- to 5-mm strip of epidermis along with papillary dermis is elevated with a razor and the mini-grafts are placed dermis down in the cavity. The flap is then folded over and secured with cyanoacrylate gel followed by transparent polyurethane dressing. Dressing removal is performed after 7 days with graft survival indicated by the presence of pigmented macules under the flap. Pigment should be assessed after 1 month. The advantages of this procedure include simplicity, lack of special equipment, even repigmentation, minimal scarring, and lack of a recipient site dressing. However, a significant amount of skill is required, it can only be performed over small areas, and is unsuitable for areas of thickened epidermis, such as the palms and soles.[14,33,34]

Hair follicle graft

Hair follicle grafts are based on the principle that the stem cell population in the bulge region of the follicle can lead to repigmentation by retrograde migration. Follicles are harvested from the occipital scalp either as a strip that is dissected into follicular units or as 1-mm punch biopsies with follicular unit extraction. The follicular units are then transplanted to the recipient site using a hair transplantation machine, a curved cutting needle, or an 18-gauge needle. Alternatively, the recipient site can be prepared using 1-mm punch biopsies approximately 3 to 10 mm apart, with the follicular units being planted in these cavities. Both the donor and recipient sites are dressed with paraffin gauze with dressing removal 5 days postoperatively. Special care should be taken to not remove hairs during dressing removal. This technique has been successful in repigmenting leukotrichia and does not require specialized equipment. However, strip grafting does leave a scar and this method does not work well in nonhairy areas.[14,35–39]

Cellular Graft

Cellular grafts involve creating a cellular suspension from a thin to ultrathin skin graft. These grafts can be either cultured or noncultured.

Cultured graft

Two types of cultured cellular grafts exist: cultured melanocyte grafts and cultured epidermal grafts.

Cultured melanocyte graft Cultured melanocyte grafts involve obtaining a graft from the donor site followed by trypsinization to separate the epidermis from the dermis. The cells are then vortexed to separate the melanocytes and keratinocytes after which the melanocytes are cultured in a medium containing melanocyte growth factors for approximately 15 to 30 days. The cells are detached from the culture plates and then applied as a suspension to the prepared recipient site at a density of approximately 1000 to 2000 melanocytes per square millimeter. The site is secured with gauze that has been soaked in culture medium followed by an occlusive dressing. Patients should remain on bed rest for approximately 8 to 10 hours, with dressing removal occurring at 1 week. Large areas can be treated with this method using a small graft from the donor site, but this method is expensive, requires specialized laboratory equipment and personnel, and requires multiple visits for completion.[14,40–42]

Cultured epidermal graft Cultured epidermal grafts are performed similarly to cultured melanocyte grafts, but both melanocytes and keratinocytes are cultured. The presence of both cell types prompts them to organize into a sheet similar to the basal layer of the skin. Once the graft from the donor site is trypsinized, the epidermis separated, and the melanocytes and keratinocytes are isolated, they are cultured with media containing growth factors for both cell types. After a few weeks of growth, an epidermal sheet is formed, which is detached using dispase and placed on paraffin gauze. The gauze is then applied to the prepared recipient site, and a secondary dressing is placed on top of the paraffin gauze. The advantages and disadvantages to this method are similar to those of the cultured melanocyte grafts, but less culture time is needed for epidermal versus melanocyte grafts.[14,43]

Noncultured Graft

Noncultured epidermal melanocyte suspension

Noncultured epidermal melanocyte suspension grafts are performed by shaving the skin and taking an ultrathin skin graft from the donor site, which is then rinsed and incubated in 0.25% trypsin for 30 minutes after which the cells are rinsed in normal saline and exposed to antitrypsin. This procedure is followed by cellular separation, which involves manual removal of the epidermis from the dermis. The epidermis is manually broken down into small fragments, which are centrifuged at 1800 rpm for 5 minutes. This process results in the formation of a cellular pellet, which is resuspended in lactated Ringer solution in a 1-mL syringe. Approximately 0.5 mL of solution is required for a treatment area of 100 cm^2. The cellular suspension is applied over the prepared recipient site and then covered with collagen, paraffin gauze, cotton gauze, and then secured with either Tegaderm or micropore tape and mastisol. Postoperatively, movement should be restricted to avoid any displacement of the dressing, but bed rest is not required. Dressing removal is performed 4 days postoperatively for the head and neck and 7 days for other areas. The advantage of this procedure is that treatment can be performed in 1 day without the resources required to culture cells. Large surface areas can also be treated, with a 1:10 donor to recipient site ratio most commonly reported in the literature; but ratios of up to 1:80 have been used. Few studies have been performed investigating the optimal treatment ratio, but results are conflicting. Another advantage is that the cellular suspension is easy to apply and the procedure yields good cosmetic results and color match (**Fig. 5**). However, some specialized equipment, such as an incubator and centrifuge, are needed in addition to a skilled team. This method is also costly and cannot be used to treat certain areas, such as the palms and soles.[3,13,15,41,44]

Noncultured follicular root sheath suspension

Noncultured follicular cell suspension grafts use the hair follicle to create a cellular suspension that is applied to the recipient site. Follicular melanocytes and their stem cell precursors are more abundant, larger, and less prone to autoimmune destruction than their counterparts in the epidermis. However, follicular melanocytes are more affected by age and have cyclical activity. Then 1-mm punch biopsies are performed to obtain approximately 15 to 25 hair follicles from the occipital scalp depending on the recipient site size. Follicular plucking can also be used but is thought to reduce the stem cell reservoir. The extracted follicles are washed in phosphate-buffered saline 3 times and then incubated in 0.25% trypsin/0.05% ethylenediaminetetraacetic acid at 37°C for 90 minutes. The follicles are transferred to a new tube of trypsin every 30 minutes for a total of 3 tubes with antitrypsin being added to the previous tube. The keratinous shafts are discarded after the third tube; the supernatants of the 3 tubes are combined and centrifuged at 1000 rpm for 5 minutes to create a cellular pellet, which is resuspended in normal saline and applied

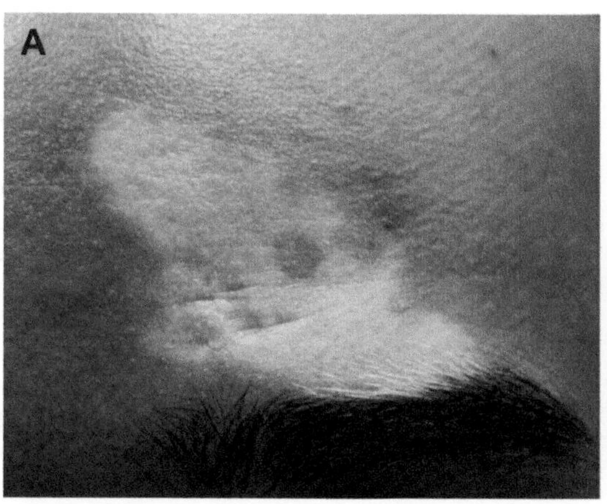

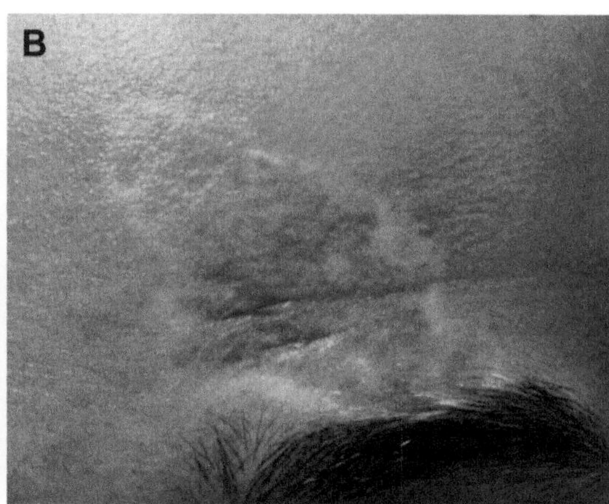

Fig. 5. (*A*) Segmental vitiligo of the left eyebrow at baseline. (*B*) Segmental vitiligo of the left eyebrow 7 months after treatment with noncultured epidermal melanocyte suspension (NCEMS).

to the prepared recipient site. The area is then dressed with collagen, paraffin gauze, cotton gauze, and secured with micropore tape or Tegaderm. The advantage of this technique is that no shave biopsy is performed and a few follicles can be used to treat large areas, with the resulting scars being camouflaged. The disadvantage is that these grafts may have changes in pigmentation due to the cyclical activity of follicular melanocytes and their accelerated aging.[14,45–47]

POSTOPERATIVE CARE

After surgery, patients should be given specific and detailed instructions on how to care for their graft. Loose clothing is worn over the treated areas to prevent any trauma or displacement of the dressing. The first postoperative 48 hours are the most crucial for graft survival, but patients are cautioned to restrict movement at the recipient site until the dressing removal is performed. The dressing is kept dry, with treated areas being elevated as much as possible to avoid edema and discomfort. Antibiotics are not routinely administered, but some practitioners prefer to give prophylactic antibiotics if large surface areas are being treated. Greenish exudates are expected and thought to be the result of myeloperoxidase release from neutrophils, but are not necessarily an indication of infection.[22] Symptoms concerning for infection include fevers, chills, excessive pain, erythema and heat surrounding the treated areas, and foul odor. Patients should inform their physician of these symptoms for evaluation and prescription of antibiotics if necessary. For pain control, over-the-counter analgesic agents, such as acetaminophen, are effective.

Dressing removal is performed gently to prevent trauma to the recipient site. Soaking the dressing with saline can increase the ease of dressing removal in areas of crusting. Collagen dressings can remain on the wound as they will either be absorbed into the skin or detach. These loose edges are trimmed to avoid catching on clothing and peeling off. Wound care after dressing removal includes using a mild cleanser to wash the treated areas, avoiding vigorous rubbing of the site, and application of petroleum jelly (Vaseline) to the treated areas until they no longer burn when dry. For 1 week after the procedure, the use of any other products on the treated site, such as cosmetics, medications, or lotions, should be avoided. Swimming should be avoided for 1 month postoperatively because of chemicals in the water. Shaving can be resumed 1 week after bandage removal and should be performed in the direction of hair growth for a month and a half after which patients can resume shaving against the grain if desired.

EVALUATION

Evaluation of repigmentation postoperatively can be performed by multiple methods, including visual evaluation, photography with or without software analysis, tracings, and validated scoring systems. These systems include the VASI, VETF, and Vitiligo Scoring Tool, which is a more comprehensive system that evaluates repigmentation, color match, and postsurgical complications.[48,49] The most common grading system for repigmentation appears in **Table 3**, with the observed patterns of repigmentation being follicular, marginal, diffuse, or combined. Color match is often graded as excellent, good, or poor and assesses postprocedural hyperpigmentation/hypopigmentation. Side effects at the donor and recipient site, such as infection, changes in pigment or

Table 3
Grading system for repigmentation after vitiligo surgery

Grade	Repigmentation (%)
Excellent	90–100
Very good	76–90
Good	51–75
Fair	26–64
Poor	0–25

texture, scarring, keloids, milia, cobblestoning, or tire-track appearance, are monitored as well.[14] Evaluation of quality of life is also important postoperatively as vitiligo has a significant psychosocial impact on patients. Changes in quality of life can be tracked using validated measures, such as the Dermatology Life Quality Index, Skindex, or Vitiligo Specific Quality of Life Instrument. This tracking allows practitioners to measure patient satisfaction and reinforces the efficacy of treatment. Because vitiligo surgery is not covered by insurance, gaining recognition that surgery is an effective treatment that improves patient productivity and quality of life is the first step in obtaining coverage for these procedures.

SUMMARY

Although vitiligo surgery is a safe and effective method of treating vitiligo, many practitioners are unaware of how to select appropriate candidates and surgical techniques and where to refer patients for treatment. By gaining a better understanding of vitiligo surgery, practitioners can identify good candidates and consider adding these techniques to their clinical skills to increase the availability of a therapy that has the potential to change the lives of patients with vitiligo.

REFERENCES

1. Haxthausen H. Studies on the pathogenesis of morphea, vitiligo, and acrodermatitis atrophicans by means of transplantation experiments. Acta Dermato-Venereologica (Stockholm) 1947;27:352.
2. Faria AR, Tarle RG, Dellatorre G, et al. Vitiligo–part 2–classification, histopathology and treatment. An Bras Dermatol 2014;89(5):784–90.
3. Mulekar SV. Melanocyte-keratinocyte cell transplantation for stable vitiligo. Int J Dermatol 2003;42(2):132–6.
4. Njoo MD, Das PK, Bos JD, et al. Association of the Kobner phenomenon with disease activity and therapeutic responsiveness in vitiligo vulgaris. Arch Dermatol 1999;135(4):407–13.
5. Falabella R. The minigrafting test for vitiligo: validation of a predicting tool. J Am Acad Dermatol 2004;51(4):672–3.
6. Falabella R, Arrunategui A, Barona MI, et al. The minigrafting test for vitiligo: detection of stable lesions for melanocyte transplantation. J Am Acad Dermatol 1995;32(2 Pt 1):228–32.
7. Li W, Wang S, Xu AE. Role of in vivo reflectance confocal microscopy in determining stability in vitiligo: a preliminary study. Indian J Dermatol 2013;58(6):429–32.
8. Gupta S, D'Souza P, Dhali TK, et al. Serum homocysteine and total antioxidant status in vitiligo: a case control study in Indian population. Indian J Dermatol 2016;61(2):131–6.
9. Cucchi ML, Frattini P, Santagostino G, et al. Catecholamines increase in the urine of non-segmental vitiligo especially during its active phase. Pigment Cell Res 2003;16(2):111–6.
10. Singh RK, Lee KM, Vujkovic-Cvijin I, et al. The role of IL-17 in vitiligo: a review. Autoimmun Rev 2016;15(4):397–404.
11. Wang X, Wang Q, Wu J, et al. Increased expression of CXCR3 and its ligands in vitiligo patients and CXCL10 as a potential clinical marker for vitiligo. Br J Dermatol 2016;174(6):1318–26.
12. Shi YL, Weiland M, Li J, et al. MicroRNA expression profiling identifies potential serum biomarkers for non-segmental vitiligo. Pigment Cell Melanoma Res 2013;26(3):418–21.
13. Mulekar SV, Isedeh P. Surgical interventions for vitiligo: an evidence-based review. Br J Dermatol 2013;169(Suppl 3):57–66.
14. Ghia D, Mulekar S. Surgical management of vitiligo. In: Hamzavi I, Mahmoud B, Isedeh P, editors. Handbook of vitiligo: basic science and clinical management. London: JP Medical Publishers; 2015. p. 111–38.
15. Huggins RH, Henderson MD, Mulekar SV, et al. Melanocyte-keratinocyte transplantation procedure in the treatment of vitiligo: the experience of an academic medical center in the United States. J Am Acad Dermatol 2012;66(5):785–93.
16. Kahn AM, Cohen MJ. Repigmentation in vitiligo patients. Melanocyte transfer via ultra-thin grafts. Dermatol Surg 1998;24(3):365–7.
17. Majid I, Imran S. Ultrathin split-thickness skin grafting followed by narrowband UVB therapy for stable vitiligo: an effective and cosmetically satisfying treatment option. Indian J Dermatol Venereol Leprol 2012;78(2):159–64.
18. Feetham HJ, Chan JL, Pandya AG. Characterization of clinical response in patients with vitiligo undergoing autologous epidermal punch grafting. Dermatol Surg 2012;38(1):14–9.
19. Gupta S, Ajith C, Kanwar AJ, et al. Surgical pearl: standardized suction syringe for epidermal grafting. J Am Acad Dermatol 2005;52(2):348–50.

20. Gupta S, Chandrashekar BS, Reddy R, et al. Rapid induction of suction blisters by intra-cavity positive pressure enhancement. Dermatol Surg 2011;37(6): 843–5.
21. Gupta S, Jain VK, Saraswat PK. Suction blister epidermal grafting versus punch skin grafting in recalcitrant and stable vitiligo. Dermatol Surg 1999; 25(12):955–8.
22. Al-Hadidi N, Griffith JL, Al-Jamal MS, et al. Role of recipient-site preparation techniques and post-operative wound dressing in the surgical management of vitiligo. J Cutan Aesthet Surg 2015;8(2): 79–87.
23. Srinivas CR, Rai R, Kumar PU. Meshed split skin graft for extensive vitiligo. Indian J Dermatol Venereol Leprol 2004;70(3):165–7.
24. Paddle-Ledinek JE, Nasa Z, Cleland HJ. Effect of different wound dressings on cell viability and proliferation. Plast Reconstr Surg 2006;117(7 Suppl): 110S–8S [discussion: 119S–20S].
25. Singh O, Gupta SS, Soni M, et al. Collagen dressing versus conventional dressings in burn and chronic wounds: a retrospective study. J Cutan Aesthet Surg 2011;4(1):12–6.
26. Fongers A, Wolkerstorfer A, Nieuweboer-Krobotova L, et al. Long-term results of 2-mm punch grafting in patients with vitiligo vulgaris and segmental vitiligo: effect of disease activity. Br J Dermatol 2009;161(5): 1105–11.
27. Ashique KT, Kaliyadan F. Long-term follow-up and donor site changes evaluation in suction blister epidermal grafting done for stable vitiligo: a retrospective study. Indian J Dermatol 2015;60(4):369–72.
28. Gou D, Currimbhoy S, Pandya AG. Suction blister grafting for vitiligo: efficacy and clinical predictive factors. Dermatol Surg 2015;41(5):633–9.
29. Lee DY, Kim JH, Park SW. A convenient method to distinguish the epidermal from the dermal side in suction-blister epidermal grafting. Dermatol Surg 2013;39(11):1731–2.
30. Agrawal K, Agrawal A. Vitiligo: repigmentation with dermabrasion and thin split-thickness skin graft. Dermatol Surg 1995;21(4):295–300.
31. Malakar S, Malakar RS. Surgical pearl: composite film and graft unit for the recipient area dressing after split-thickness skin grafting in vitiligo. J Am Acad Dermatol 2001;44(5):856–8.
32. Krishnan A, Kar S. Smashed skin grafting or smash grafting - a novel method of vitiligo surgery. Int J Dermatol 2012;51(10):1242–7.
33. McGovern TW, Bolognia J, Leffell DJ. Flip-top pigment transplantation: a novel transplantation procedure for the treatment of depigmentation. Arch Dermatol 1999;135(11):1305–7.
34. Sharma S, Garg VK, Sarkar R, et al. Comparative study of flip-top transplantation and punch grafting in stable vitiligo. Dermatol Surg 2013;39(9):1376–84.
35. Sardi JR. Surgical treatment for vitiligo through hair follicle grafting: how to make it easy. Dermatol Surg 2001;27(7):685–6.
36. Thakur P, Sacchidanand S, Nataraj HV, et al. A study of hair follicular transplantation as a treatment option for vitiligo. J Cutan Aesthet Surg 2015;8(4):211–7.
37. Na GY, Seo SK, Choi SK. Single hair grafting for the treatment of vitiligo. J Am Acad Dermatol 1998; 38(4):580–4.
38. Mapar MA, Safarpour M, Mapar M, et al. A comparative study of the mini-punch grafting and hair follicle transplantation in the treatment of refractory and stable vitiligo. J Am Acad Dermatol 2014;70(4):743–7.
39. Malakar S, Dhar S. Repigmentation of vitiligo patches by transplantation of hair follicles. Int J Dermatol 1999;38(3):237–8.
40. Chen YF, Yang PY, Hu DN, et al. Treatment of vitiligo by transplantation of cultured pure melanocyte suspension: analysis of 120 cases. J Am Acad Dermatol 2004;51(1):68–74.
41. Hong WS, Hu DN, Qian GP, et al. Ratio of size of recipient and donor areas in treatment of vitiligo by autologous cultured melanocyte transplantation. Br J Dermatol 2011;165(3):520–5.
42. Hong WS, Hu DN, Qian GP, et al. Treatment of vitiligo in children and adolescents by autologous cultured pure melanocytes transplantation with comparison of efficacy to results in adults. J Eur Acad Dermatol Venereol 2011;25(5):538–43.
43. Guerra L, Primavera G, Raskovic D, et al. Erbium:YAG laser and cultured epidermis in the surgical therapy of stable vitiligo. Arch Dermatol 2003;139(10):1303–10.
44. Tegta GR, Parsad D, Majumdar S, et al. Efficacy of autologous transplantation of noncultured epidermal suspension in two different dilutions in the treatment of vitiligo. Int J Dermatol 2006;45(2):106–10.
45. Kumar A, Gupta S, Mohanty S, et al. Stem cell niche is partially lost during follicular plucking: a preliminary pilot study. Int J Trichology 2013;5(2):97–100.
46. Kumar A, Mohanty S, Sahni K, et al. Extracted hair follicle outer root sheath cell suspension for pigment cell restoration in vitiligo. J Cutan Aesthet Surg 2013; 6(2):121–5.
47. Mohanty S, Kumar A, Dhawan J, et al. Noncultured extracted hair follicle outer root sheath cell suspension for transplantation in vitiligo. Br J Dermatol 2011;164(6):1241–6.
48. Gupta S, Honda S, Kumar B. A novel scoring system for evaluation of results of autologous transplantation methods in vitiligo. Indian J Dermatol Venereol Leprol 2002;68(1):33–7.
49. Henderson MD, Huggins RH, Mulekar SV, et al. Autologous noncultured melanocyte-keratinocyte transplantation procedure in an African American man with postburn leukoderma. Arch Dermatol 2011;147(9):1025–8.

Repigmentation through Melanocyte Regeneration in Vitiligo

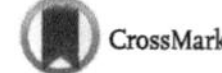

Stanca A. Birlea, MD, PhD[a,*],
Nathaniel B. Goldstein, BA, MA[a], David A. Norris, MD[a,b]

KEYWORDS

- Vitiligo • Repigmentation • Melanocyte stem cell • Bulge • Hair follicle • Proliferation • Migration • Differentiation

KEY POINTS

- Repigmentation is an active process during epidermal crisis reversing the loss of epidermal melanocytes.
- It usually develops in hair-bearing areas.
- The most common clinical presentation is the perifollicular pattern.
- The initiating event is the activation of melanocyte precursors from the hair follicle and of immature melanocytes from the basal epidermis.
- It is induced by different stimuli: UV light, drugs (steroids, calcineurin inhibitors).

INTRODUCTION

The loss of epidermal mature melanocytes in vitiligo depends on melanocyte-specific CD8+ cytotoxic T lymphocytes. It is reversed by halting the immune attack and by activating melanocyte precursors in the bulge and hair follicle infundibulum, to proliferate, migrate, and differentiate through the process called repigmentation.[1–4] Although repigmentation refers to the replenishment of pigment cells only, keratinocytes in vitiligo skin demonstrate architectural abnormalities and are also likely to be directly involved in repigmentation. Changes of the keratinocytes architecture seem to appear in the absence of basal melanocytes, in the sun-exposed skin. Therefore, significant increase in thickness of both stratum corneum and viable epidermis in vitiligo-depigmented skin, as compared with the adjacent, normal-appearing skin, was reported.[5] This increase likely occurs as an adaptive response to lack of melanin that can minimize and counteract the harmful UV effects on the skin.

Based on current knowledge, vitiligo repigmentation depends on available melanocytes from 2 sources:

- The hair follicle, which is the main source of pigment cells and is often unaffected by the T cell–mediated attack, likely because the hair follicle bulge is an immune privileged location[6]
- The epidermis at the lesional borders, which contains a pool of functional melanocytes and represents a secondary source for repigmentation

Melanocyte activation, followed by migration, proliferation, and differentiation is triggered by several stimuli, such as UV radiation (delivered as treatment or by natural sunlight) and drugs

Disclosure Statement: The authors do not have any commercial or financial conflicts of interest.
This work was supported by an American Skin Association Research Scholar Award in Vitiligo/Pigment Cell Disorders to Stanca Birlea.

[a] Department of Dermatology, University of Colorado Anschutz Medical Campus, 12801 17th Avenue, Aurora, CO 80045, USA; [b] Department of Dermatology, Denver Department of Veterans Affairs Medical Center, 1055 Clermont Street, Denver, CO 80220, USA
* Corresponding author.
E-mail address: Stanca.Birlea@ucdenver.edu

Dermatol Clin 35 (2017) 205–218
http://dx.doi.org/10.1016/j.det.2016.11.015
0733-8635/17/Published by Elsevier Inc.

(systemic and topical steroids and topical calcineurin inhibitors).

CLINICAL PATTERNS OF REPIGMENTATION AND THE REPIGMENTATION SOURCES

There are 4 classic repigmentation patterns observed on clinical examination[7–9]: perifollicular (most common) (**Fig. 1**A-i), marginal (see **Fig. 1**A-ii),[9] diffuse (see **Fig. 1**A-iv),[7] and combined, which includes more than one pattern (an example of marginal combined with perifollicular pattern is provided in **Fig. 1**A-v).[9] A fifth newly described repigmentation pattern, the medium-spotted patern,[10] is presented in **Fig. 1**A-vi.[11]

The perifollicular pattern presents as small, round, pigmented macules around the hair follicles (see **Fig. 1**A-i). This clinical observation was confirmed by numerous previous *in vivo* studies[12–16] that identified amelanotic, inactive, 3,4-dihydroxy-L-phenylalanine (DOPA)(−) melanocytes in the infundibulum outer root sheath of hair follicles collected from healthy individuals[12,13,16,17] or from vitiligo patients.[14,15,18] The origin of DOPA(−) melanocytes was later identified as the hair follicle bulge (both in the transgenic mouse model[19] and then in human skin).[20] From this location melanocyte precursors ascend to repopulate the depigmented epidermis (**Fig. 1**B, right side) in the ultraviolet radiation (UVR)-treated vitiligo. Activation by UV treatment or ionizing radiation induces these precursors to migrate, proliferate, and differentiate, finally expressing the full pigmentation pathway in the interfollicular

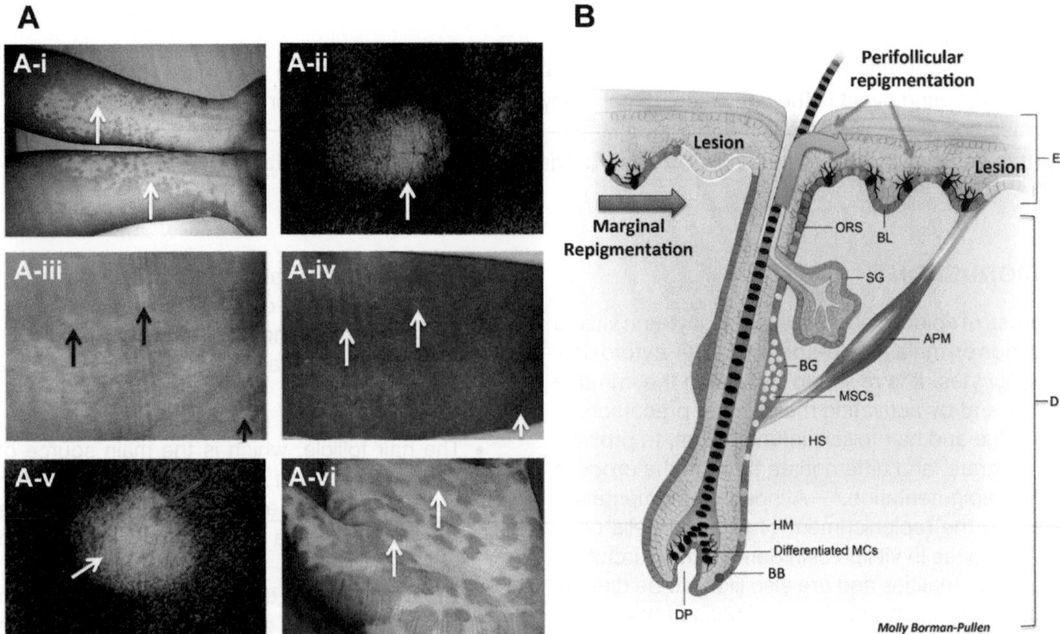

Fig. 1. (*A*) Clinical patterns of repigmentation. (*A-i*) Perifollicular pattern-multiple black dots of pigment are seen around the hair follicles (*white arrows*) in a patient with vitiligo treated with narrow band UVB (NBUVB). (*A-ii*) Marginal repigmentation pattern presented as a pigmented rim at the borders of the lesions (*white arrow*). (*A-iii*) Depigmented spots (*blue arrows*) treated 12 weeks with NBUVB repigment the skin following a diffuse repigmentation pattern, as indicated in (*A-iv*) by white arrows. (*A-v*) Combined repigmentation pattern including marginal pattern (*white arrow*) and perifollicular pattern (*red arrow*). (*A-vi*) Medium-spotted repigmentation pattern[10] in a patient who underwent psoralen plus UVA treatment. Repigmentation of palmar surface presents as round brown macules (*white arrows*). (*B*) Cellular mechanism of perifollicular repigmentation (*right side, blue arrows*) and marginal repigmentation (*left side, red arrow*) in human vitiligo. APM, arrector pili muscle; BB, bulb; BG, bulge; BL, basal layer; D, dermis; DP, dermal papilla; E, epidermis; HM, hair matrix; HS, hair shaft; MCs, melanocytes; MSCs, melanocyte stem cells; ORS, outer root sheath; SG, sebaceous gland. ([*A-i, ii, v*] *From* Gan EY, Gahat T, Cario-André M, et al. Clinical repigmentation patterns in paediatric vitiligo. Br J Dermatol 2016;175:555–60, with permission; and [*A-iii, iv*] Yang YS, Cho HR, Ryou JH, et al. Clinical study of repigmentation patterns with either narrow-band ultraviolet B (NBUVB) or 308 nm excimer laser treatment in Korean vitiligo patients. Int J Dermatol 2010;49(3):317–23, with permission; and [*A-vi*] Davids LM, du Toit E, Kidson SH, et al. A rare repigmentation pattern in a vitiligo patient: a clue to an epidermal stem-cell reservoir of melanocytes? Clin Exp Dermatol 2009;34(2):246–8, with permission; and [*B*] This cartoon was drawn by Molly Borman-Pullen, biomedical illustrator, Fort Collins, CO.)

epidermis.[4,17] Data confirming the follicular reservoir also came from animal and human models of pigmentation, which is revisited in this review.

The marginal pattern is observed as a repigmentation rim at the borders of the lesions[7] (see **Fig. 1**A-ii).[9] It is the result of activation of functional epidermal melanocytes in the lesional borders.[3] Some investigators have proposed an epidermal repigmentation reservoir,[21,22] consisting of more immature melanocyte precursors with supposed migratory, differentiation, and perhaps proliferative abilities (see **Fig. 1**B, left side).

The diffuse repigmentation pattern appears as generalized darkening across the patches of vitiligo[3] (see **Fig. 1**A-iv),[7] whereas, in the combined pattern (see **Fig. 1**A-v),[9] the repigmentation does not fit into any single type or where more than one pattern contributes to the repigmentation process.[7] The diffuse pattern suggests that repigmentation can arise from interfollicular melanocyte precursors either in the dermis or interfollicular epidermis (by reactivation of DOPA(−) melanocytes, which are hypothesized to persist in the center of the lesions).[3]

A very recent study reported in pediatric vitiligo patients a medium-spotted repigmentation pattern, located in non–hair-bearing to minimal hair-bearing sites, such as the palms, soles, lips, ankles, and anterior wrists.[10] This uncommon pattern begins as larger spots that are not centered on any particular hair follicle. Consistent with these findings, a previous study[11] reported a rare pattern of repigmentation on the palms of a patient, consisting of irregular brown macules developed after a course of psoralen plus UVA (PUVA) therapy (see **Fig. 1**A-vi).[11] Tyrosinase (TYR)(+) melanocytes were found along the basement membrane of the repigmenting lesions, in contrast to the adjacent vitiliginous skin, which lacked these cells. Based on observation of repigmentation that occurred in the center of an initially fully depigmented lesion on the palm (a region devoid of hair follicles), the investigators hypothesized that the melanocyte precursors/stem cells can remain in vitiliginous lesions serving as repigmentation reservoir. The pattern seen in this case seems to support medium-spotted repigmentation, recently reported in children with vitiligo.[10]

Other reports identified melanocytes within the depigmented vitiligo,[23–25] and one of them claimed that melanocytes in depigmented epidermis were "never completely absent."[24] The investigators hypothesized that these melanocytes can recover their functionality *in vivo* and *in vitro* on the removal of hydrogen peroxide,[24] which they propose is the major mediator of cytotoxicity.

Interestingly, in some of the frozen epidermal sections of depigmented untreated skin collected from vitiligo patients of skin types II and III, the authors' group observed large cells, with fragmented bodies, and diminished and abnormal, fragmented dendrites, expressing a Premelanosome protein (PMEL)(+)/Tyrosine kinase receptor (C-KIT)(−) phenotype (**Fig. 2**A). The authors noticed similar aspects in paraffin sections of depigmented skin, in which epidermal cells carried a dopachrome tautomerase (DCT)(+)/C-KIT(−) phenotype (see **Fig. 2**B). These rare cells were amelanotic (Fontana-Masson(−) staining, see **Fig. 2**B) and located not only close to lesional borders but also within the lesions. It was previously proposed[26] that these cells might be residual nonfunctional, senescent cells (progressing toward apoptosis)[26] rather than poorly differentiated melanocyte precursors with potential to form functional melanocytes. Loss of C-KIT expression is an interesting and expected finding, knowing the major implication of stem cell factor (SCF)/c-kit in melanocyte survival and migration.[27] The authors think that acquisition of C-KIT expression is essential in the repigmentation process associated with the migratory, proliferative, and differentiating phenotype of post–stem cell melanoblasts.[4]

Based on indirect evidence of stem cell markers, tissue culture studies, and repigmentation patterns observed in patients with vitiligo, another previous report hypothesized[28] the existence of a pool of extrafollicular melanocyte stem cells in a well-protected area of the dermis with the ability to replace any damaged melanocytes in the basal layer of the epidermis. More recently, a dermal source of melanoblasts (DCT(+)) was identified in the secretory portion of the eccrine sweat glands after skin exposure to ionizing radiation.[29] It seems that the precursors of these cells colonize sweat glands during development, being maintained in an immature, slow-cycling state; they were shown to renew themselves in response to genomic stress (eg, ionizing radiation) having the capacity to provide their differentiating progeny to the epidermis. It has been hypothesized that these melanoblasts can provide an anatomic niche for melanocyte-melanoma precursor cells[29]; however, their implication in regeneration of vitiligo epidermis awaits investigation.

CLINICAL PARTICULARITIES OF REPIGMENTATION AND THEIR CORRELATION WITH CELLULAR AND MOLECULAR CHANGES

The Lag Time Between Initiation of Stimulus (Ultraviolet) and Visible Repigmentation

Repigmentation is unpredictable, not proportional to the magnitude of the lesions, and often cosmetically insufficient.[30] Curiously, in the same patient,

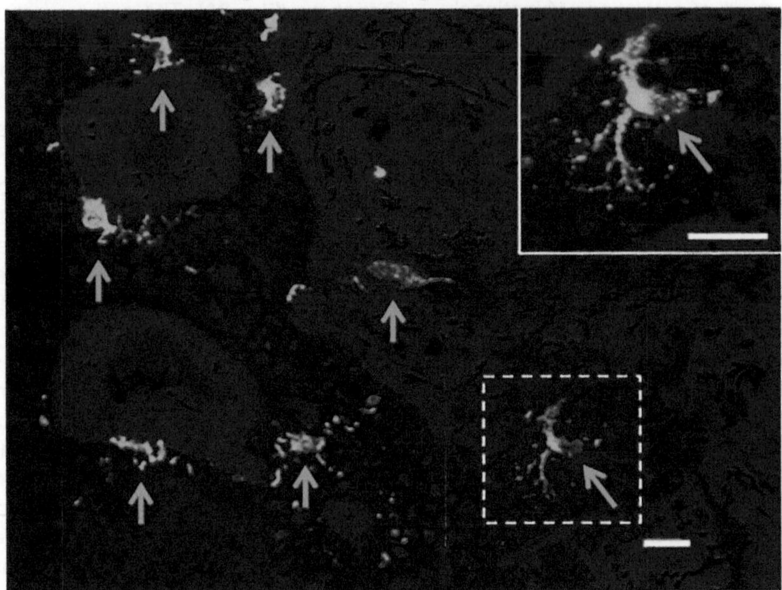

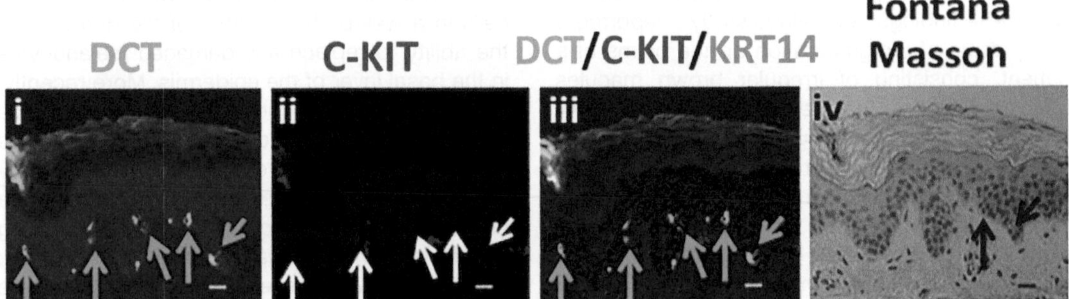

Fig. 2. (*A*) Longitudinal paraffin sections of interfollicular epidermis of depigmented vitiligo (immunostained with combination of anti-human C-KIT [*red*], anti-human K14 [*blue*], and anti-human PMEL [NKI-beteb antibody] [*green*]). NKI-beteb(+)/C-KIT(−) melanocytes (*green arrows*) can be seen with abnormal morphology, consisting of fragmented and distorted bodies, diminished dendricity, and cell debris. White dotted lines indicate area of higher magnification (*inset*). Scale bars = 20 μm. (*B*) Transverse paraffin sections of interfollicular epidermis of depigmented vitiligo (immunostained with combination of [*i*] anti-human DCT [*green*], [*ii*] anti-human C-KIT [*red*], and [*iii*] anti-human K14 [*blue*]). DCT(+) (*green arrows*) and C-KIT(−) (*white arrows*) melanocytes can be seen with abnormal morphology, consisting of fragmented and distorted bodies and diminished dendricity. None of the melanocytes exhibit pigmentation in Fontana-Masson staining (*iv, black arrows*). Scale bars = 20 μm.

vitiligo repigmentation in some regions can commonly parallel active depigmentation of other regions.[1] Neither sex nor skin type are associated with differences in onset or pace of repigmentation following UVR treatment of vitiligo.[4] Patients' clinical response to narrow band UVB (NBUVB) exposure, applied twice weekly, has a lag time ranging between 4 weeks and 4 months, variable between body areas and from patient to patient. This lag time may depend on the integrity of the bulge stem cell reservoir, on the melanocyte precursors susceptibility to activation, and on their migratory and proliferative abilities. If there is a lack of any visible repigmentation after 6 months of treatment, further therapy is discouraged, in both adult and pediatric patients,[31] and consideration of a different alternative can be advised.

Interestingly, in animal models, the cellular response to UVB seems to appear shortly after exposure. Therefore, in the C57BL/6 mouse, an increase of Tyrosinase protein 1 (TRP1)(+) epidermal melanocytes was first identified on the 5th day after UVB (one exposure of 0.18 J/cm^2 of energy, corresponding to 1.5 minimal erythema dose for the C57BL mice) and reached a cellularity 4 times as great as that of the normal control on the 14th day.[32]

Repigmenting Versus Treatment-Resistant Lesions

- Repigmentation develops best in the hair-bearing regions. Areas with a higher density of hair follicles (face, arms, forearms, thighs, legs, abdomen, back) respond more rapidly to treatment, and those with lower density (dorsum of hands, fingers, feet, and toes) respond more slowly.[1]
- Depigmented areas where hair follicles are absent or in low density (palms, soles, volar wrists, genital sites, mucosal or semimucosal surfaces) rarely respond to treatment; the response, if present, is slow and incomplete. The potential treatment response relies on the epidermal source of melanocytes from the lesional borders (that can migrate ~ 4–5 mm into the depigmented area),[2] on epidermal melanocytes that are hypothesized to persist in the center of the depigmented lesions,[10] or on melanocytes with extrafollicular dermal origin.[28]
- Depigmented areas with white terminal hairs (leukotrichia) are poor responders to medical treatment[33] with minimal chances of repigmentation. Leukotrichia is perhaps an indicator of more severe, long-lasting, and active CD8+ T-cell immune-mediated attack on melanocytes, which progresses gradually downward, from the epidermis to the bulge. Depletion of the bulge melanocyte stem cells leads to exhaustion of secondary hair germ in the bulb, which is composed of melanocytes precursors more committed to melanocyte differentiation.

Cellular and Molecular Changes of Repigmented Skin

The sequences of repigmentation process

There has been surprisingly limited research addressing the repigmentation process in vitiligo, despite impressive progress studying the mechanisms of vitiligo immunology[34,35] and genetics.[36] It is known that the UV-induced repigmentation process includes keratinocyte stimulation and melanocyte activation by UV light (**Fig. 3**A)[37,38] melanocyte migration, proliferation, and differentiation (differentiation implies cell melanization). Melanocyte migration involves the following steps: melanocyte decoupling from the basement membrane and from keratinocytes, cell movement, and recoupling to the basement membrane and to keratinocytes. The intimate melanocyte-keratinocyte anatomic and functional interactions in the hair follicle and epidermis are essential for epidermal repopulation in vitiligo. However, how these processes develop during repigmentation and the triggers that initiate one process in favor of the other have not yet been identified.

There are 2 major pathways, p53 and Wnt/β-catenin, that strongly activate the pigmentation process. It has been clearly shown that cellular and DNA damage[39,40] by UVR induces p53 activation. In normal skin repeatedly exposed to UVR, p53 orchestrates melanocyte activation by coordinating the release of keratinocyte-paracrine/growth factors with melanogenic activity, which induces microphthalmia-associated transcription factor (MITF) expression in melanocytes[37,41] (see **Fig. 3**A).[37,38] Similarly, in vitiligo, repigmentation occurs following melanocyte activation by NBUVB orchestrated by p53 and its downstream effector, α-melanocyte stimulating hormone, which is a potent inducer of MITF.

The Wnt/β-catenin signaling pathway has also been implicated in the pigmentation process. UVB irradiation of the mouse F1 of HR-1 × HR/De induced robust expression of Wnt7a and subsequent β-catenin translocation into the nucleus in the melanocyte stem cells[42] (the model is presented in the *Transgenic mouse models* section). In the same model, intradermal injection of inhibitor of Wnt response 1(IWR-1) (a chemical inhibitor of β-catenin activation), and small interfering RNA against Wnt7a inhibited the proliferation of epidermal melanocytes. It was demonstrated that Wnt7a triggered melanocyte stem cell differentiation through β-catenin activation.[42] The Wnt/β-catenin pathway seemed to be modulated by the UVB treatment in the mouse model, but the effects of UVB on the Wnt/β-catenin pathway on melanocytes and keratinocytes in the bulge of human vitiligo skin await to be studied. Wnt signaling is essentially required for melanocyte development; its activation results in stabilization of β-catenin/lymphoid enhancer factor (Lef) complex, which leads to transactivation of downstream target genes, such as *Mitf*, to promote melanocyte-fate specification and melanocyte

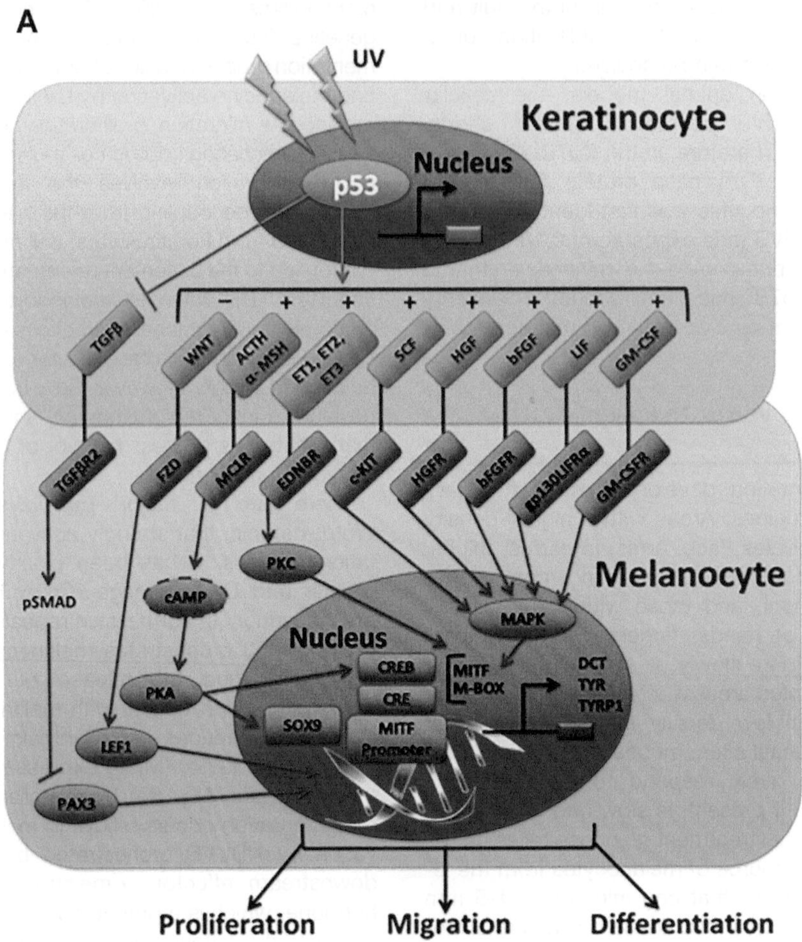
A
UV
Keratinocyte
Nucleus
p53
TGFβ
WNT
ACTH α- MSH
ET1, ET2, ET3
SCF
HGF
bFGF
LIF
GM-CSF
TGFβR2
FZD
MC1R
EDNBR
c-KIT
HGFR
bFGFR
gp130LIFRα
GM-CSFR
PKC
Melanocyte
pSMAD
cAMP
MAPK
Nucleus
CREB
CRE
MITF M-BOX
DCT
TYR
TYRP1
PKA
SOX9
MITF Promoter
LEF1
PAX3
Proliferation
Migration
Differentiation

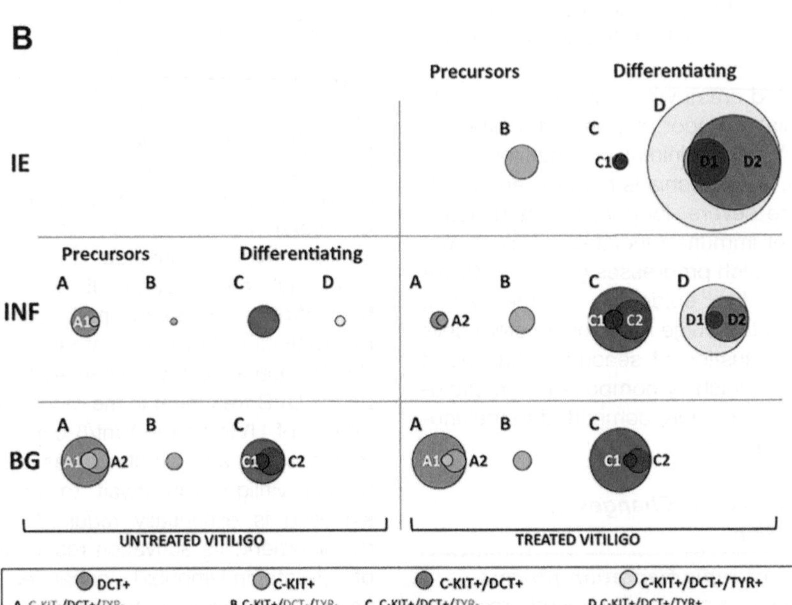
B
Precursors
Differentiating
IE
INF
BG
A
A1
A2
B
C
C1
C2
D
D1
D2
UNTREATED VITILIGO
TREATED VITILIGO
DCT+
C-KIT+
C-KIT+/DCT+
C-KIT+/DCT+/TYR+
A C-KIT-/DCT+/TYR-
A1 C-KIT-/DCT+/TYR-/KI-67+/MCAM-
A2 C-KIT-/DCT+/TYR-/KI-67-/MCAM+
B C-KIT+/DCT-/TYR-
C C-KIT+/DCT+/TYR-
C1 C-KIT+/DCT+/TYR-/KI-67+/MCAM-
C2 C-KIT+/DCT+/TYR-/KI-67-/MCAM+
D C-KIT+/DCT+/TYR+
D1 C-KIT+/DCT+/TYR+/KI-67+/MCAM+
D2 C-KIT+/DCT+/TYR+/KI-67-/MCAM+

differentiation.[43] Moreover, epidermal Wnt controls hair follicle induction by orchestrating dynamic signaling crosstalk between the epidermis and dermis.[44] Epithelial Wnt/β-catenin signaling is required for hair matrix cell proliferation, and β-catenin is required in bulge stem cells and also for epidermal proliferation.[45]

More recently, transcriptome analysis on lesional, perilesional, and nondepigmented skin from patients with vitiligo and from matched skin of healthy subjects identified decreased Wnt activation in depigmented vitiligo skin.[46] In addition, using *ex vivo* explants of depigmented human vitiligo skin, the authors found that treatment with Wnt agonists or glycogen synthase kinase 3 β (GSK3β) inhibitors induce increased expression of melanocyte-specific markers, triggering the differentiation of resident melanocyte stem cells in pre-melanocytes expressing paired box protein-3 (PAX3) and DCT. All these findings raise the possibility that Wnt normalization is important for the repigmentation process.

p53 seems to crosstalk with β-catenin in several cell lines, including the hair follicle stem cells. It has been reported that β-catenin and pygopus homolog 2 (Pygo2) (the latter with regulatory roles on Wnt/β-catenin target genes) converge to induce p53 in cultured keratinocytes and in cycling hair follicles. These findings identify Pygo2 as an important regulator of Wnt/β-catenin function in skin epithelia and p53 activation as a prominent downstream event of β-catenin/Pygo2 action in stem cell activation.[47] Whether p53-β-catenin crosstalk intervenes during the repigmentation process awaits further study.

Human and animal models to study repigmentation

There are several mouse models and few human models used to study repigmentation, which the authors summarize later. They have revealed valuable information about the sequence of melanocyte proliferation, migration and differentiation.

Transgenic mouse models

SLFTg1-1 mice injected with anti-c-Kit monoclonal antibody ACK2 Investigation using this model has revealed the melanocyte precursors in the hair follicle, their migratory capacity, and participation to the repigmentation process.[48] This model is a nonvitiligo repigmentation model, using the *SLFTg1-1* humanized mouse, expressing steel factor (SLF) in the basal layer, under control of the Keratin *(Krt)14* promoter. Treatment with the anti–c-Kit (ACK2) antibody eliminated the c-Kit(+) melanoblasts in the hair follicle and induced complete skin and hair depigmentation. In the next hair cycles, perifollicular repigmentation occurred, based on a population of residual melanocyte stem cells Dct(+)/c-Kit(−) maintained in the hair follicle, which showed migratory abilities.

K14-SLF/+; Dct-lacZ/+ transgenic mouse model The experiments done on this model identified the melanocyte precursors in the bulge, their

Fig. 3. Summary of the UV effects in normal and vitiligo skin. (*A*) UV-induced pigmentation pathways in normal skin. p53 is stimulated by UV light and induces the release of melanogenic paracrine growth factors and cytokines by keratinocytes. The keratinocyte factors further interact with their corresponding receptors on melanocytes and induce melanocyte activation, with subsequent stimulation of microphthalmia-associated transcription factor (MITF) and its downstream targets, the melanogenic enzymes TYR, tyrosinase-related protein 1 (TYRP1), and DCT, leading to synthesis of melanin and melanocyte differentiation. (*B*) Melanocyte precursors and more differentiated phenotypes in treated and untreated vitiligo. The precursors and more differentiated phenotypes are represented with different colors in the bulge (BG), infundibulum (INF), and interfollicular epidermis (IE). The relative diameter of each circle in each study region represents the estimated percent of melanocytes exhibiting particular phenotypes in each study region, normalized to the average number of melanocytes in each region. ACTH, adrenocorticotropic hormone; Alpha-MSH, alpha-melanocyte-stimulating hormone; bFGF, basic fibroblastic growth factor; bFGFR, basic fibroblastic growth factor receptor; cAMP, cyclic adenosine monophosphate; c-KIT, tyrosine kinase receptor; CREB, cAMP response element-binding protein; CRE, cAMP response element; EDNBR, endothelin receptor beta; ET, Endothelin; FZD, frizzled; GM-CSF, granulocyte-macrophage colony-stimulating factor; gp130 LIFR-alpha, leukocyte inhibitory factor receptor-alpha; GM-CSFR, granulocyte-macrophage colony-stimulating factor receptor; HGF, hepatocyte growth factor; HGFR, hepatocyte growth factor receptor; LEF1, lymphoid enhancer binding factor 1; LIF, leukocyte inhibitory factor; MAPK, mitogen activated protein kinase; MC1R, melanocortin receptor 1; MSH, melanocyte-stimulating hormone; PAX3, paired box 3; PKC, protein kinase C; SCF, stem cell factor; SOX9, SRY-Box9; TGFb, transforming growth factor; TGFbR2, transforming growth factor b receptor 2; TGF-β, transforming growth factor-β. ([*A*] *Adapted from* Costin GE, Hearing VJ. Human skin pigmentation: melanocytes modulate skin color in response to stress. FASEB J 2007;21(4):976–94; and Hirobe T. How are proliferation and differentiation of melanocytes regulated? Pigment Cell Melanoma Res 2011;24(3):462–78, with permission; and [*B*] *From* Goldstein NB, Koster MI, Hoaglin LG, et al. Narrow band ultraviolet B treatment for human vitiligo is associated with proliferation, migration, and differentiation of melanocyte precursors. J Invest Dermatol 2015;135(8):2068–76, with permission.)

migratory capacity under SLF stimulation, and their differentiation ability.[19] This model is a non-vitiligo repigmentation model that, in addition to the *SLFTg1-1* mutation,[48] expresses the lacZ reporter gene under the control of the Dct promoter. Histologic examination of this mouse skin demonstrated that the progeny of surviving melanoblasts in the bulge could migrate upward to the epidermis in the presence of SLF, indicating that bulge stem cells are the source of melanocytes in the epidermis. Increasing numbers of lacZ+ cells appeared in the epidermis as pigmented spots in a concentric pattern around the terminal hairs.

F1 hairless HR-1 x HR/De mouse model The experiments done on this model reveal the differentiation ability of melanocyte precursors in the bulge, their ability to migrate along the hair follicle outer root sheath, and also to repigment the interfollicular epidermis following UVB stimulation.[42] This model is also a non-vitiligo model, in which homozygous mutants (Hr^{hr}/Hr^{hr}) show normal development of the first hair cycle. They become completely hairless at 3 weeks of age; at 4 weeks of age they become depigmented. In this model, delayed pigmented spots are induced long after UV irradiation. Following UVB exposure, the melanocyte precursors were observed to proliferate in the bulge and differentiate to melanoblasts that migrated to the epidermis and became melanotic cells.

Dct-LacZ+ mouse model The experiments done on this model revealed the migratory ability of bulge melanocyte precursors along the hair follicle outer root sheath, achieving proliferative and differentiation ability only after they reached interfollicular epidermis.[49] This model is a non-vitiligo transgenic mouse model, expressing the lacZ reporter gene under the control of the *Dct* promoter. Following exposure to UVB or on induction of a wound on the back of the mouse, melanocyte stem cells were shown to exit the bulge and migrate along the outer root sheath infundibulum without proliferation; they proliferated and differentiated in the epidermis.

$Mc1r^{e/e}$ transgenic mouse model The experiments done on this model revealed the migratory ability of melanocyte precursors along the hair follicle outer root sheath under melanocortin 1 receptor (Mc1r) stimulation.[49] This mouse is a non-vitiligo, non-humanized mouse expressing a non-functional Mc1r. After wounding on the back of $Mc1r^{e/e}$ mice, a lower number of epidermal melanocytes were noticed as compared with their control littermate, $Mc1r^{+/+}$ mice; the difference in melanocyte number in the epidermis was caused by impaired melanocyte migration from the bulge to the interfollicular epidermis, which was attributed to the lack of Mc1r function in the mouse expressing the defective gene.

Human models of repigmentation

Human vitiligo model using punch grafts Punch grafts were performed on depigmented vitiligo lesions, and then they were exposed to khellin and UV light.[50] Immunostaining experiments revealed the migratory capacity of melanocytes (horizontal migration to depigmented areas).

Human vitiligo model using punch biopsies The experiments done on this model revealed the proliferative, migratory, and differentiation ability of melanocyte precursors in both hair follicle and interfollicular epidermis.[4] Skin biopsies taken from patients with untreated vitiligo and from patients treated with NBUVB for 3 and 6 months were immunostained with melanocyte markers (DCT, C-KIT, TYR, or PAX3), markers of proliferation (KI-67), and/or of migration (melanoma cell adhesion molecule [MCAM]), and a keratinocyte specific marker (K14). NBUVB was associated with a significant increase in the number of melanocytes in the infundibulum and with restoration of the normal melanocyte population in the epidermis (see **Fig. 3**B).[4]

Repigmented narrow band ultraviolet treated–skin versus normal skin and untreated vitiligo skin

Using immunostaininig techniques coupled with collection of skin biopsies from patients with vitiligo, the authors showed that in the hair follicle bulge, NBUVB treatment stimulated a slight increase of 2 populations of immature melanocytes, a stem cell population C-KIT(–)/DCT(+), and a melanoblast population C-KIT(+)/DCT(+) (see **Fig. 3**B).[4] The targeted immature melanocyte in the hair follicle bulge and infundibulum of untreated vitiligo contained only amelanotic melanocytes (ie, they expressed the melanocyte markers DCT and/or C-KIT and/or PAX3, but they were TYR(–) and Fontana-Masson(–)); these immature populations remained amelanotic in the bulge after 3 to 6 months of NBUVB treatment. Fontana-Masson(+) cells and TYR(+) cells were seen only in the upper infundibulum and epidermis after treatment. NBUVB treatment was associated with significantly increased expression of melanocyte markers in the vitiligo treated skin, the most striking contrast being observed between the untreated depigmented epidermis (devoid of melanocytes) and the treated pigmented epidermis, which was heavily DCT(+), C-KIT(+), PAX3(+), TYR(+), and strongly Fontana-Masson(+).

Melanocyte proliferation after NBUVB was indirectly supported by the observation of increased melanocyte numbers in all regions tested and was directly quantified by KI-67 coexpression with C-KIT, DCT, and TYR. The authors identified a presumed migratory population of melanocytes (DCT(+)/MCAM(+)) that was minimally expressed in the bulge but showed increased expression in the infundibulum and epidermis. The melanocyte precursors showed differentiation abilities in the upper infundibulum by gradually exhibiting TYR expression, a process that paralleled proliferation and migration and that continued in the epidermis (population TYR(+)/MCAM(+)/KI-67(+)). The authors found no significant difference in melanocyte marker expression between NBUVB-treated vitiligo skin and normal skin, which suggested that NBUVB exposure for 3 to 6 months returns depigmented skin to a normal status in respect to pigmentation.

REPIGMENTATION INDUCED BY ULTRAVIOLET LIGHT AND BY DRUGS

The key principle of vitiligo therapy is to stabilize depigmentation (by halting the immune response) and to stimulate the melanocyte precursors to repigment the skin.[1] Most treatment alternatives (UV, steroids, calcineurin inhibitors) seem to act on both steps, although at present, it is not clearly understood to what extent these alternatives must suppress the autoimmune process versus stimulate melanocyte repopulation of the epidermis to provide maximum efficacy.

The clinical observation that pigmented terminal hairs are present within depigmented spots of most patients with vitiligo suggested that the human bulge melanocyte precursors are preserved in the depigmented skin. These bulge precursors constitute a source for bulb secondary hair germ to provide immature melanocytes for normal hair shaft pigmentation but also for epidermal regeneration (perifollicular repigmentation). The authors' immunostaininig study of vitiligo depigmented skin showed that the melanocyte precursors in the hair follicle bulge are present (**Fig. 4**A), in similar proportions with the normal skin[4] ready to be activated by UV or drugs. These precursors consist of melanocyte stem cells (DCT(−)/C-KIT(−)) and melanoblasts (DCT(−)/C-KIT(−)).[4]

The authors discuss later the repigmentation outcome of few meta-analyses of vitiligo treatment presented in the literature and of reviews of literature data. The most recent meta-analysis, including 4512 participants,[51] reflected the need of new methodology to assess permanence of repigmentation as well as the need for better designed studies: high-quality randomized trials using standardized measures and also addressing quality of life. None of the studies were able to demonstrate long-term benefits.

Repigmentation and Ultraviolet Light

The strongest stimulator of melanocyte precursors is UVR (delivered mainly as NBUVB light, broad band UVB [BBUVB] light, or PUVA). The deep penetration of NBUVB to the level of the human hair follicle bulge was indirectly suggested by the authors' immunostaining studies.[52] The authors found increased expression of DNA damage markers in the bulge keratinocyte stem cells of skin exposed for 3 months to twice-weekly NBUVB treatment (**Fig. 4**B-i), as compared with the bulge of skin unexposed to UV (see **Fig. 4**B-ii).

An earlier meta-analysis of all vitiligo therapies showed that the highest mean repigmentation rate was achieved with NBUVB, BBUVB, and PUVA.[53] NBUVB therapy was considered the most effective and safest alternative for generalized and localized vitiligo. The most recent meta-analysis of vitiligo therapies showed that marked repigmentation (of >75%) appeared more often in the NBUVB-treated patients as compared PUVA-treated patients.[51] The repigmentation induced by NBUVB was also reported to be more stable than that induced by PUVA.[54]

In a review of published clinical studies about excimer laser in vitiligo, the repigmentation induced by the UVB-excimer laser was described as marked and relatively fast (≤15 weeks in most studies analyzed).[55]

Repigmentation and Steroids

The role of steroids on pigmentation is mainly informed by clinical studies. Melasma, commonly seen on the face during pregnancy (a state accompanied by high levels of the sex steroid hormones like estrogens and progesterone often coexist with increased pigmentation in other areas [areolae, linea alba, and perineal skin]. Pigmentation of all these areas fades following parturition.[56] This clinical observation suggests that steroids stimulate melanocyte differentiation. Oral contraceptives containing estrogens can also result in hyperpigmentation of the face; ointments containing estrogens can produce intense pigmentation of the genitals, mammary areola, and linea alba of the abdomen in male and female infants.[56] Moreover, experimental data support the hypothesis that a decrease in the antibody-mediated cytotoxicity against melanocytes in patients with vitiligo treated with systemic steroids improves depigmentation.[57] The most recent meta-analysis of

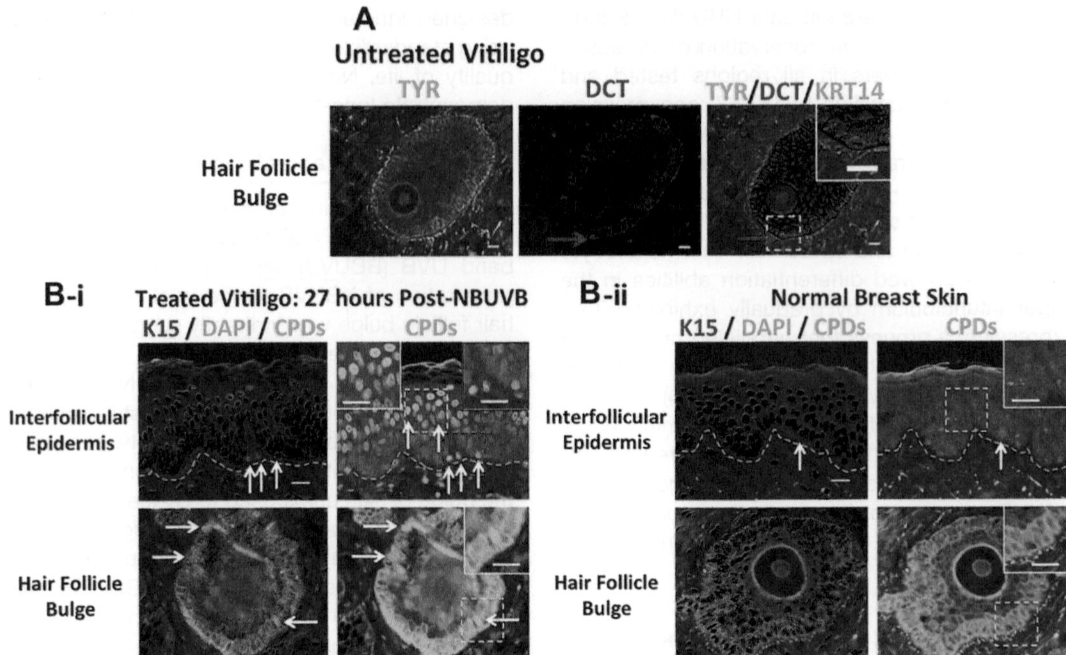

Fig. 4. (*A*) Triple fluorescent immunostaining of untreated vitiligo skin, showing absence of TYR expression in the hair follicle bulge (TYR being a marker of differentiated melanocytes, *green channel*). An immature, DCT(+) melanocyte (*red arrows*) with very low TYR expression can be seen in the hair follicle bulge outer root sheath. (*B-i*) Transverse paraffin sections of bulge of NBUVB-treated human vitiligo (immunostained with combination of anti-chicken K15 [*red*], anti-human cyclobutan pyrimidine dimers (CPDs) [*green*], and DAPI ([*blue*]). CPDs staining showed that CPD(+) cells were mainly located in the interfollicular epidermis (*green cells, white arrows*) 27 hours after UV exposure in an Ultralite Phototherapy Chamber source (NBUVB phototherapy lamps 311 nm). Sporadic CPD(+) cells, both K15(+) or K15(−) cells, are also seen in the hair follicle bulge (*white arrows*). (*B-ii*) Normal breast skin showing very few CPD(+) cells in the interfollicular epidermis (*green cells, white arrow*) and no visible staining in the hair follicle bulge. Blue dotted lines highlight epidermal boundary. White dotted lines indicate area of higher magnification (*inset*). The bulge regions were mapped by K15 staining in consecutive sections (*not shown*). Scale bars = 20 μm.

vitiligo therapy[51] showed that repigmentation induced by:

- Topical corticosteroids were better than that induced by PUVA sol.
- Topical hydrocortisone plus laser light was better than that induced by laser light alone.
- Oral mini-pulse of prednisolone (OMP) plus NBUVB was better than that induced by OMP alone.
- Topical clobetasol propionate was better than that induced by PUVA sol.

An earlier meta-analysis of nonsurgical vitiligo therapies[53] showed that among randomized controlled trials on localized vitiligo, the repigmentation with topical class 2 corticosteroids was highly significant as compared with placebo; they were considered, together with NBUVB, the most effective and safest treatment of generalized and localized vitiligo. The highest mean success repigmentation rates in the patients' series were produced by topical classes 1 and 2 corticosteroids.

Repigmentation and Calcineurin Inhibitors

Topical calcineurin inhibitors can be effective in vitiligo therapy because of their ability to restore the altered cytokine network. Tacrolimus has been shown to inhibit T-cell activation by downregulating transcription of genes encoding proinflammatory cytokines interleukin (IL)-2, IL-3, IL-4, IL-5, interferon (IFN)-γ, tumor necrosis factor (TNF)-α, and granulocyte-macrophage colony-stimulating factor in T cells.[58] In addition, direct effects of tacrolimus on melanocyte migration[59] and differentiation[60] during repigmentation have been reported, although the roles on cell growth/proliferation remain controversial.[59,61]

A recent meta-analysis of the effect of topical calcineurin inhibitors (tacrolimus, pimecrolimus) in vitiligo[62] showed that:

- Repigmentation with calcineurin inhibitors is significantly higher than with placebo.
- Repigmentation with calcineurin inhibitors is significantly higher when these compounds are combined with NBUVB as compared with their use as monotherapy.

In addition, an earlier review of literature data on calcineurin inhibitors in vitiligo[63] showed that:

- Repigmentation obtained in a double-blind study with combination tacrolimus 0.1% ointment and excimer laser is superior to placebo, especially for UV-resistant areas (eg, bony prominences).
- Repigmentation obtained with tacrolimus 0.1% ointment monotherapy is almost as effective as clobetasol propionate 0.05% ointment.

Repigmentation and Vitamin D Analogues

Topical vitamin D analogues could restore pigmentation in vitiligo by inducing skin immunosuppression, which halts the local autoimmune process, and via direct activation of melanocytic precursors and melanogenic pathways.[64] However, a comprehensive review of the literature[30] reported the lack of consistent evidence to support the stimulatory effect of calcipotriol/tacalcitol monotherapy on vitiligo repigmentation, although at both the cellular and molecular level experimental data suggest a stimulatory effect of vitamin D compounds on human and animal melanocyte pigmentation.[64] The therapeutic effect of vitamin D analogues seems to be obtained in combination with phototherapy[30,51,65] or with topical steroids.[65]

Repigmentation and JAK Inhibitors

JAK inhibitors can be a promising treatment of human vitiligo; besides their anti–IFN-γ effect, they also seem to activate the hair follicle melanocyte stem cells.[66]

However, their effect in inducing repigmentation was reported in a very limited number of studies, and their safety and efficacy need to be explored in depth in the future.

- Good repigmentation on all depigmented areas (more visible on the face) was observed in one case using oral ruxolitinib (given for alopecia areata), until the medication was discontinued.[67]
- Repigmentation of 5% body surface area, described as nearly complete on the forehead and hands, was observed in another vitiligo case (with generalized, progressive disease resistant to topicals or NBUVB), after oral intake of JAK 1/3 inhibitor tofacitinib citrate.[68]

Repigmentation and Afamelanotide

The synthetic analogue of α-melanocyte-stimulating hormone, afamelanotide, is a promising treatment alternative for vitiligo, currently in phase III clinical trials. Repigmentation generated by the combination of afamelanotide and NBUVB has been shown to be superior to that obtained with NBUVB monotherapy and being seen significantly earlier on the face and upper extremities in a significantly higher percent of patients, as compared with NBUVB monotherapy. Repigmentation with combination therapy was significantly superior at day 84 as compared with day 56 for patients of darker skin types (IV–VI), as measured using the Vitiligo Area Scoring Index.[69]

Repigmentation and Simvastatin

The 3-hydroxy-3-methyl-glutaryl coenzyme A reductase inhibitor simvastatin, approved by the Food and Drug Administration for treatment of hypercholesterolemia, was shown to inhibit IFN-γ-induced signal transducer and activator of transcription 1 (STAT1) activation *in vitro*.[70] High-dose simvastatin administrated in a patients with vitiligo with hypercholesterolemia resulted in rapid repigmentation of the skin, supporting simvastatin as a potential therapy for vitiligo.[71] Simvastatin given 3 times per week for 5 weeks in therapeutic doses used for human patients with hypercholesterolemia prevented and reversed depigmentation in the Krt14-Kitl* transgenic mice and reduced the number of CD8+ T cells in the skin.[72] Studies of safety and efficacy of this drug should be explored in depth in the future in vitiligo clinical trials. Its effect in inducing repigmentation in humans, observed only at high doses, suggests its utility as an adjuvant therapeutic alternative.

Repigmentation and Biologics

The effects of anti-TNF-α agents on repigmentation have been studied on a limited number of patients and have shown inconsistent results. Repigmentation following disease stabilization was reported after treatment with etanercept[73,74] or infliximab[75] or with the anti-CD20 monoclonal antibody-rituximab.[76] Repigmentation was not observed in a small number of patients with greater than 5% body surface area affected taking infliximab, or etanercept, or adalimumab,[75] whereas other studies actually reported spreading/onset of vitiligo after taking adalimumab[77–80] or infliximab.[75–79]

SUMMARY

- Both hair follicle and epidermal melanocyte precursors have the ability to proliferate, migrate, and differentiate in NBUVB-treated vitiligo, serving as a source for repigmentation, most commonly resulting in perifollicular and marginal patterns.
- Clinical observation of repigmentation in the glabrous skin, recently described as a medium-spotted pattern, suggests that melanocyte precursors/stem cells can remain in vitiliginous lesions, serving as a repigmentation reservoir. Confirmatory experimental work at the cellular and molecular levels is necessary.
- A reservoir of immature melanocytes was identified in the sweat gland ducts. Nevertheless, the role of an extrafollicular dermal source in vitiligo repigmentation needs further studies for clarification.
- Two signaling pathways, Wnt/β-catenin and p53, have been implicated in NBUVB-induced pigmentation. Further research is essential to identify in detail the cellular and molecular pathways governing the complex repopulation process.
- The treatments summarized earlier can provide acceptable results in hair-bearing areas and are typically unsatisfactory in areas devoid of hair follicles. To improve treatment outcomes in vitiligo repigmentation, we need to design new pharmacologic compounds that provide more robust stimulation of melanocyte precursors in the hair follicle and epidermis.

ACKNOWLEDGMENTS

The authors thank the National Disease Research Institute for providing human skin samples.

REFERENCES

1. Birlea SA, Spritz RA, Norris DA. Vitiligo. In: Wolff K, Goldsmith LA, Katz SI, et al, editors. Fitzpatrick's dermatology in general medicine. 8th edition. New York: McGraw-Hill; 2012. p. 792–803.
2. Falabella R. Vitiligo and the melanocyte reservoir. Indian J Dermatol 2009;54(4):313–8.
3. Kanwar AJ, Parsad D. Understanding the mechanism of repigmentation in vitiligo. In: Gupta S, Olsson MJ, Kanwar AJ, et al, editors. Surgical management of vitiligo. 1st edition. MA: John Wiley & Sons; 2007. p. 14–9.
4. Goldstein NB, Koster MI, Hoaglin LG, et al. Narrow band ultraviolet B treatment for human vitiligo is associated with proliferation, migration and differentiation of melanocyte precursors. J Invest Dermatol 2015;135(8):2068–76.
5. Jung SE, Kang HY, Lee ES, et al. Changes of epidermal thickness in vitiligo. Am J Dermatopathol 2015;37(4):289–92.
6. Meyer KC, Klatte JE, Dinh HV, et al. Evidence that the bulge region is a site of relative immune privilege in human hair follicles. Br J Dermatol 2008;159(5):1077–85.
7. Yang YS, Cho HR, Ryou JH, et al. Clinical study of repigmentation patterns with either narrow-band ultraviolet B (NBUVB) or 308 nm excimer laser treatment in Korean vitiligo patients. Int J Dermatol 2010;49(3):317–23.
8. Kim DY, Cho SB, Park YK. Various patterns of repigmentation after narrowband UVB monotherapy in patients with vitiligo. J Dermatol 2005;32(9):771–2.
9. Parsad D, Pandhi R, Dogra S, et al. Clinical study of repigmentation patterns with different treatment modalities and their correlation with speed and stability of repigmentation in 352 vitiliginous patches. J Am Acad Dermatol 2004;50(1):63–7.
10. Gan EY, Gahat T, Cario-André M, et al. Clinical repigmentation patterns in paediatric vitiligo. Br J Dermatol 2016;175:555–60.
11. Davids LM, du Toit E, Kidson SH, et al. A rare repigmentation pattern in a vitiligo patient: a clue to an epidermal stem-cell reservoir of melanocytes? Clin Exp Dermatol 2009;34(2):246–8.
12. Staricco RG, Miller-Milinska A. Activation of the amelanotic melanocytes in the outer root sheath of the hair follicle following ultra violet rays exposure. J Invest Dermatol 1962;39:163–4.
13. Staricco RG. Amelanotic melanocytes in the outer sheath of the human hair follicle and their role in the repigmentation of regenerated epidermis. Ann N Y Acad Sci 1963;100:239–55.
14. Ortonne JP, Schmitt D, Thivolet J. PUVA-induced repigmentation of vitiligo: scanning electron microscopy of hair follicles. J Invest Dermatol 1980;74(1):40–2.
15. Arrunátegui A, Arroyo C, Garcia L, et al. Melanocyte reservoir in vitiligo. Int J Dermatol 1994;33(7):4847.
16. Tobin DJ, Colen SR, Bystryn JC. Isolation and long-term culture of human hair-follicle melanocytes. J Invest Dermatol 1995;104(1):86–9.
17. Horikawa T, Norris DA, Johnson TW, et al. DOPA-negative melanocytes in the outer root sheath of human hair follicles express premelanosomal antigens but not a melanosomal antigen or the melanosome-associated glycoproteins tyrosinase, TRP-1, and TRP-2. J Invest Dermatol 1996;106(1):28–35.
18. Cui J, Shen LY, Wang GC. Role of hair follicles in the repigmentation of vitiligo. J Invest Dermatol 1991;97(3):410–6.
19. Nishimura EK, Jordan SA, Oshima H, et al. (2002) Dominant role of the niche in melanocyte stem-cell fate determination. Nature 2002;416(6883):854–60.

20. Nishimura EK, Granter SR, Fisher DE. Mechanisms of hair graying: incomplete melanocyte stem cell maintenance in the niche. Science 2005;307(5710): 720–4.
21. Medic S, Ziman M. PAX3 expression in normal skin melanocytes and melanocytic lesions (naevi and melanomas). PLoS One 2010;5(4):e9977.
22. Grichnik JM, Ali WN, Burch JA, et al. KIT expression reveals a population of precursor melanocytes in human skin. J Invest Dermatol 1996;106(5):967–71.
23. Husain I, Vijayan E, Ramaiah A, et al. Demonstration of tyrosinase in the vitiligo skin of human beings by a sensitive fluorometric method as well as by 14C(U)-L-tyrosine incorporation into melanin. J Invest Dermatol 1982;78(3):243–52.
24. Tobin DJ, Swanson NN, Pittelkow MR, et al. Melanocytes are not absent in lesional skin of long duration vitiligo. J Pathol 2000;191(4):407–16.
25. Dogra S, Kumar B. Repigmentation in vitiligo universalis: role of melanocyte density, disease duration, and melanocytic reservoir. Dermatol Online J 2005; 11(3):30.
26. Bellei B, Pitisci A, Ottaviani M, et al. Vitiligo: a possible model of degenerative diseases. PLoS One 2013;8(3):e59782.
27. Yoshida H, Kunisada T, Grimm T, et al. Review: melanocyte migration and survival controlled by SCF/c-kit expression. J Investig Dermatol Symp Proc 2001; 6(1):1–5.
28. Hoerter JD, Bradley P, Casillas A, et al. Extrafollicular dermal melanocyte stem cells and melanoma. Stem Cells Int 2012;2012:407079.
29. Okamoto N, Aoto T, Uhara H, et al. A melanocyte-melanoma precursor niche in sweat glands of volar skin. Pigment Cell Melanoma Res 2014;27(6):1039–50.
30. Birlea SA, Costin GE, Norris DA. New insights on therapy with vitamin D analogs targeting the intracellular pathways that control repigmentation in human vitiligo. Med Res Rev 2009;29(3):514–46.
31. Parsad D, Bhatnagar A, De D, et al. Vitiligo: treatment with narrowband ultraviolet B: side effects of NBUVB in vitiligo patients: short & long term. 2010. Available at: http://www.medscape.org/viewarticle/725936_5.
32. Kawaguchi Y, Mori N, Nakayama A. Kit(+) melanocytes seem to contribute to melanocyte proliferation after UV exposure as precursor cells. J Invest Dermatol 2001;116(6):920–5.
33. Parsad D. Natural history and prognosis. In: Vitiligo. Picardo M, Taïeb A, editors. Heidelberg (Germany): Springer; 2010. p. 139–42.
34. Mosenson JA, Zloza A, Nieland JD, et al. Mutant HSP70 reverses autoimmune depigmentation in vitiligo. Sci Transl Med 2013;5(174):174.
35. Rashighi M, Harris JE. Interfering with the IFN-γ/CXCL10 pathway to develop new targeted treatments for vitiligo. Ann Transl Med 2015;3(21):343.
36. Spritz RA. Modern vitiligo genetics sheds new light on an ancient disease. J Dermatol 2013;40(5):310–8.
37. Costin GE, Hearing VJ. Human skin pigmentation: melanocytes modulate skin color in response to stress. FASEB J 2007;21(4):976–94.
38. Hirobe T. How are proliferation and differentiation of melanocytes regulated? Pigment Cell Melanoma Res 2011;24(3):462–78.
39. Burren R, Scaletta C, Frenk E, et al. Sunlight and carcinogenesis: expression of p53 and pyrimidine dimers in human skin following UVA I, UVA I + II and solar simulating radiations. Int J Cancer 1998; 76(2):201–26.
40. Will K, Neben M, Schmidt-Rose T, et al. p53-dependent UVB responsiveness of human keratinocytes can be altered by cultivation on cell cycle-arrested dermal fibroblasts. Photochem Photobiol 2000; 71(3):321–6.
41. Murase D, Hachiya A, Amano Y, et al. The essential role of p53 in hyperpigmentation of the skin via regulation of paracrine melanogenic cytokine receptor signaling. J Biol Chem 2009;284(7):4343–53.
42. Yamada T, Hasegawa S, Inoue Y, et al. Wnt/β-catenin and kit signaling sequentially regulate melanocyte stem cell differentiation in UVB-induced epidermal pigmentation. J Invest Dermatol 2013; 133(12):2753–62.
43. Osawa M. Melanocyte stem cells. In: Girard L, editor. Stem book. 1st edition. Cambridge (MA): 2009. p. 11–12. Available at: https://www.ncbi.nlm.nih.gov/books/NBK27077/. Accessed February 8, 2017.
44. Fu J, Hsu W. Epidermal Wnt controls hair follicle induction by orchestrating dynamic signaling crosstalk between the epidermis and dermis. J Invest Dermatol 2013;133(4):890–8.
45. Choi YS, Zhang Y, Xu M, et al. Distinct functions for Wnt/β-catenin in hair follicle stem cell proliferation and survival and interfollicular epidermal homeostasis. Cell Stem Cell 2013;13(6):720–33.
46. Regazzetti C, Joly F, Marty C, et al. Transcriptional analysis of vitiligo skin reveals the alteration of WNT pathway: a promising target for repigmenting vitiligo patients. J Invest Dermatol 2015;135(12): 3105–14.
47. Sun P, Watanabe K, Fallahi M, et al. Pygo2 regulates β-catenin-induced activation of hair follicle stem/progenitor cells and skin hyperplasia. Proc Natl Acad Sci U S A 2014;111(28):10215–20.
48. Kunisada T, Yoshida H, Yamazaki H, et al. Transgene expression of steel factor in the basal layer of epidermis promotes survival, proliferation, differentiation and migration of melanocyte precursors. Development 1998;125(15):2915–23.
49. Chou WC, Takeo M, Rabbani P, et al. Direct migration of follicular melanocyte stem cells to the epidermis after wounding or UVB irradiation is dependent on Mc1r signaling. Nat Med 2013;19(7):924–9.

50. Kovacs D, Abdel-Raouf H, Al-Khayyat M, et al. Vitiligo: characterization of melanocytes in repigmented skin after punch grafting. J Eur Acad Dermatol Venereol 2015;29(3):581–90.
51. Whitton ME, Pinart M, Batchelor J, et al. Interventions for vitiligo. Cochrane Database Syst Rev 2015;24(2):CD003263.
52. White RA, Neiman JM, Reddi A, et al. Epithelial stem cell mutations that promote squamous cell carcinoma metastasis. J Clin Invest 2013;123(10): 4390–404.
53. Njoo MD, Spuls PI, Bos JD, et al. Nonsurgical repigmentation therapies in vitiligo. Meta-analysis of the literature. Arch Dermatol 1998;134(12): 1532–40.
54. Parsad D, Kanwar AJ, Kumar B. Psoralen-ultraviolet A vs. narrow-band ultraviolet B phototherapy for the treatment of vitiligo. J Eur Acad Dermatol Venereol 2006;20(2):175–7.
55. Mouzakis JA, Liu S, Cohen G. Rapid response of facial vitiligo to 308 nm excimer laser and topical calcipotriene. J Clin Aesthet Dermatol 2011;4(6):41–4.
56. Stevenson S, Thornton J. Effect of estrogens on skin aging and the potential role of SERMs. Clin Interv Aging 2007;2(3):283–97.
57. Hann SK, Kim HI, Im S, et al. The change of melanocyte cytotoxicity after systemic steroid treatment in vitiligo patients. J Dermatol Sci 1993; 6(3):201–5.
58. Sisti A, Sisti G, Oranges CM. Effectiveness and safety of topical tacrolimus monotherapy for repigmentation in vitiligo: a comprehensive literature review. An Bras Dermatol 2016;91(2):187–95.
59. Lan CC, Chen GS, Chiou MH, et al. FK506 promotes melanocyte and melanoblast growth and creates a favourable milieu for cell migration via keratinocytes: possible mechanisms of how tacrolimus ointment induces repigmentation in patients with vitiligo. Br J Dermatol 2005;153(3): 498–505.
60. Jung H, Chung H, Chang SE, et al. FK506 regulates pigmentation by maturing the melanosome and facilitating their transfer to keratinocytes. Pigment Cell Melanoma Res 2016;29(2):199–209.
61. Kang HY, Choi YM. FK506 increases pigmentation and migration of human melanocytes. Br J Dermatol 2006;155(5):1037–40.
62. Dang YP, Li Q, Shi F, et al. Effect of topical calcineurin inhibitors as monotherapy or combined with phototherapy for vitiligo treatment: a meta-analysis. Dermatol Ther 2016;29(2):126–33.
63. Wong R, Lin AN. Efficacy of topical calcineurin inhibitors in vitiligo. Int J Dermatol 2013;52(4):491–6.
64. Birlea SA, Costin GE, Norris DA. Cellular and molecular mechanisms involved in the action of vitamin D analogs targeting vitiligo depigmentation. Curr Drug Targets 2008;9(4):345–59.
65. Picardo M. Vitamin D analogs. In: Picardo M, Taïeb A, editors. Vitiligo. Heidelberg (Germany): Springer; 2010. p. 339–42.
66. Harel S, Higgins CA, Cerise JE, et al. Pharmacologic inhibition of JAK-STAT signaling promotes hair growth. Sci Adv 2015;1(9):e1500973.
67. Harris JE, Rashighi M, Nguyen N, et al. Rapid skin repigmentation on oral ruxolitinib in a patient with coexistent vitiligo and alopecia areata (AA). J Am Acad Dermatol 2016;74(2):370–1.
68. Craiglow BG, King BA. Tofacitinib citrate for the treatment of vitiligo: a pathogenesis-directed therapy. JAMA Dermatol 2015;151(10):1110–2.
69. Lim HW, Grimes PE, Agbai O, et al. Afamelanotide and narrowband UV-B phototherapy for the treatment of vitiligo: a randomized multicenter trial. JAMA Dermatol 2015;151(1):42–50.
70. Zhao Y, Gartner U, Smith FJ, et al. Statins downregulate K6a promoter activity: a possible therapeutic avenue for pachyonychia congenita. J Invest Dermatol 2011;131(5):1045–52.
71. Noël M, Gagné C, Bergeron J, et al. Positive pleiotropic effects of HMG-CoA reductase inhibitor on vitiligo. Lipids Health Dis 2004;3:7.
72. Agarwal P, Rashighi M, Essien KI, et al. Simvastatin prevents and reverses depigmentation in a mouse model of vitiligo. J Invest Dermatol 2015;135(4): 1080–8.
73. Rigopoulos D, Gregoriou S, Larios G, et al. Etanercept in the treatment of vitiligo. Dermatology 2007; 215(1):84–5.
74. Kim NH, Torchia D, Rouhani P, et al. Tumor necrosis factor-a in vitiligo: direct correlation between tissue levels and clinical parameters. Cutan Ocul Toxicol 2011;30(3):225–7.
75. Alghamdi KM, Khurrum H, Taieb A, et al. Treatment of generalized vitiligo with anti-TNF-a agents. J Drugs Dermatol 2012;11(4):534–9.
76. Ruiz-Argüelles A, García-Carrasco M, Jimenez-Brito G, et al. Treatment of vitiligo with a chimeric monoclonal antibody to CD20: a pilot study. Clin Exp Immunol 2013;174(2):229–36.
77. Jung JM, Lee YJ, Won CH, et al. Development of vitiligo during treatment with adalimumab: a plausible or paradoxical response? Ann Dermatol 2015; 27(5):620–1.
78. Maruthappu T, Leandro M, Morris SD. Deterioration of vitiligo and new onset of halo naevi observed in two patients receiving adalimumab. Dermatol Ther 2013;26(4):370–2.
79. Posada C, Flórez A, Batalla A, et al. Vitiligo during treatment of Crohn's disease with adalimumab: adverse effect or co-occurrence? Case Rep Dermatol 2011;3(1):28–31.
80. Smith DI, Heffernan MP. Vitiligo after the resolution of psoriatic plaques during treatment with adalimumab. J Am Acad Dermatol 2008;58(2 Suppl):S50–2.

Depigmentation Therapies for Vitiligo

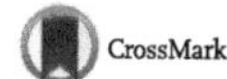

Pearl E. Grimes, MD[a,b,*], Rama Nashawati, BS, MSGM[a]

KEYWORDS

- Depigmentation • Vitiligo • Pigmentary disorders • Disorders of appearance
- Monobenzyl ether of hydroquinone • MBEH • 4-Methoxyphenol • Mequinol

KEY POINTS

- The general goals of medical management of vitiligo are to repigment affected areas of skin and to stabilize the progression of depigmentation.
- However, for some patients with vitiligo affecting extensive body surface areas who are unresponsive to repigmentation therapies, depigmentation of the remaining normal skin may be a better choice.
- Candidates for depigmentation therapy should be carefully screened and patient education is essential.
- Permanent topical therapies used for depigmentation include monobenzyl ether of hydroquinone, 4-methoxyphenol, and 88% phenol. Physical modalities, such as cryotherapy and lasers, are also being used successfully.

INTRODUCTION

Vitiligo is a common acquired disorder of the epidermis and hair follicles that manifests clinically as progressive depigmentation due to loss of functioning melanocytes. It affects 1% to 2% of the global population.[1] Studies suggest an equal incidence in all racial-ethnic groups. However, because of the highly visible contrast between the constitutive skin color and the white patches, vitiligo can be particularly disfiguring in darker-complexioned skin types.[2,3] Given the disfiguring aspect of the disease, vitiligo can profoundly impact the quality of life in children and adults.[4,5]

Multiple theories have been proffered for the pathogenesis of vitiligo, including autoimmune, biochemical, oxidative stress, neural, melanocytorrhagy and viral mechanisms.[2] However, multiple recent studies document the expanding role of immune mechanisms in the pathogenesis of vitiligo.[6,7]

In general, therapies for vitiligo address stabilization of the disease and repigmentation of affected sites. Stabilization agents include systemic corticosteroids, oral mini-pulse corticosteroid therapy, minocycline, and methotrexate. First-line therapies for repigmentation are calcineurin inhibitors, topical corticosteroids, and narrow band (NB)-UVB phototherapy. Although many patients achieve successful repigmentation outcomes, others develop progressive disease affecting extensive body surface areas and fail to respond to repigmentation protocols. The goal for such patients with extensive disease would be to create a uniform skin tone by depigmenting the remaining pigmented skin sites.

CANDIDATES FOR DEPIGMENTATION THERAPY

Depigmentation therapy can be a viable therapeutic alternative in patients with extensive disease

[a] Vitiligo & Pigmentation Institute of Southern California, 5670 Wilshire Boulevard #650, Los Angeles, CA 90036, USA; [b] Division of Dermatology, David Geffen School of Medicine, University of California, Los Angeles, 10833 Le Conte Avenue, Los Angeles, CA 90095, USA
* Corresponding author. 5670 Wilshire Boulevard #650, Los Angeles, CA 90036.
E-mail address: pegrimesmd@aol.com

Dermatol Clin 35 (2017) 219–227
http://dx.doi.org/10.1016/j.det.2016.11.010
0733-8635/17/

affecting greater than 30% to 40% of body surface areas.[2,3,8]

Most patients who choose depigmentation have failed to achieve optimal repigmentation. Depigmentation therapy can be used in all skin types devastated by the contrasting areas of normal and vitiliginous skin. Patient selection is of paramount importance, given the permanency of depigmentation therapy (**Box 1**). Prospective patients should be carefully screened. A detailed medical history should be obtained including any history of psychiatric illness portending unrealistic therapeutic outcomes.[9] An extended consultation should be conducted with patients and their families when possible. Issues that should be discussed in depth are included in **Box 2**. It is imperative that potential patients thoroughly understand the permanent nature of the process. It is important with younger patients and their families to explain that if medical advances provide new therapies for repigmentation, they may not be candidates for such therapies if they have undergone depigmentation.[10] All patients treated at the Vitiligo & Pigmentation Institute of Southern California sign an informed consent before initiating depigmentation therapy. A sample template of the authors' informed consent is included in **Box 3**.

The decision to undergo depigmentation of areas of normal skin is especially complex. For example, the decision may be more complicated for African Americans and Asians by the continued presence of secondary racial characteristics, such as facial features and hair texture. Thus, the potential sociocultural issues should be thoroughly explored with patients before initiating therapy.

TOPICAL DEPIGMENTATION THERAPIES

The most readily available depigmenting agents include monobenzyl ether of hydroquinone (MBEH), 4-methoxyphenol (4MP, mequinol or p-hydroxyanisole) and phenol (**Table 1**). In addition, physical therapies, such as lasers and cryotherapy, both as monotherapy and as adjuncts to topical treatments, are also used for depigmentation.

Depigmentation is a gradual process characterized by gradual progressive fading of patients' unaffected normal pigmentation. Complete depigmentation may require 1 to 3 years of treatment. In the authors' experience, most patients are satisfied with the therapeutic outcomes.

Box 1
General indications and inclusion criteria for depigmentation therapy

- Patients with severe disease affecting greater than 30% or 40% body surface areas who have failed repigmentation therapies
- Patients with severe disease affecting greater than 30% or 40% depigmentation who are unable to undergo the time and rigors of repigmentation therapies
- Emotionally stable patients
- Patients willing to adhere to photoprotection
- A willingness to accept the inability to tan

Box 2
Issues for discussion with prospective patients

- Permanency of the treatment
- Realistic expectations
- Color match with areas of depigmentation
- Treatment time and cost
- Mechanism of action of the drug, including depigmentation at sites distal to areas of use
- Drug-related side effects
- The potential for patchy repigmentation
- Consort depigmentation with inappropriate use

Monobenzyl Ether of Hydroquinone

MBEH (p-benzyloxy-phenol, monobenzone) is the only topical depigmenting agent that is currently approved for vitiligo by the Food and Drug Administration. Moreover, the only indication for use of the drug is in patients with vitiligo (**Figs. 1** and **2**). It is a hydroquinone (HQ) derivative. MBEH was ushered into the realm of dermatology in the late 1930s following seminal observations by McNally[11] and Oliver and colleagues.[12,13] They reported that workers exposed to MBEH, which was used as an antioxidant in the rubber tannery industry, developed depigmentation. Tannery workers developed white patches at the site of chemical contact from their rubber gloves that contained Agerite Alba (MBEH). Depigmentation also developed at sites distal to exposure to the chemical.

Although MBEH is structurally related to HQ, commonly used as a hypopigmenting agent, it has not been associated with the development of exogenous ochronosis. This condition is a rare but serious complication of prolonged use of HQ frequently seen in users of over-the-counter skin bleaching creams. MBEH remains the first-line agent for depigmentation in patients with vitiligo.

Box 3
Consent form for treatment with monobenzyl ether of hydroquinone

I have been informed by ____________________ of the benefits, risks, possible alternative methods of treatment, and possible consequences involved in depigmentation therapy with monobenzyl ether of hydroquinone (MBEH, monobenzone) for the relief of vitiligo.

Depigmentation therapy for vitiligo has been explained to me in detail. The benefits include evening out of my skin tone by removing the remaining pigmentation with MBEH cream 20%. Higher concentrations can also be used (30%, 40%).

MBEH cream is a depigmenting agent whose mechanism of action is not fully understood. MBEH may cause destruction of melanocytes (skin cells that produce pigment) and permanent depigmentation. It may take 1 to 4 months before lightening begins to appear. When applied to my skin, this drug induces progressive and diffuse depigmentation of the normal pigmented skin. After several months, depigmentation also commonly develops on areas of normal skin where the drug has never been applied. Exposure to sunlight reduces the depigmenting (fading) effect of the drug. The appearance of the skin when examined under a microscope after depigmentation with topical monobenzone is the same as that seen in vitiligo; the skin is normal except for the absence of identifiable melanocytes.

Potential side effects include recurrence of pigmentation after depigmentation, severe allergic reactions of the skin, alopecia, dermatitis, dry skin, redness of the skin, itching, premature graying, and vitiligolike pigment loss in a spouse or other individuals if intimate contact occurs. My skin must be protected from sun exposure at all times. Sun exposure can cause depigmented areas to repigment. My treated skin will not tan.

In a small minority of patients, intense hyperpigmentation (darken of the skin) can occur after use of MBEH.

Understanding that stated above, I hereby authorize the above doctor, or whomever he or she may designate, to administer such treatment to me. If I had any questions regarding this treatment, I have asked the doctor and have received all needed answers.

____

Name of patient

____

Signature of patient

____

Signature of witness

MBEH has been shown to be selectively cytotoxic toward melanocytes. The drug's dependence on melanocytes is evidenced in patients who selectively develop irritation from MBEH only in pigmented areas of skin[14–16] (**Fig. 3**). This selective action may be due to its structural homology with tyrosine. When combined with tyrosinase, which is rate limiting for melanogenesis, MBEH is converted into reactive quinones that may react with enzymatic compounds within the melanosome. Reactive quinones can act as potent skin sensitizers. MBEH-induced melanocyte necrosis has shown a negative correlation with cellular melanin content suggesting that melanin may protect against MBEH-induced necrosis.[15] These data correlate with the authors' clinical experience of observing severe rebound pigmentation in primarily darker racial ethnic groups.

Table 1
Agents for depigmentation

First-Line Therapies	Emerging Therapies
MBEH/monobenzone	Imatinib
Monomethyl ether of hydroquinone/4-methoxyphenol	Imiquimod
88% Phenol	Diphencyprone
Cryotherapy	
Lasers	
Q-switched ruby	
Q-switched alexandrite	

MBEH is converted into a reactive quinone product (4-benzoxy-1,2-benzoquinone) that binds as a quinone-hapten to cysteine residues in the tyrosinase protein, hence, generating neoantigens in the tyrosinase peptide chain. The formation of neoantigens stimulates a systemic immune

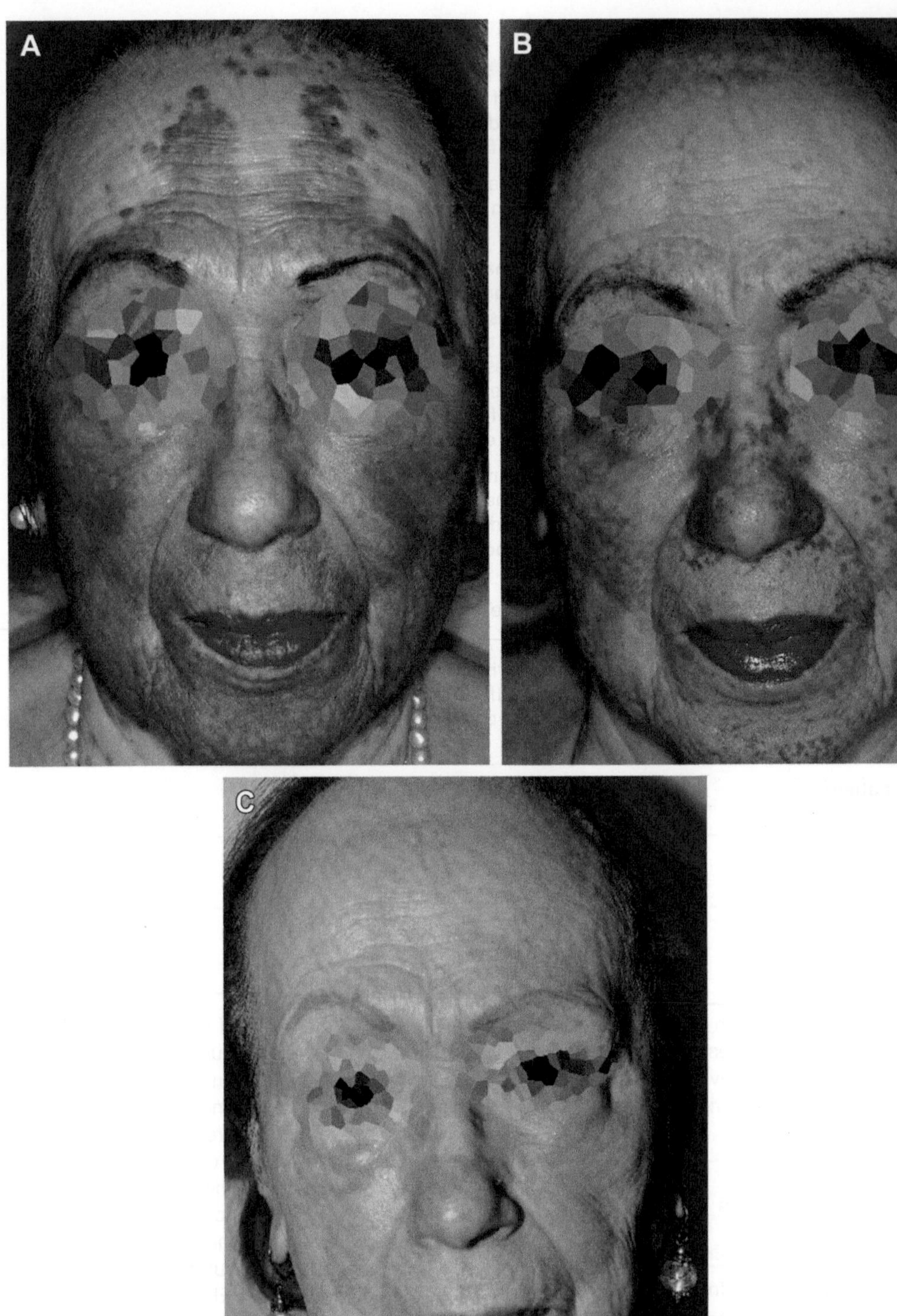

Fig. 1. A 72-year-old woman with extensive vitiligo unresponsive to repigmentation therapies. (*A*) Before MBEH. (*B*) After 3 months of daily treatment with MBEH 20%. (*C*) After 1 year of treatment with MBEH 20%.

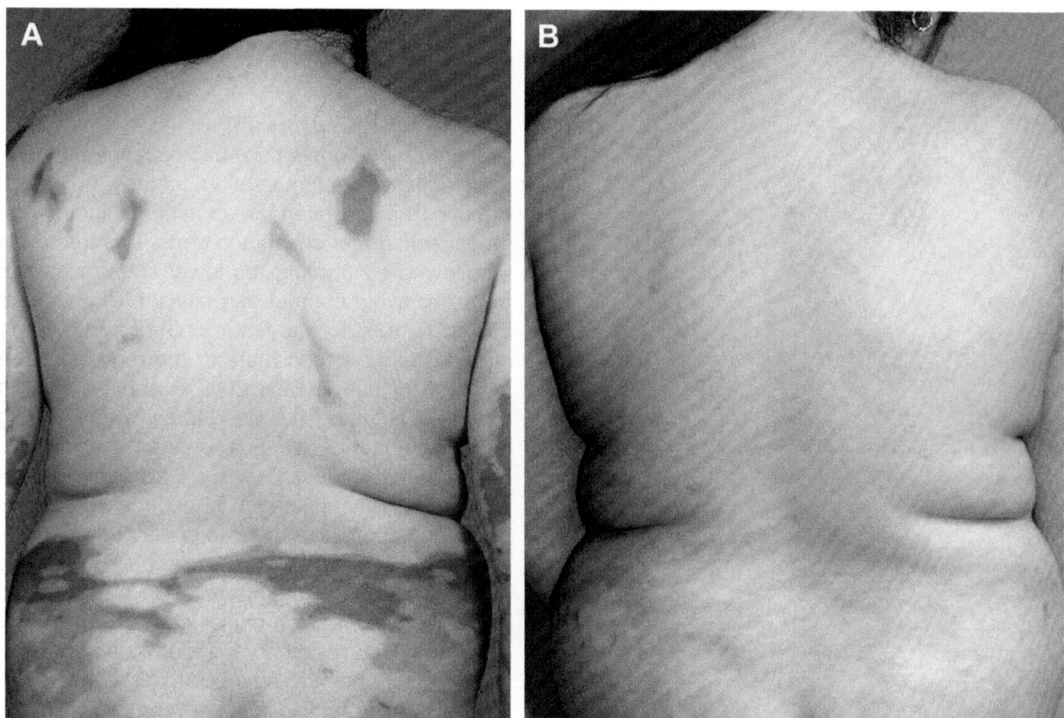

Fig. 2. A 21-year-old woman with severe generalized vitiligo; minimal response to NB-UVB phototherapy. (*A*) Before MBEH. (*B*) After 6 months of daily treatment with MBEH 20%.

T-cell–mediated destruction of melanocytes.[15–17] The conversion of MBEH by tyrosinase also generates reactive oxygen species (ROS), which induce lysosomal destruction of melanosomes, autophagy, and tyrosinase ubiquitination.[17] These changes eventuate in surface presentation of melanosome-derived antigens in surface major histocompatibility complex class I and II molecules, stimulating antigen-specific T-cell responses. ROS generation also promotes the excretion of exosomes, which activate the innate immune response.[17]

MBEH induces chemical vitiligo. Therefore, it is paramount that all users understand that the only indication for use of this agent is in vitiligo, given its ability to induce depigmentation at sites distal to drug application. It should NEVER be prescribed as a hypopigmenting agent. The authors have evaluated several patients in which MBEH was prescribed as a skin-lightening agent for hyperpigmentation and vitiligo ensued. One case occurred in a 35-year-old woman who was given MBEH by a relative in the medical profession for treatment of postinflammatory hyperpigmentation of the face. After 6 months of use, the patient developed disseminated depigmented patches affecting the face, trunk, and extremities.

Mosher and colleagues[18] treated 18 patients with severe vitiligo with 20% MBEH. Fifteen were women. Sixteen were Caucasian and 2 were black. Eight achieved complete depigmentation after 10 months or more of use. Three experienced significant but not complete depigmentation. Three patients had no response. They used MBEH for less than 4 months. Three experienced some pigment loss; one patient developed contact dermatitis, which prevented further use of MBEH. Depigmentation began to appear after 2 to 3 months of using the drug. All patients achieving complete depigmentation were pleased with the outcome. Other side effects included burning, itching, erythema, and dryness.

A retrospective study reviewed all cases of vitiligo treated with MBEH at a London hospital over a 6.5-year period.[19] The study population consisted of 53 subjects (79% female), with a mean age of 42.3 years. Most subjects had either olive or darker Asian skin color (23% and 62%, respectively). The mean vitiligo duration was 18.5 years (range 2–60 years). More than half of the subjects had greater than 75% body surface area involvement. The most frequently treated areas were the face (89%) and upper limbs (64%), followed by the trunk, lower limbs, hands, and neck. The highest tolerated concentration of MBEH was 20% for most patients, although tolerated concentrations ranged from 5% to 50% MBEH. The mean duration of application was 6.4 years (range 0.5–30.0

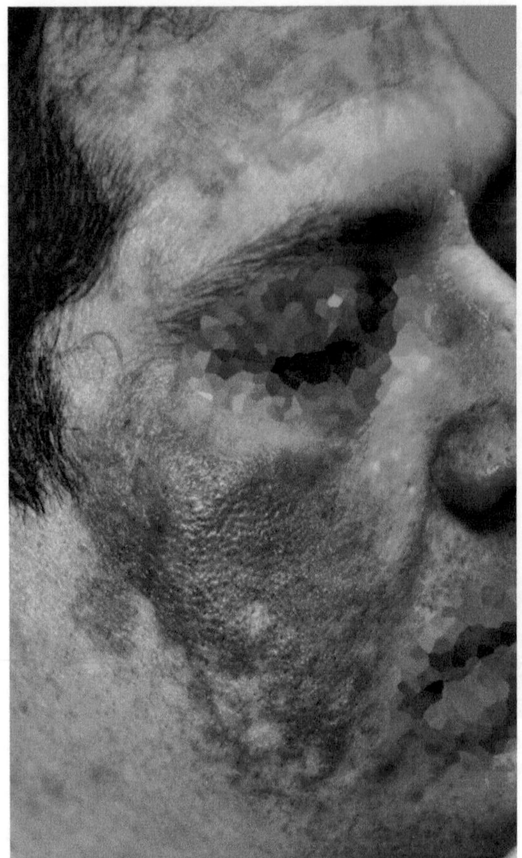

Fig. 3. Allergic contact dermatitis from MBEH. Note edema and erythema only affecting the pigmented areas of skin.

years). In 34% of the subjects, depigmentation was noted to be "marked but incomplete" with a mean time to depigmentation of 9.7 months. The investigators underscored the high (78%) repigmentation rate of successfully depigmented areas, which, they noted, was most often caused by sun exposure. Nearly half the subjects had dose-dependent skin irritation, which was resolved with a reduction in MBEH concentration.

The depigmenting efficacy of MBEH has been demonstrated in the black guinea pig model to be synergistically enhanced by the addition of retinoic acid (RA), which can inhibit glutathione-s-transferase protection of melanocytes, increasing melanocyte susceptibility to depigmenting agents.[20] When 10% MBEH was combined with RA 0.025%, the combination produced complete depigmentation in 4 of 6 treated areas and moderate depigmentation in 2 areas after 10 days of treatment, which was significantly better than that achieved with MBEH alone ($P = .002$). Unlike with the latter, the depigmentation that occurred with the combination was almost always uniform. The combination also reduced the average number of melanocytes to 6 ($\pm$6) per field versus 42 $\pm$ 6 per field with MBEH alone.

Depigmentation protocol

After informed consent has been obtained, the authors initiate depigmentation therapy in stages treating the exposed areas first, including the face, neck, upper chest, and arms. This treatment is followed by treating the lower extremities and trunk. To avoid contact dermatitis, MBEH 20% is diluted to 10% for the first month of treatment to allow patients to acclimate to the regimen. After 1 month of use, MBEH 20% is applied daily. If tolerated, it can be increased to twice daily during the third month of use. For some patients xerosis mitigates twice-daily use. By 3 to 6 months of use, most patients begin to experience loss of pigmentation at sites distal to areas of drug application. If the treated areas are unresponsive to MBEH 20%, the concentration can be increased to 30% or 40%. Such higher concentration may offer enhanced results for the elbows and knees.[8]

Given its potential for ocular irritation, MBEH should not be applied to the eyelid area. Broad-spectrum high sun-protection-factor sunscreens must be worn daily along with photo-protective clothing. Current data suggest that MBEH only destroys epidermal melanocytes. Follicular melanocytes, in general, may remain intact. Hence, sun exposure can often trigger follicular and confluent areas of repigmentation.

Complications

In general, depigmentation is tolerated well by most patients. Some experience mild to moderate xerosis; hence, additional use of emollients is essential during treatment. Irritant contact dermatitis and less common allergic reactions can be mitigated by initiating treatment with a lower concentration (10%) of MBEH. Other reactions include erythema, pruritus, and unmasking preexisting telangiectases.[8,18] The authors have observed 2 cases of alopecia and premature graying in patients using excessive quantities of MBEH. In addition, the authors have had 3 cases of depigmentation occurring in consorts of individuals undergoing depigmentation. In 2 cases, the spouse of the patient undergoing depigmentation developed vitiligo as a result of MBEH exposure following bedtime application of MBEH in the patient. In another instance, a child developed vitiligo following exposure from the mother who was undergoing depigmentation therapy. Hence, very detailed instructions must be provided to patients to avoid this complication, including avoiding immediate contact with the spouse or other intimate relationships following application of the drug. Showers or baths should be taken before intimate connubial relations. Protective clothing can also be worn to minimize exposures. Rare cases of corneal and conjunctival melanoses have also been reported.[21]

4-Methoxyphenol

4MP (mequinol) acts similarly to MBEH.[8] 4-MP is usually applied twice daily until complete depigmentation is achieved. Mequinol 20% cream as monotherapy and, in combination with Q-switched ruby laser (QSR), was studied in 16 patients with vitiligo universalis.[22] Of these, 13 were treated with both therapies, although not at the same time. Three patients used only the 4-MP cream. Of the 16 patients, 11 (69%) achieved total depigmentation. Onset of depigmentation was between 4 and 12 months with the cream. The relapse rate in the 11 patients who had responded to the cream was 36% after a treatment-free period of 2 to 36 months. Total depigmentation was achieved in 9 of 13 patients treated with QSR. Onset of depigmentation was 7 to 14 days after laser treatment. Between 2 and 10 treatments were required to achieve total depigmentation. Of patients who achieved total depigmentation, there was a 44% relapse rate after 2 to 18 months of no treatment. Pigment returned particularly on facial areas. The efficacy of 4-MP is correlated with duration of drug use.

Other studies have used topical depigmenting therapies in combination with physical methods inducing rapid and complete depigmentation such as cryotherapy and lasers. Di Nuzzo and Masotti[23] reported on a single patient with a 45-year history of vitiligo whose residual facial pigmentation was successfully treated with one session of cryotherapy, using 2 freeze-thaw cycles followed, after 3 weeks, by twice-daily application of 20% mequinol for 14 months. The pigment cleared successfully with no side effects, although small areas of repigmentation that developed 6 months after discontinuation of topical therapy required one further session of cryotherapy.

Complications

Side effects are mild and include burning, pruritus, and contact dermatitis.[22] Compared with MBEH, 4-MP may necessitate a longer duration of treatment to achieve optimal outcomes.

Phenol

Phenol 88% is a medium-depth peeling agent generally used for treatment of rhytids and photodamage. The melanotoxic effects of phenol are well documented.[24–26] Phenol suppresses melanogenesis and induces protein coagulation in the epidermis.[27] Zanini and Machado Filho[26] reported the efficacy of an 88% phenol solution for treatment of residual pigmentation of the neck in a 62-year-old woman with vitiligo. After 2 sessions, 45 days apart, there was total elimination of residual pigmentation. Kavuossi[25] used cryotherapy along with 88% phenol on a 13 year old with residual facial pigmentation. After one session the patient had complete clearing of the pigmented areas.

Complications

Cardiotoxicity and other systemic toxicities have been reported in patients treated with medium and deep phenol peeling.[24] However, its use in limited areas in patients with vitiligo has been well tolerated with minimal complications, including scarring.[8]

PHYSICAL DEPIGMENTATION THERAPIES

Cryotherapy achieves rapid and permanent depigmentation via irreversible tissue damage resulting from intracellular ice ball formation. Inflammation occurs within 24 hours of treatment, which also augments lesion destruction. Cryotherapy is particularly effective in areas of koebnerization.[8] Cryotherapy is advantageous because of its low cost and excellent side-effect profile. Anesthesia, sedatives, dressings, and antibiotics are not required. Physician experience is essential for optimum results, but experienced dermatologists can perform the procedure without scarring.

Lasers cause depigmentation by selectively targeting melanocytes. As with cryotherapy, lasers are particularly effective in patients with a positive Koebner status and can produce rapid depigmentation. Large areas of skin can be treated at one time with expeditious outcomes.[8] The effective wavelengths of the QSR laser are between 600 nm and 800 nm and are more easily absorbed by melanin than by hemoglobin.[28,29] The Q-switched alexandrite laser has a faster pulse frequency than the QSR, which permits more rapid therapy and has a higher wavelength (755 nm vs 694 nm), which may provide better tissue penetration.[30] In one study of 15 patients, the Nd:YAG laser was used at a wavelength of 532 nm to target only epidermal pigment and to encourage koebnerization of vitiliginous lesions. Excellent response, defined as greater than or equal to 90% depigmentation, was achieved by 13 of 15 patients, whereas 2 patients showed a poor response with less than 50% depigmentation. The number of sessions required to treat each site ranged between 1 and 3. None of the patients reported any significant adverse events.[31]

A retrospective study included 27 patients with widespread vitiligo who were treated with QSR depigmentation.[32] After a mean follow-up of 13 months, 48% showed greater than 75% depigmentation. Patients with active disease (63%) showed significantly greater depigmentation than those with stable disease (*P*<.05). From these findings, the authors recommend postponing treatment until the disease flares.

A recent retrospective study that compared depigmentation in 22 patients with generalized vitiligo who had previously been treated with cryotherapy or alexandrite 755 nm laser therapy found no significant difference in depigmentation activity after 1 treatment.[33] The study did find significant differences in percentage of depigmentation by area, with best results obtained on the trunk, followed by arms, face, and neck. No serious side effects were noted with either treatment, although mild hyperpigmentation was noted in a small number of cases with cryotherapy.

EMERGING THERAPIES

Other emerging therapies include imatinib, imiquimod, and diphencyprone. Imatinib (imatinib mesylate), used to treat a variety of conditions, including leukemias and gastrointestinal stromal tumors, interferes with the production of melanin through its inhibition of tyrosine kinase.[34,35] Patients treated with imatinib for chronic myelogenous leukemia have been reported to develop generalized hypopigmentation or depigmentation.[35] Imiquimod, usually used for the topical treatment of anogenital warts and basal cell carcinomas, is an imidazoquinoline immune response modifier that directly and indirectly influences cells to induce vitiligolike depigmented lesions.[36–38] Multiple cases of depigmentation at sites of imiquimod use have been reported. Diphencyprone can induce depigmentation as a side effect when used to treat alopecia areata.[39]

SUMMARY

Vitiligo can be psychologically devastating and socially stigmatizing, particularly for patients with darker skin types in whom the contrast between the bleached vitiliginous lesions and uninvolved skin can be especially apparent and disfiguring. In cases whereby vitiligo affects greater than 30% to 40% of the body, or has proven resistant to standard topical and light-based therapies, depigmentation therapy should be considered. Moreover, it can be considered in severe cases in which patients have no interest in repigmentation therapies. In addition to careful patient selection, patient education and counseling are key elements for positive long-term outcomes.

REFERENCES

1. Grimes PE. White patches and bruised souls: advances in the pathogenesis and treatment of vitiligo. J Am Acad Dermatol 2004;51:S5–7.
2. Grimes PE. Vitiligo: pathogenesis, clinical features, and diagnosis. In: Tsao H, editor. UpToDate; 2016. Available at: http://www.uptodate.com/contents/vitiligo-pathogenesis-clinical-features-and-diagnosis?source=search_result&search=grimes+vitiligo&selectedTitle=4%7E88.
3. Grimes PE. Vitiligo: management and prognosis. In: Tsao H, editor. UpToDate; 2016. Available at: http://www.uptodate.com/contents/vitiligo-management-and-prognosis?source=search_result&search=grimes+vitiligo&selectedTitle=2%7E88.
4. Kruger C, Schallreuter KU. Stigmatisation, avoidance behaviour and difficulties in coping are common among adult patients with vitiligo. Acta Derm Venerol 2015;95:553.
5. Silverberg JI, Silverberg NB. Quality of life impairment in children and adolescents with vitiligo. Pediatr Dermatol 2014;31:309.
6. Richmond JM, Frisoli ML, Harris JE. Innate immune mechanisms in vitiligo: danger from within. Curr Opin Immunol 2013;25(6):676–82.
7. van den Boorn JG, Konijnenberg D, Dellemijn TA, et al. Autoimmune destruction of skin melanocytes by perilesional T cells from vitiligo patients. J Invest Dermatol 2009;129(9):2220–32.
8. Gupta D, Kumari R, Thappa D. Depigmentation therapies in vitiligo. Indian J Dermatol Venereol Leprol 2012;78:49–58.
9. Grau C, Silverberg NB. Vitiligo patients seeking depigmentation therapy: a case report and guidelines for psychological screening. Cutis 2013;91:248–52.
10. Black W, Russell N, Cohen G. Depigmentation therapy for vitiligo in patients with Fitzpatrick skin type VI. Cutis 2012;89:57–60.
11. McNally W. A depigmentatioin of the skin. Industrial Med 1939;8:405–10.
12. Oliver EA, Schwartz L, Warren LH. Occupational leukoderma: preliminary report. JAMA 1939;113:927.
13. Oliver EA, Schwartz L, Warren LH. Occupational leukoderma. Arch Derm Syphilol 1940;42:993.
14. Nordlund JJ, Forget B, Kirkwood J, et al. Dermatitis produced by applications of monobenzone in patients with active vitiligo. Arch Dermatol 1985;121(9):1141–4.

15. Hariharan V, Toole T, Klarquist J, et al. Topical application of bleaching phenols: in vivo studies and mechanism of action relevant to melanoma treatment. Melanoma Res 2011;21:115–26.
16. Hariharan V, Klarquist J, Reust MJ, et al. Monobenzyl ether of hydroquinone and 4-tertiary butyl phenol activate markedly different physiological responses in melanocytes: relevance to skin depigmentation. J Invest Dermatol 2010;130:211–20.
17. Van doon Boom JG, Melief CJ, Luiten RM. Monobenzone induced depigmentation: from enzymatic blockade to autoimmunity. Pigment Cell Melanoma Res 2011;24:673–9.
18. Mosher DB, Parrish JA, Fitzpatrick TB. Monobenzylether of hydroquinone. Br J Dermatol 1977;97(6):669–79.
19. Tan ES-T, Sarkany R. Topical monobenzyl ether of hydroquinone is an effective and safe treatment for depigmentation of extensive vitiligo in the medium term: a retrospective cohort study of 53 cases. Br J Dermatol 2015;172:1662–4.
20. Kasraee B, Fallahi MR, Arekani GS, et al. Retinoic acid synergetically enhances the melanocytic and depigmenting effects of monobenzylether of hydroquinone in black guinea pig skin. Exp Dermatol 2006;15:509–14.
21. Hedges TR, Kenyon KR, Hanninen LA, et al. Corneal and conjunctival effects of monobenzone in patients with vitiligo. Arch Ophthalmol 1983;101(1):64–8.
22. Njoo MD, Vodegel RM, Westerhof W. Depigmentation therapy in vitiligo universalis with topical 4-methoxyphenol and the Q-switched ruby laser. J Am Acad Dermatol 2000;42(5 pt. 1):760–9.
23. Di Nuzzo S, Masotti A. Depigmentation therapy in vitiligo universalis with cryotherapy and 4-hydroxyanisole. Clin Exp Dermatol 2010;35:215–6.
24. Brody HJ. Variations and comparisons in medium-depth chemical peeling. J Dermatol Surg Oncol 1989;15(9):953–63.
25. Kavuossi H. Induction of depigmentation in a universal vitiligo patient with combination of cryotherapy and phenol. J Pak Assoc Dermatol 2009;19:112–4.
26. Zanini M, Machado Filho CD. Depigmentation therapy for generalized vitiligo with topical 88% phenol solution. An Bras Dermatol 2005;80(4):415–6.
27. Toosi S, Orlow SJ, Manga P. Vitiligo-inducing phenols activate the unfolded protein response in melanocytes resulting in upregulation of IL6 and IL8. J Invest Dermatol 2012;132(11):2601–9.
28. Alghamdi KM, Kumar A. Depigmentation therapies for normal skin in vitiligo universalis. J Eur Acad Dermatol Venereol 2011;25:749–57.
29. Nelson JS, Applebaum J. Treatment of superficial cutaneous pigmented lesions by melanin-specific selective photothermolysis using the Q-switched ruby laser. Ann Plast Surg 1992;29:231–7.
30. Rao J, Fitzpatrick RE. Use of the Q-switched 755 nm alexandrite laser to treat recalcitrant pigment after depigmentation therapy for vitiligo. Dermatol Surg 2004;30:1043–5.
31. Majid I, Imran S. Depigmentation therapy with Q-switched Nd:YAG laser in universal vitiligo. J Cutan Aesthet Surg 2013;6:93–6.
32. Komen L, Zwertbroek L, Burger SJ, et al. Q-switched laser depigmentation in vitiligo, most effective in active disease. Br J Dermatol 2013;169:1246–51.
33. Van Geel N, Depaepe L, Speeckaert R. Laser (755 nm) and cryotherapy as depigmentation treatments for vitiligo: a comparative study. J Eur Acad Dermatol Venereol 2015;29:1121–7.
34. Leong KW, Lee TC, Goh AS. Imatinib mesylate causes hypopigmentation in the skin. Cancer 2004;100:2486–7.
35. Aleem A. Hypopigmentation of the skin due to imatinib mesylate in patients with chronic myeloid leukemia. Hematol Oncol Stem Cell Ther 2009;2(2):358–61.
36. Zirvi TB, Costarelis G, Gelfand JM. Vitiligo-like hypopigmentation associated with imiquimod treatment of genital warts. J Am Acad Dermatol 2005;52:715–6.
37. Kang HY, Park TJ, Jin SH. Imiquimod, a toll-like receptor 7 agonist, inhibits melanogenesis and proliferation of human melanocytes. J Invest Dermatol 2009;129:243–6.
38. Kim CH, Ahn JH, Kang SU, et al. Imiquimod induces apoptosis of human melanocytes. Atch Dermatol Res 2010;302:301–6.
39. Duhra P, Foulds IS. Persistent vitiligo induced by diphencyprone. Br J Dermatol 1990;123:415–6.

Special Considerations in Children with Vitiligo

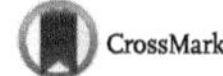

Alain Taïeb, MD, PhD[a,b,*], Julien Seneschal, MD, PhD[a,b], Juliette Mazereeuw-Hautier, MD, PhD[c]

KEYWORDS

• Child • Vitiligo • Hypopigmentation • Differential diagnosis • Therapy

KEY POINTS

- Childhood vitiligo differs from adult-onset vitiligo for several features including more segmental forms, higher prevalence of halo nevi, and more common family history for autoimmune diseases and atopic diathesis.
- The major differential diagnoses are the postinflammatory hypomelanoses for nonsegmental vitiligo and nevus depigmentosus for segmental vitiligo.
- From the therapeutic standpoint, early awareness of the diagnosis seems to correlate with a good treatment outcome in this age group.

INTRODUCTION, EPIDEMIOLOGY, AND CLASSIFICATION

Childhood vitiligo differs from adult-onset vitiligo for several features, but is basically the same disease, with a potentially better regenerative capacity of the melanocytic lineage. The exact prevalence of vitiligo in the pediatric age group is unknown but the figure of approximately 25% of onset of vitiligo before the age of 10 years obtained in Denmark seems correct.[1] The mean age of onset in pediatric series varied among different studies from 4 to 8 years,[2] but very early onset, as young as 3 months, is acknowledged, whereas congenital vitiligo is usually piebaldism misdiagnosed as vitiligo. The existence of true congenital vitiligo remains controversial. In fair-skinned individuals, vitiligo patches are usually detected only after the first exposure of the skin to sunlight, following the first summer of life. Girls predominate in reported pediatric series, but population-based studies do not confirm a sex bias.

The most common form of vitiligo in children is the nonsegmental type or "vitiligo" based on the international consensus.[3] Nevertheless, the percentage of segmental vitiligo (SV) is higher in children compared with adults, whatever the ethnic background, and suggests a mosaic skin developmental predisposition.[4] The prevalence of SV in childhood varies from 4.6% to 32.5% in published reports (reviewed in Ref.[2]). Mixed vitiligo is a more recently described, mostly pediatric subtype, with segmental involvement preceding typical generalized vitiligo.[5,6] This presentation may exist in adults but is probably more frequently masked by widespread bilateral lesions.

The authors have no commercial or financial conflict of interest related to this article. They received no funding for writing this article.

[a] Service de Dermatologie Adulte et Pédiatrique, Centre de Référence des Maladies Rares de la Peau, Hôpital Saint André, 1 rue Jean Burguet, Bordeaux 33075, France; [b] INSERM 1035, University of Bordeaux, Bordeaux 33000, France; [c] Centre de Référence des Maladies Rares de la Peau Hôpital Larrey - Service de Dermatologie 24, Chemin de Pouvourville TSA 30030, Toulouse Cedex 9 31059, France

* Corresponding author. Service de Dermatologie Adulte et Pédiatrique, Centre de Référence des Maladies Rares de la Peau, Hôpital Saint André, 1 rue Jean Burguet, Bordeaux 33075, France.

E-mail address: alain.taieb@chu-bordeaux.fr

Dermatol Clin 35 (2017) 229–233
http://dx.doi.org/10.1016/j.det.2016.11.011

PERSONAL AND FAMILIAL PREDISPOSING FACTORS

Pajvani and colleagues[7] reported that among children with vitiligo, those with a family history of vitiligo were more likely to have an earlier age of onset of the disease than those with a negative family history. The incidence for autoimmunity found in families of childhood vitiligo patients across different reported studies ranges from 3.3% to 27.3%.[8–11] Halder and colleagues[12] showed that a family history of autoimmunity was more frequently reported in children with vitiligo, as compared with adults with vitiligo. Mazereeuw-Hautier and colleagues[13] found a similar percentage of familial autoimmune diseases in children with SV and non-SV.

A so far neglected finding has been the association of vitiligo with atopic dermatitis, a common finding at vitiligo pediatric clinics, with either associated/ongoing atopic dermatitis or with a well-documented personal history of atopic dermatitis or other atopic manifestations. This association has been confirmed in larger series[14,15] and simultaneously genome-wide association studies have shown predisposing genes common to atopy and vitiligo, such as thymic stromal lymphopoietin.[16]

CLINICAL CHARACTERISTICS

Knees, elbows, shins, arms, and hands are often the sites of initial involvement in children. Such locations are frequently scraped and scratched in this age group, but it is not known if this phenomenon occurs more or less commonly than in adults. The recently developed K-VSCOR indicates a correlation between rapid spread and koebnerization.[17]

At diagnosis, the most common location of SV is the face, followed by the trunk, neck, and limbs (**Fig. 1**). The face is also the most common location of vitiligo, especially around the eyes and neck, followed by the lower limbs, trunk, neck, and upper limbs. A burning sensation of the eyelids is a clue to the onset of vitiligo in fair-skinned children during outdoor activities. Involvement of the perineum and in particular perianal and buttocks skin is a common onset location of vitiligo in toddlers, suggesting a role of the Koebner phenomenon triggered by nappies and hygiene care (**Fig. 2**).

Leukotrichia in the scalp area, sometimes preceding the onset of vitiligo by several months or years, is noticed occasionally including probably some cases of halo nevi more difficult to detect in this location. Independent of interfollicular skin involvement, premature diffuse graying of the hair is sometimes observed, which may correspond to the recently delineated follicular vitiligo.[18]

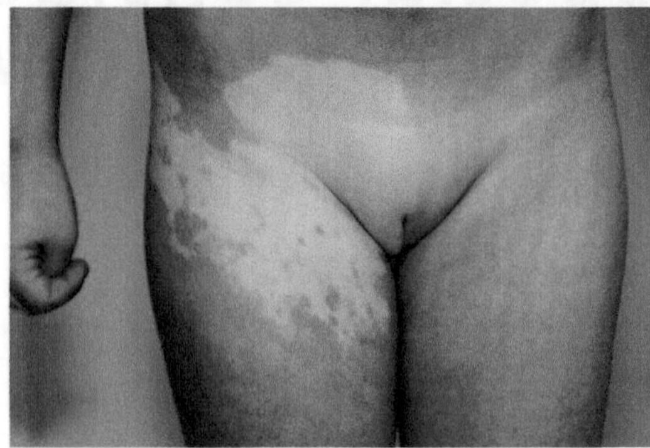

Fig. 1. Segmental vitiligo, note sharp midline demarcation.

The presence of halo nevi, and leukotrichia, in a patient with SV may be a risk for mixed vitiligo.[19] The significance of isolated halo nevi as a clinical marker of risk for vitiligo is frequently debated. A comparison with the general pediatric population is difficult because the prevalence of halo nevi is not well known, possibly around 1%. Prcic and colleagues[20] found that there are more halo nevi in children with vitiligo, compared with children without vitiligo (34% vs 3.3%). The prevalence of halo nevi in children with vitiligo varies widely according to series, from 2.5% to 34% (reviewed in Ref.[2]), and based on personal experience some cases would have gone undetected without Wood lamp examination. It is also unclear whether the prevalence of halo nevi in children with vitiligo is different from that found in adult vitiligo, but in general they are more easy to detect, without a background of skin aging. Vitiligo may develop within or around congenital nevi, and unusually on Becker nevus (**Fig. 3**).

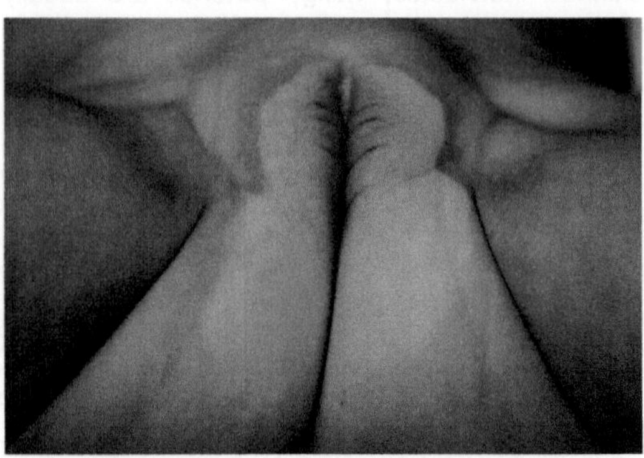

Fig. 2. Napkin vitiligo, a common mode of revelation of the disease in infants.

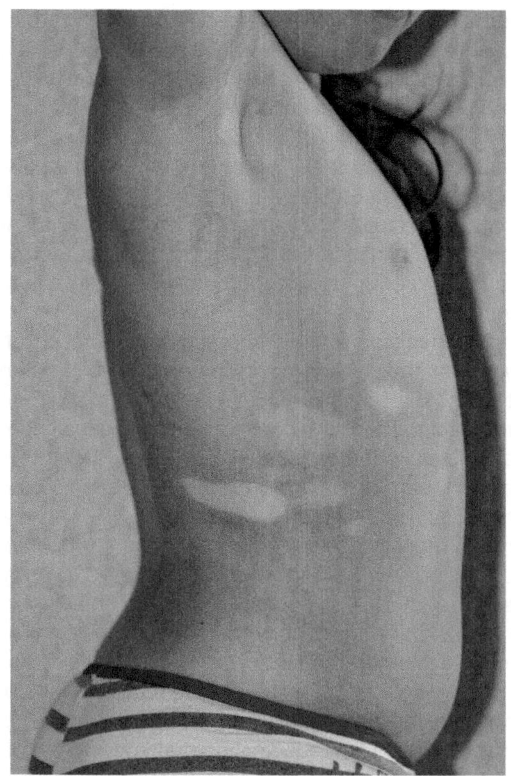

Fig. 3. Unusual onset of vitiligo on Becker nevus.

Mucosal vitiligo is rare in childhood, the most common being vulval vitiligo in girls, which needs to be distinguished from lichen sclerosus.

There is a paucity of studies on the evolution of childhood vitiligo and on the impact of early treatment, but our experience suggests that early and aggressive intervention may halt the process and help repigmentation, even in SV cases. Concerning repigmentation patterns, mixed patterns are the most common in childhood, and a new type has been recently delineated in glabrous skin, the "medium spotted" pattern.[21]

LABORATORY INVESTIGATIONS, INCLUDING AUTOIMMUNE SCREENING

Children suffering from vitiligo are mostly in good health. Nevertheless, as in adult vitiligo, other autoimmune diseases are associated. The most common is thyroiditis. The prevalence of thyroid dysfunction in childhood vitiligo is variable according to reports (0%–25%) (reviewed in Ref.[2]). Based on a large study, female patients, and patients with longer duration of disease and greater body surface involvement, are more likely to present with autoimmune thyroid disease and should thus be monitored for thyroid function and antithyroid antibodies on a regular basis.[22] The other autoimmune diseases reported in children with vitiligo include alopecia areata, diabetes mellitus, and Addison disease isolated or within the autoimmune polyglandular syndrome type I. The prevalence of these other diseases is very low.

Antinuclear antibodies may be found in children with vitiligo, but not in segmental forms.[13] This is considered a marker of the general autoimmune status of the child with vitiligo.

In clinical practice, it seems appropriate to perform a routine initial thyroid screening in children with vitiligo, which should include antithyroperoxidase (TPO) antibodies and thyroid-stimulating hormone determinations. If there is a strong family history of autoimmunity or in case of baseline detection of anti-TPO antibodies, repeated annual assessment and/or endocrinologic visit should be performed.

DIFFERENTIAL DIAGNOSIS

In children, the most common causes of hypomelanoses are the postinflammatory hypomelanoses for vitiligo and nevus depigmentosus for SV. Other rarer diseases, such as tuberous sclerosis, need to be occasionally ruled out. Wood lamp examination is particularly helpful in difficult situations, because the ultraviolet enhancement of vitiligo lesions lacks in postinflammatory lesions and nevus depigmentosus. In nevus depigmentosus, there is also a slight ability to tan in the depigmented area and depigmentation is not more marked under Wood lamp irradiation.

Considering genital lichen sclerosus, some cases may precede true vitiligo (Fig. 4) with usually acrofacial distribution.

PSYCHOSOCIAL ISSUES

There is a lack of specific studies on psychological effects of vitiligo in children, but negative experiences from childhood vitiligo may influence adult life.[23] Nevertheless, although vitiligo is not a

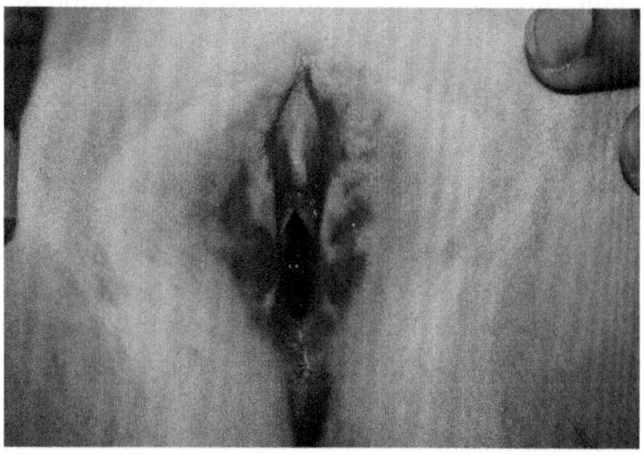

Fig. 4. Vulvar lichen sclerosus and vitiligo.

life-threatening disease, it can be a life-altering disease. Children are probably affected differently, depending on the location, extent, and course of the disease; their age; individual capacities; and social environment. It is important to assess as early as possible without too much parental influence how the children cope with their disease to make appropriate treatment plans.

THERAPEUTIC ISSUES

There are minor differences in the management of childhood versus adult vitiligo mostly because of feasibility and aesthetic demand of treatment. The major difference comes from the parent's behavior and coping with the disease, especially in vitiligo families. One important unsolved issue is the possible impact of early aggressive treatment on disease outcome in severe rapidly progressive disease in children.

It is crucial to avoid undertreatment of common conditions in childhood, especially in skin disorders, such as atopic dermatitis and psoriasis, but also in vitiligo where early intervention is helpful before a widespread loss of skin melanocytes and the melanocyte niche. The reasons for undertreatment of skin disorders in children are not always clear, but the reluctance to treat because of age first, assuming that children are less hardy than adults, or because of interference with growth and development, is usually not scientifically founded. Parents may also not adhere to the management plans because of personal beliefs or neglect. In contrast, aggressive parents seeking to have a "perfect child" may push the physician to intervene because of a minor cosmetic disfigurement (eg, focal vitiligo). The dictum *primum non nocere* should always be kept in mind. Overtreatment of benign cutaneous conditions is a difficult problem, but physicians must be persuasive, and parental management through good quality information is a key issue.

A request for treatment by the child is usually not common until the age of 6, when entering primary school. However, earlier unformulated harm to self-image may remain undetected during early development. Early intervention, whatever the type of vitiligo in the child, is preferable to limit disease extension. However, the benefits/risks of the treatment should be weighed cautiously, in terms of time needed to apply topicals or more importantly in case of deciding for phototherapy. Many dermatologists are uncomfortable treating children with phototherapy and deny treatment in many instances. The chronic use of calcineurin inhibitors is debated in children, but there is little evidence of induction of local/systemic immunosuppression,[24] especially in a disorder, such as vitiligo, which is not associated with an increased skin permeability. Currently, in our pediatric clinic, tacrolimus is prescribed for face and neck, and potent topical corticosteroids are prescribed on extrafacial areas, with a discontinuous regimen to avoid skin atrophy (once daily 1 week out of 2). We use the same maintenance treatment as in adults (twice weekly applications of tacrolimus ointment or topical corticosteroid, alternating weeks).[25]

The decision to start phototherapy is based on whether topical options are unrealistic and when the child is believed to be able to stand alone in the cabin. The duration of sessions is usually not a problem but the distance and time to treatment station can be limiting. Currently, we advocate hand devices for home phototherapy, which are much more practical to deliver treatment in case of limited involvement (less than 5%–10% body surface area). For counseling issues, the importance of the Koebner phenomenon should be clinically evaluated respective to the activities of the child. The K-VSCOR is easy to perform and helpful for making a rapid assessment.[17] There is increasing evidence indicating that koebnerization reflects disease flares and the best intervention is systemic administration of corticosteroids as minipulses (8 mg methylprednisolone on Saturday and Sundays for 3 months <30 kg, 16 mg >30 kg). Particular attention should be given to uncontrolled repeated movements and tics, which may be avoidable with motivation. Guidance through educational slides is helpful. Surgical procedures are rarely attempted in children. Most would need repeated general anesthesia, which is questionable if the disfigurement is limited. Generally, surgery is started at adolescence when better tolerated by the patient. Camouflage should be discussed in children handicapped by disfiguring lesions, especially when bullying at school is noticed and when surgery is not yet possible. Camouflage workshops are organized at some centers and nurses can provide information following the visit.

REFERENCES

1. Howitz J, Brodthagen H, Schwartz M, et al. Prevalence of vitiligo. Epidemiological survey of the Isle of Bornholm, Denmark. Arch Dermatol 1997;113: 47–52.
2. Mazereeuw-Hautier J, Taïeb A. Vitiligo in childhood. In: Picardo M, Taieb A, editors. Vitiligo. Berlin: Springer; 2010. p. 117–25.
3. Ezzedine K, Lim HW, Suzuki T, et al, Vitiligo Global Issue Consensus Conference Panelists. Revised

classification/nomenclature of vitiligo and related issues: the Vitiligo Global Issues Consensus Conference. Pigment Cell Melanoma Res 2012;25:E1–13.
4. Taïeb A, Morice-Picard F, Jouary T, et al. Segmental vitiligo as the possible expression of cutaneous somatic mosaicism: implications for common non-segmental vitiligo. Pigment Cell Melanoma Res 2008;21:646–52.
5. Gauthier Y, Cario André M, Taïeb A. A critical appraisal of vitiligo etiologic theories. Is melanocyte loss a melanocytorrhagy? Pigment Cell Res 2003; 16:322–32.
6. Ezzedine K, Gauthier Y, Léauté-Labrèze C, et al. Segmental vitiligo associated with generalized vitiligo (mixed vitiligo): a retrospective case series of 19 patients. J Am Acad Dermatol 2011;65:965–71.
7. Pajvani U, Ahmad N, Wiley A, et al. Relationship between family medical history and childhood vitiligo. J Am Acad Dermatol 2006;55:238–44.
8. Cho S, Kang HC, Hahn JH. Characteristics of vitiligo in Korean children. Pediatr Dermatol 2000;17: 189–93.
9. Hu Z, Liu JB, Ma SS, et al. Profile of childhood vitiligo in China: an analysis of 541 patients. Pediatr Dermatol 2006;23:114–6.
10. Jaisankar TJ, Baruah MC, Garg BR. Vitiligo in children. Int J Dermatol 1992;31:621–3.
11. Pagovich OE, Silverberg JI, Freilich E, et al. Thyroid anomalies in pediatric patients with vitiligo in New York city. Cutis 2008;81:463–6.
12. Halder RM, Grimes PE, Cowan CA, et al. Childhood vitiligo. J Am Acad Dermatol 1987;16:948–54.
13. Mazereeuw-Hautier J, Bezio S, Mahe E, et al, Groupe de Recherche Clinique en Dermatologie Pédiatrique (GRCDP). Segmental and nonsegmental childhood vitiligo has distinct clinical characteristics: a prospective observational study. J Am Acad Dermatol 2010;62:945–9.
14. Ezzedine K, Diallo A, Léauté-Labrèze C, et al. Pre- vs. post-pubertal onset of vitiligo: multivariate analysis indicates atopic diathesis association in pre-pubertal onset vitiligo. Br J Dermatol 2012;167: 490–5.
15. Ezzedine K, Le Thuaut A, Jouary T, et al. Latent class analysis of a series of 717 patients with vitiligo allows the identification of two clinical subtypes. Pigment Cell Melanoma Res 2014;27:134–9.
16. Birlea SA, Jin Y, Bennett DC, et al. Comprehensive association analysis of candidate genes for generalized vitiligo supports XBP1, FOXP3, and TSLP. J Invest Dermatol 2011;131:371–81.
17. Diallo A, Boniface K, Jouary T, et al. Development and validation of the K-VSCOR for scoring Koebner's phenomenon in vitiligo/non-segmental vitiligo. Pigment Cell Melanoma Res 2013;26:402–7.
18. Gan EY, Cario-André M, Pain C, et al. Follicular vitiligo: a report of 8 cases. J Am Acad Dermatol 2016;74(6):1178–84.
19. Ezzedine K, Diallo A, Léauté-Labrèze C, et al. Halo naevi and leukotrichia are strong predictors of the passage to mixed vitiligo in a subgroup of segmental vitiligo. Br J Dermatol 2012;166:539–44.
20. Prcic S, Djuran V, Poljacki M. Vitiligo in childhood. Med Pregl 2002;55:475–80.
21. Gan EY, Gahat T, Cario-André M, et al. Clinical repigmentation patterns in paediatric vitiligo. Br J Dermatol 2016;175(3):555–60.
22. Gey A, Diallo A, Seneschal J, et al. Autoimmune thyroid disease in vitiligo: multivariate analysis indicates intricate pathomechanisms. Br J Dermatol 2013;168:756–61.
23. Homan MWL, de Korte J, Grootenhuis MA, et al. Impact of childhood vitiligo on adult life. Br J Dermatol 2008;159:915–20.
24. Legendre L, Barnetche T, Mazereeuw-Hautier J, et al. Risk of lymphoma in patients with atopic dermatitis and the role of topical treatment: a systematic review and meta-analysis. J Am Acad Dermatol 2015;72:992–1002.
25. Cavalié M, Ezzedine K, Fontas E, et al. Maintenance therapy of adult vitiligo with 0.1% tacrolimus ointment: a randomized, double blind, placebo-controlled study. J Invest Dermatol 2015;135:970–4.

The Role of Diet and Supplements in Vitiligo Management

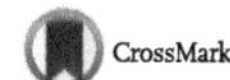

Pearl E. Grimes, MD[a,b,*], Rama Nashawati, BS, MSGM[b]

KEYWORDS

• Vitiligo • Autoimmune disease • Oxidative stress • Vitamin D • Vitamins • Polypodium leucotomos • Ginkgo biloba • EGCG

KEY POINTS

- Vitiligo is an autoimmune disorder that involves the interplay between oxidative stress and the immune system.
- Preliminary observations suggest that the presence of gluten in the diet may play a role in vitiligo development in some patients, but to date vitiligo-specific diets have not been studied.
- The role of oral supplements, including vitamins, minerals, and botanicals, is increasingly being investigated as adjuncts to conventional medical treatment due to their antioxidant and immunomodulatory activity.
- Studies suggest that many of these agents may have some efficacy as monotherapy, but are more often as adjuncts to topical agents and phototherapy.

INTRODUCTION

Vitiligo is an acquired disorder of pigmentation characterized by well-defined depigmented patches of skin. Biopsies of lesional skin classically reveal an absence of epidermal melanocytes.[1–3]

Multiple theories have been proffered for melanocyte destruction, including genetic, autoimmune, biochemical, viral, and melanocyte detachment mechanisms. Current research data suggest that autoimmune aberrations and oxidative stress are the key pathways mediating the destruction of melanocytes in vitiligo.[4,5] Oxidative stress may initiate the cycle of destruction of melanocytes.[4] An altered intracellular redox status and depletion of enzymatic and nonenzymatic antioxidants has been documented in the epidermis of patients with vitiligo.[6–8] Hence, the generation of reactive oxygen species (ROS) may begin the cycle of destruction of melanocytes in genetically susceptible individuals by activation of the innate and adaptive immune response.[1,2,6]

A variety of humoral and cell-mediated immune defects are reported in patients with vitiligo.[2,5,9] However, multiple studies now document the role of activated cytotoxic CD8+ T lymphocytes and the interferon gamma–induced chemokine CXCL10 as key immune mediators of melanocyte destruction.[10–12] Therefore, the interplay between oxidative stress and the immune system may represent critical pathways in vitiligo. Hence, it is a novel and rational strategy to address the role of diet, lifestyle modifications, and oral supplementation with vitamins, minerals, and botanicals as adjunctive approaches in the therapeutically challenging vitiligo arena.

[a] Division of Dermatology, Vitiligo & Pigmentation Institute of Southern California, David Geffen School of Medicine, University of California, Los Angeles, 10833 Le Conte Avenue, Los Angeles, CA 90095, USA; [b] Vitiligo & Pigmentation Institute of Southern California, 5670 Wilshire Boulevard, #650, Los Angeles, CA 90036, USA
* Corresponding author.
E-mail address: pegrimesmd@aol.com

Dermatol Clin 35 (2017) 235–243
http://dx.doi.org/10.1016/j.det.2016.11.012
0733-8635/17/

THE ROLE OF DIET IN VITILIGO MANAGEMENT

A review of the literature revealed no controlled studies assessing the role of diet in the prevention or management of patients with vitiligo. However, there are multiple books, web sites, and lay publications recommending unsubstantiated diets and supplements for myriad autoimmune diseases, including vitiligo. In some countries, such as India, patients with vitiligo are cautioned to avoid citrus fruits, sour yogurt, vitamin C products, milk, and fish; however, this is not substantiated in controlled studies (see Vitamin C section).

Although food per se may not appear to play an important role in vitiligo management, there are general dietary recommendations based on the antioxidant, vitamin, and micronutrient composition of foods. For example, vegetable oils that are high in omega-6 may increase the production of ROS and proinflammatory cytokines that may play a role in vitiligo.[13] Dietary choices are also relevant in avoiding foods that could lead to allergic reactions or irritation that could trigger or worsen vitiligo.[14] Celiac disease (CD) is frequently comorbid with myriad other autoimmune diseases, including vitiligo. This disorder is characterized by a general gluten intolerance, whereby gluten ingestion leads to inflammation in the small intestine and malabsorption over time. In a case control study of 64 patients with vitiligo and 64 controls, immunoglobulin (Ig)A anti-endomysial antibodies and IgA antiglutaminase antibodies, which are diagnostic markers for CD, were measured.[15] Two female subjects with vitiligo were found to be seropositive for these antibodies versus none of the controls. The investigators suggest that both CD and vitiligo may be triggered by a common immune system signal associated with a high-gluten diet. Alternatively, both diseases may share similar genetic risks. The author is observing an increasing frequency of CD in her vitiligo patient population at the Vitiligo and Pigmentation Institute of Southern California.

Two case reports in patients with vitiligo who had not responded to topical agents and phototherapy showed some degree of repigmentation with a gluten-free diet.[16,17] In one patient, who continued on oral dapsone, it was noted that significant repigmentation began within 1 month after initiation of a gluten-free diet. Maximal improvement was achieved by 3 months.[15] In the other study, there was progressive repigmentation over 3 years despite no conventional therapy. Pigmentation was maintained with the gluten-free diet at 7-year follow-up.

A recent study sought to examine the relationship between exposure to a number of thyroid disruptors and toxins and the presence of thyroid hormone antibodies to T3 and T4 in 70 white patients with vitiligo. It was found that 95.7% of the subjects had thyroid hormone antibodies and most had both T3 and T4 antibodies. A significant association was noted between intake of foods containing nitrates (leafy green vegetables), thiocyanate (broccoli, cabbage, and other brassicas), and soy isoflavones and the presence of T3 antibodies.[18]

Oral Supplements

Because many diets do not provide vitamins and minerals in sufficient quantities or types to counter oxidative stress or modulate the immune system, there is increasing interest in supplementation (**Table 1**). Unfortunately, many patients who seek consultation at the Vitiligo and Pigmentation Institute of Southern California use unreliable sources as a guide for supplementation, ingesting more than 10 agents daily (**Fig. 1**).

Vitamin B12 and folic acid

Vitamin B12, also known as cobalamin, is a water-soluble vitamin that exerts hematological and neurologic effects. It is 1 of 8 B vitamins. Folic acid (vitamin B9) is the synthetic form of B9 where folate occurs naturally in food.

Humans cannot synthesize folates, hence it must be obtained via diet. Folates are needed for DNA repair, synthesis, and methylation of DNA. They are crucial for cell growth, division, and brain function. Montes and colleagues[19] reported diminished blood levels of vitamin B12, folic acid, and ascorbic acid in a group of 15 patients with vitiligo. Prolonged supplementation with oral folic acid, parental B12, and oral ascorbic acid was associated with repigmentation of vitiliginous patches.[19]

Evidence for vitamin B12 and/or folic acid supplementation, either alone or as an adjuvant to light therapy, is mixed. The rationale for their use is their possible role in melanin synthesis and the possible association of vitiligo and pernicious anemia in which vitamin B12 is insufficiently absorbed.[20] Several groups found no association between serum B12 and folate levels and vitiligo.[20–22] In one study, 100 patients with vitiligo were treated with 1 mg vitamin B12 and 5 mg folic acid twice daily for 3 months.[23] Patients were also encouraged to expose their skin to sunlight or UVB irradiation. Total repigmentation of sun-exposed skin was achieved in 6 patients. Repigmentation was clearly apparent in 52 patients and was more common in patients younger than 26 years and those with vitiligo of less than 10 years'

Table 1
Vitamins and supplements for vitiligo

Supplement	Properties In Vivo	Effect on Vitiligo Management
Vitamin B12/folic acid	DNA repair, synthesis, methylation of DNA	May be used alone or with phototherapy for repigmentation
Vitamin C	Antioxidant/immunomodulatory	0.5–2 g per day leads to high antioxidant activity
Vitamin D	Melanocyte/keratinocyte growth and differentiation Inhibits T-cell activation Increases melanogenesis Immunomodulatory	High levels of vitamin D may reduce disease activity
Vitamin E	Free radical scavenger/inhibits platelet coagulation/ antioxidant/anti-inflammatory	Alone or with phototherapy leads to rapid repigmentation with photoprotective effects Decreases oxidative stress and increases effectiveness of phototherapy
Zinc	Antioxidant/regulates gene expression/cofactor for superoxide dismutase	May offer a slight benefit when combined with topical steroids
Phyllanthus emblica (amla fruit)	Antioxidant/anti-inflammatory/ antimicrobial/antiviral	Decreased phototoxicity from phototherapy and enhances repigmentation
Gingko biloba	Antioxidant/anti-inflammatory platelet-activating factor antagonist	Slows progression of disease
Polypodium leucotomos	Protection, antioxidant, inhibition of apoptosis, immune modulation, decreases proinflammatory cytokines	Increased repigmentation in the head and neck areas with phototherapy use
Piperine (animal studies)	Stimulates melanocyte replication Induces formation of melanocytic dendrites	Pigmentation in newly formed melanocytes Effective when phototherapy is not concurrent to prevent photoisomerization of piperine
Green tea (epigallocatechin-3-gallate) (animal studies)	Antioxidant/anti-inflammatory/ anti-atherogenic/anticancer	Decreases proinflammatory cytokines Immune modulation

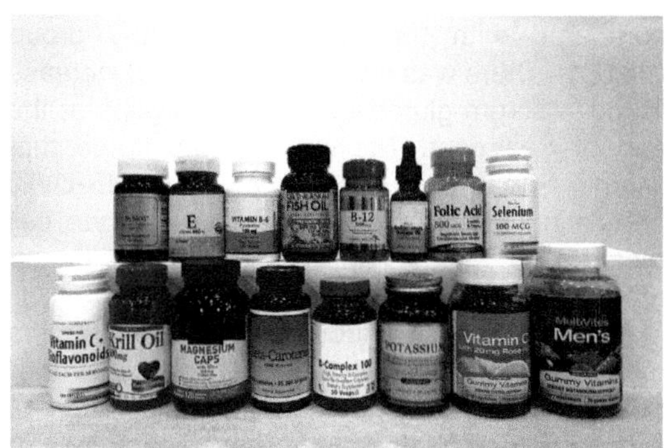

Fig. 1. Vitamins and supplements.

duration. Vitiligo progression was halted in 64% of patients. The investigators concluded that B12/ folic acid supplementation combined with sun exposure was better in inducing repigmentation than either treatment alone. However, another study showed no advantage to adding B12 and folic acid supplements to narrow-band UVB phototherapy (NB-UVB).[24]

Vitamin C (ascorbic acid)

Vitamin C is a water-soluble vitamin found abundantly in citrus fruits and a variety of leafy vegetables. Multiple studies have documented the beneficial health effects of vitamin C, including its antioxidant and immunomodulatory properties.

It has been suggested that vitamin C supplementation is contraindicated in vitiligo, because of its skin-lightening activity. However, Yoon and colleagues[14] suggested that its antioxidant benefits override this risk. They recommend vitamin C supplementation at a dosage of 0.5 to 2 g per day.

The efficacy and safety of ascorbic acid was assessed in 188 Indian patients with vitiligo. The patients were stratified to 3 groups. Given societal myths regarding ascorbic acid use in vitiligo, 75 avoided vitamin C products. The second group of 113 patients consumed vitamin C daily in their diet and/or medicinal products. A third group of 12 patients ingested vitamin C 1000 mg daily for 6 months. Statistical analysis of the 3 groups showed no difference in the progression of the disease.[25]

Vitamin D

Vitamin D3 binding to vitamin D receptors in the skin affects melanocyte and keratinocyte growth and differentiation and inhibits T-cell activation.[26,27] Additionally, melanocytes are believed to express 1-alpha-dihydroxyvitamin D3 receptors, which may have a role in stimulating melanogenesis.[26] Moreover, vitamin D is believed to exert immunomodulatory effects by inhibiting the expression of proinflammatory and proapoptotic cytokines.[28,29] Vitamin D supplementation has been shown to be effective in several animal models of autoimmune diseases.[28] Although it is unknown whether vitamin D deficiency plays a role in human vitiligo, it is reasonable to suggest that vitamin D may be useful as an immunomodulator in this disorder.[28]

Multiple recent studies have addressed vitamin D deficiency in patients with vitiligo. Silverberg and coworkers[29] showed that serum 25(OH) D levels were normal (>30 ng/mL) in 31% of patients, whereas 55.6% were insufficient and 13.3% were very low (<15 ng/mL). Very low levels were associated with comorbid autoimmune diseases. Insufficient levels were associated with increasing Fitzpatrick phototype but not with ethnicity. The investigators suggest that very low 25(OH) D may be a useful screening tool for comorbid autoimmunity in vitiligo. This recommendation was supported by findings of a more recent study that showed lower serum 25 (OH) D levels in patients with vitiligo with autoimmune disease than in those without a comorbid autoimmune disorder.[30] In one study from China, both subjects with vitiligo and controls were found to be universally vitamin D insufficient.[31]

There are a dearth of studies showing the effects of oral vitamin D supplementation in vitiligo. Finamor and colleagues[32] treated 16 patients with 35,000 IU vitamin D3 daily for 6 months in association with a low-calcium diet and adequate hydration for safety. At baseline, 100% of subjects had serum 25 (OH) D3 $\leq$30 ng/mL. After 6 months of supplementation, levels increased from 18.4 $\pm$ 8.9 to 132.5 $\pm$ 37.0 ng/mL ($P<.0005$). Fourteen of 16 patients with vitiligo achieved 25% to 75% repigmentation. Whenever present, standard treatments were not changed; however, such treatments were not defined. The investigators concluded that this level of supplementation is safe in patients with vitiligo in the setting of calcium restriction and might be effective for reducing disease activity.

Vitamin E

Vitamin E is a fat-soluble vitamin exerting multiple biologic effects, including potent scavenging of free radicals and inhibition of platelet coagulation.[33] Ramadan and coworkers[34] examined levels of vitamin E and paraoxonase (PON1), an important free radical scavenger, in 3 autoimmune disorders, including vitiligo. They found statistically significantly lower tissue and serum levels of both substances in patients with vitiligo compared with controls ($P<.001$). Vitamin E supplementation was studied as an adjunct to NB-UVB in 24 patients with stable vitiligo. Patients received either 400 IU vitamin E per day, beginning 2 weeks before the initiation of light therapy or NB-UVB monotherapy.[35] After 6 months of treatment, the combination therapy group showed marked repigmentation in 72.7% versus 55.6% of those receiving NB-UVB monotherapy. Mild erythema was noted in 70% of those receiving combination therapy and 85% receiving light therapy alone, suggesting a UVB-protective effect of vitamin E. The mean number of treatments needed to achieve 50% repigmentation was significantly less with combination therapy.[22] Mean plasma malondialdehyde (MDA), a marker of lipid peroxidation, and reduced glutathione were measured before and after treatment. The combination group showed a significant reduction in plasma MDA compared with the light monotherapy group ($P<.001$). There was also a nonsignificant increase in mean serum glutathione in both groups at the end of treatment. The investigators noted that vitamin E may be a useful adjuvant to NB-UVB, preventing lipid peroxidation of melanocyte cell membranes and improving light treatment efficacy.[35]

A small Turkish study of 30 patients who received either 900 IU vitamin E and PUVA or PUVA monotherapy found that the addition of vitamin E to light therapy improved repigmentation.[36] In the combination treatment group, 60%

achieved ≥75% repigmentation whereas 20% had 24% to 74% repigmentation. In the PUVA monotherapy group, a combined total of 67% showed these levels of repigmentation.

Vitamin E was also studied as a component of a mixed antioxidant supplement regimen. Dell'Anna and colleagues[37] examined the use of a balanced antioxidant supplement combining vitamins C, E, alpha-lipoic acid, and polyunsaturated fatty acids versus placebo in 35 patients undergoing NB-UVB treatment for vitiligo. Alpha-lipoic acid, also known as lipoic acid, is vital for mitochondrial energy production. It is a powerful antioxidant that stimulates the synthesis of glutathione, a key intracellular antioxidant.[38] Supplementation was administered for 2 months before treatment as well as for the 6 months of light therapy. Area and number of lesions, and redox status of peripheral blood mononuclear cells (PBMCs) were estimated at several time points. After 2 months of the active treatment regimen, catalase activity was 121% of baseline values and the production of ROS was reduced to 57% of baseline ($P<.05$ and $P<.02$ vs placebo). The antioxidant supplement also appeared to improve the efficacy of the NB-UVB in that 47% of the active treatment group achieved greater than 75% repigmentation versus 18% of the placebo group ($P<.05$). In PBMCs, there was an increase in catalase activity to 114% of baseline ($P<.05$ vs placebo) and a decrease of up to 60% in ROS ($P<.02$ vs placebo). The authors concluded that oral supplementation with a mixed antioxidant containing alpha-lipoic acid before and during treatment with NB-UVB enhances the effectiveness of the light therapy and reduced oxidative stress associated with vitiligo.

Zinc

Zinc is an essential mineral that functions as a cofactor for at least 3000 proteins, including enzymes, nuclear factors, and hormones. It regulates gene expression and acts as a cofactor for superoxide dismutase, an antioxidant in the skin.[39] Zinc plays a key role in melanogenesis.[40] Shameer and colleagues[41] assessed zinc levels in 60 patients and found deficiencies in 21.6% of patients with vitiligo compared with controls. In a study by Yaghoobi and colleagues,[42] 35 patients were treated with a topical steroid regimen with and without 440 mg per day of oral zinc supplementation, 16 of whom received no zinc. No difference was noted with zinc levels at baseline. However, at 4 months, there was greater improvement in the group of patients treated with corticosteroids plus zinc. Zinc may offer some benefit when used in combination with other modalities.[43] Gastrointestinal irritation was common.[42]

Herbal Supplements

Other supplements that have been used in the management of vitiligo include a number of botanicals that have been shown to have antioxidant, anti-inflammatory, and immune-modulating properties.

Phyllanthus emblica fruit extract, vitamin E, and carotinoid combination

Phyllanthus emblica, also known as amla fruit or Indian gooseberry, has antioxidant, anti-inflammatory, antimicrobial, and antiviral properties. It contains vitamin C, tannins, and polyphenols.[44–46]

Colucci and colleagues evaluated the efficacy of an oral supplement containing *Phyllanthus emblica* fruit extract 100 mg, vitamin E 10 mg, and carotenoids 4.7 mg taken 3 times daily for 6 months. Patients with vitiligo were stratified into 2 groups of 65 patients each. Both groups A and B received the same concomitant topical or phototherapy treatment, whereas only group A received the daily supplement. At 6 months, there was a statistically greater response in group A patients receiving the oral supplement. Compared with group B, greater repigmentation responses were observed on the head, neck, and trunk regions. Group B patients showed statistically significant greater inflammation, erythema, and progression of the disease. Minimal changes were noted in the control group receiving no supplementation.[47]

Ginkgo biloba

Ginkgo biloba (GB) contains bioflavonoids, proanthocyanidens, flavonoids, and trilactonic diterpenes. It exerts multiple antioxidant and anti-inflammatory effects including its antagonizing effects on platelet-activating factor, causing vasodilation. Other mechanisms include its effects on neurotransmission by improving alpha-2-adrenoreceptor activity.[48]

GB extract 40 mg administered 3 times daily for 6 months was shown in a placebo-controlled double-blind study to be effective in arresting the spread of vitiligo in the active treatment group ($P = .006$). Ten patients in the GB group achieved marked to complete repigmentation.[49]

A more recent 12-week study showed that 60 mg of standardized GB extract twice per day resulted in improvement in the Vitiligo Area Scoring Index (VASI) and Vitiligo European Task Force (VETF), validated outcome measures of disease area and intensity of depigmentation in 11 of 12 subjects.[50] No other treatments were permitted. VASI scores improved by a mean of 15% with 2 participants showing greater than 30% improvement. VETF scores for total lesion area showed a decrease of 0.36, indicating a 6%

decrease in lesion size. The staging scores showed a nonsignificant trend toward improvement in all body areas. GB significantly stopped the spread of vitiligo ($P<.001$). Although concern has been raised regarding the effect of GB on coagulation, clotting parameters including serum platelet count, prothrombin, and partial thromboplastin times were similar between baseline and study end.

Polypodium leucotomos

Polypodium leucotomos (PL) is a tropical fern that has been shown to protect against UV radiation–induced damage.[51] Other mechanisms of action of PL include its immunomodulatory effects and inhibition of proinflammatory cytokines.[52,53] In 1989, Mohammad ushered PL into the realm of dermatology. Anapsos is a lipid-soluble derivative of PL. Mohammad treated 22 patients with Anapsos, and 100% repigmented. The study was conducted in the summer months so the patients were also exposed to daily sunlight.[54]

In a randomized, double-blind, placebo-controlled pilot study, PL + PUVA treatment produced significantly more patients who achieved greater than 50% repigmentation compared with PUVA + placebo ($P<.01$).[55,56] Repigmentation was inversely correlated with decreases in CD3+CD25 + T cells.

In another study, 50 patients undergoing NB-UVB twice weekly were randomized to receive either PL 250 mg or placebo 3 times per day for 25 to 26 weeks.[57] Repigmentation in the head and neck area was higher in the active treatment group than in the placebo group ($P = .06$). Subjects in the PL group who attended more than 80% of the required phototherapy sessions showed more repigmentation in the head and neck than those in the placebo group (50% vs 19%, $P<.002$).[58]

Piperine

Piperine, the major alkaloid of black pepper, has been shown to stimulate the replication of melanocytes and induce formation of melanocytic dendrites in vitro. Piperine has therefore been suggested as a possible treatment for vitiligo in the setting of UV exposure to induce pigmentation in newly formed melanocytes.[58–60] Soumyanath and colleagues assessed the effects of UV irradiation on melanocytes stimulated by piperine. In a mouse cell line (called melan-a), piperine stimulated melanocyte proliferation and dendrite formation only when not in combination with UVA. The investigators noted that the UV-induced photoisomerization of the piperine molecule resulted in the loss of protein binding and melanocyte stimulatory activity.[58] In their study of hairless pigmented mice, animals were treated with dimethyl sulfoxide (DMSO) solution or piperine dissolved in DMSO solution for 9 weeks, piperine and DMSO plus simulated solar UVA 3 times per week just before piperine application from weeks 5 to 9, or UVA only for 5 weeks. The melanocyte stimulatory effect of piperine was retained and pigmentation was greater in mice treated with both piperine and ultraviolet radiation (UVR) than with either as monotherapy. The investigators note than when UVR and piperine are used to treat vitiligo, they should be used at different times to avoid photoisomerization of piperine.

Another animal study tested twice-daily application of piperine or 1 of 3 of its analogs or vehicle without or without UVR for 3 days per week.[61] After 4 weeks of treatment, all but one of the analogs produced greater levels of pigmentation than vehicle with low levels of inflammation. The addition of UVR produced darker pigmentation than either treatment alone. The pigmentation achieved with combination therapy was more even than the speckled perifollicular pattern achieved with UVR alone. When treatment was discontinued, pigmentation decreased but did not disappear and could be restarted with piperine analogs or UVR or the combination.

Green tea epigaollocalechin-3-galate

Multiple studies now document the beneficial effects of green tea (GT). Catechins contained in GT are responsible for its myriad biological effects. GT catechins include epigallocatechin, epicatechin, epicatechin-3-gallate, and epigallocatechin-3-gallate (EGCG). EGCG is the most abundant and biologically active compound in GT. EGCG has antioxidant, anti-inflammatory, anti-atherogenic, and anticancer properties. EGCG modulates multiple T-cell–mediated immune responses.[62] Zhu and colleagues[63] assessed the therapeutic effects of EGCG in vitiligo induced by monobenzone in mice. EGCG delayed the time of onset, prevalence, and surface area of monobenzone-induced depigmentation on use. Moreover, treatment with EGCG significantly decreased the production of proinflammatory cytokines, including tumor necrosis factor-α, interferon γ, and interleukin-6.[63] These findings suggest that antioxidant and immunomodulatory effects of GT should be further assessed in clinical trials.

SUMMARY

There is enormous interest among patients regarding complementary and alternative medical approaches for treatment of vitiligo. Given our current knowledge of oxidative stress and autoimmune mechanisms in the pathogenesis of vitiligo, it is reasonable to suggest that agents with immunomodulatory and/or antioxidant properties can be beneficial for patients with the disease. Such agents are likely to play a role as adjuncts to conventional therapy with the aim of achieving stabilization and repigmentation of vitiliginous lesions. To date, the results of oral supplementation studies are promising, and deserve further study in larger, well-designed trials.

REFERENCES

1. Ezzedine K, Eleftheriadou V, Whitton M, et al. Vitiligo. Lancet 2015;386:74.
2. Mohammed GF, Gomaa AH, Al-Dhubaibi MS. Highlights in pathogenesis of vitiligo. World J Clin Cases 2015;3:221.
3. Ezzedine K, Lim HW, Suzuki T, et al. Revised classification/nomenclature of vitiligo and related issues: the vitiligo global issues consensus conference. Pigment Cell Melanoma Res 2012;25:E1.
4. Grimes PE. White patches and bruised souls: advances in the pathogenesis and treatment of vitiligo. J Am Acad Dermatol 2004;51(1 Suppl):S5–7.
5. Grimes PE. Vitiligo: pathogenesis, clinical features, and diagnosis. In: Tsao H, editor. UpToDate; 2016. Available at: http://www.uptodate.com/contents/vitiligo-pathogenesis-clinical-features-and-diagnosis?source=search_result&search=grimes+vitiligo&selectedTitle=4%7E88.
6. Dell'Anna ML, Maresca V, Briganti S, et al. Mitochondrial impairment in peripheral blood mononuclear cells during the active phase of vitiligo. J Invest Dermatol 2001;117(4):908–13.
7. Picardo M, Grammatico P, Roccella F, et al. Imbalance in the antioxidant pool in melanoma cells and normal melanocytes from patients with melanoma. J Invest Dermatol 1996;107(3):322–6.
8. Morrone A, Picardo M, Luca CD, et al. Catecholamines and vitiligo. Pigment Cell Res 1992;5(2): 65–9.
9. Ongenae K, Van Geel N, Naeyaert JM. Evidence for an autoimmune pathogenesis of vitiligo. Pigment Cell Res 2003;16(2):90–100.
10. Rashighi M, Agarwal P, Richmond JM, et al. CXCL10 is critical for the progression and maintenance of depigmentation in a mouse model of vitiligo. Sci Transl Med 2014;6(223):223ra23.
11. Ortonne JP. Pathogenesis of vitiligo. In: Gupta S, Olsson MJ, Kanwar AJ, et al, editors. Surgical Management of Vitiligo 2008; p. 4–10.
12. Mandelcorn-Monson RL, Shear NH, Yau E, et al. Cytotoxic T lymphocyte reactivity to gp100, MelanA/MART-1, and tyrosinase, in HLA-A2-positive vitiligo patients. J Invest Dermatol 2003; 121(3):550–6.
13. Namazi MR, Chee Leok GOH. Vitiligo and diet: a theoretical molecular approach with practical implications. Indian J Dermatol Venereol Leprol 2009; 75:116–8.
14. Yoon J, Kim TH, Sun YW. Complementary and alternative medicine for vitiligo. In: Park KK, Murase JE, editors. Vitiligo: management and therapy. INTECH Open Access Publisher; 2011.
15. Shahmoradi Z, Najafian J, Naeini FF, et al. Vitiligo and autoantibodies of celiac disease. Int J Prev Med 2013;4:200–3.
16. Khandavala BN, Nirmalraj MC. Rapid partial repigmentation of vitiligo in a young female adult with a gluten-free diet. Case Rep Dermatol 2014;6:283–7.
17. Rodriguez-Garcia C, Gonzalez-Hernandez S, Perez-Robayna N, et al. Repigmentation of vitiligo lesions in a child with celiac disease after a gluten-free diet. Pediatr Dermatol 2011;28:209–10.
18. Colucci R, Lotti F, Arunachalam M, et al. Correlation of serum thyroid hormones autoantibodies with self-reported exposure to thyroid disruptors in a group of nonsegmental vitiligo patients. Arch Environ Contam Toxicol 2015;69:181–90.
19. Montes LF, Diaz ML, Lajous J, et al. Folic acid and vitamin B12 in vitiligo: a nutritional approach. Cutis 1992;50(1):39–42.
20. Kim SM, Kim YK, Hann S-Y. Serum levels of folic acid and vitamin B12 in Korean patients with vitiligo. Yonsei Med J 1999;40:195–8.
21. Gonul M, Cakmak SK, Soylu S, et al. Serum vitamin B12, folate, ferritin, and iron levels in Turkish patients with vitiligo. Indian J Dermatol Venereol Leprol 2010; 76:448.
22. Balci DD, Yonden Z, Yenin JZ, et al. Serum homocysteine, folic acid, and vitamin B12 levels in vitiligo. Eur J Dermatol 2009;19:382.
23. Juhlin L, Olsson MJ. Improvement of vitiligo after oral treatment with vitamin B12 and folic acid and the importance of sun exposure. Acta Derm Venereol 1977;77:460–2.
24. Tijoe M, Gerritsen MJP, Juhlin L, et al. Treatment of vitiligo vulgaris with narrow band UVB (311 nm) for one year and the effect of addition of folic acid and vitamin B12. Acta Derm Venereol 2002;82:369–72.
25. Bhattacharya SK, Dutta AK, Mandal SB, et al. Ascorbic acid in vitiligo. Indian J Dermatol 1981;26(3):4.
26. Grimes PE. New insights and new therapies in vitiligo. JAMA 2005;293(6):730–5.
27. Dusso AS, Thadhani R, Slatopolsky E. Vitamin D receptor and analogs. Semin Nephrol 2004;24(1):10–6.
28. AlGhamdi K, Kumar A, Moussa N. The role of vitamin D in melanogenesis with an emphasis on vitiligo. Indian J Dermatol Venereol Leprol 2013;79(6):750.
29. Silverberg JI, Silverberg AI, Malka E, et al. A pilot study assessing the role of 25 hydroxy vitamin D

levels in patients with vitiligo vulgaris. J Am Acad Dermatol 2010;62(6):937–41.
30. Saleh H, Fattah A, Nermeen SA, et al. Evaluation of serum 25-hydroxyvitamin D levels in vitiligo patients with and without autoimmune diseases. Photodermatol Photoimmunol Photomed 2013;29(1):34–40.
31. Xu X, Fu WW, Wu WY. Serum 25-hydroxyvitamin D deficiency in Chinese patients with vitiligo: a case-control study. PLoS One 2012;7(12):e52778.
32. Finamor DC, Sinigaglia-Coimbra R, Neves LC, et al. A pilot study assessing the effect of prolonged administration of high daily doses of vitamin D on the clinical course of vitiligo and psoriasis. Dermatoendocrinol 2013;5(1):222–34.
33. Burton GW, Ingold KU. Autoxidation of biological molecules. 1. Antioxidant activity of vitamin E and related chain-breaking phenolic antioxidants in vitro. J Am Chem Soc 1981;103(21):6472–7.
34. Ramadan S, Tawdy A, Hay RA, et al. The antioxidant role of paraoxonase 1 and vitamin E in three autoimmune diseases. Skin Pharmacol Physiol 2013;26:2–7.
35. Elgoweini M, El Din NN. Response of vitiligo to narrowband ultraviolet B and oral antioxidants. J Clin Pharmacol 2009;49:852–5.
36. Akyol M, Celik VK, Ozcelik S, et al. The effects of vitamin E on the skin lipid peroxidation and the clinical improvement in vitiligo patients treated with PUVA. Eur J Dermatol 2001;12(1):24–6.
37. Dell'Anna ML, Mastrofrancesco A, Sala R, et al. Antioxidants and narrow band-UVB in the treatment of vitiligo: a double-blind placebo controlled trial. Clin Exp Dermatol 2007;32(6):631–6.
38. Lipoic Acid | Linus Pauling Institute | Oregon State University [Internet]. Lpi.oregonstate.edu. 2016. Available at: http://lpi.oregonstate.edu/mic/dietary-factors/lipoic-acid. Accessed June 15, 2016.
39. Andreini C, Banci L, Bertini I, et al. Counting the zinc-proteins encoded in the human genome. J Proteome Res 2006;5(1):196–201.
40. Prasad AS. Zinc: an overview. Nutrition 1994;11(1 Suppl):93–9.
41. Shameer P, Prasad PV, Kaviarasan PK. Serum zinc level in vitiligo: a case control study. Indian J Dermatol Venereol Leprol 2005;71(3):206.
42. Yaghoobi R, Omidian M, Bagherani N. Comparison of therapeutic efficacy of topical corticosteroid and oral zinc sulfate-topical corticosteroid combination in the treatment of vitiligo patients: a clinical trial. BMC Dermatol 2011;11:7.
43. Bagherani N, Yaghoobi R, Omidian M. Hypothesis: zinc can be effective in treatment of vitiligo. Indian J Dermatol 2011;56(5):480.
44. Dang GK, Parekar RR, Kamat SK, et al. Antiinflammatory activity of *Phyllanthus emblica*, *Plumbago zeylanica* and *Cyperus rotundus* in acute models of inflammation. Phytother Res 2011;25(6):904–8.
45. Arunabh Bhattacharya AC, Ghosalc S, Bhattacharyac SK. Antioxidant activity of active tannoid principles of *Emblica officinalis* (amla). Indian J Exp Biol 1999;37:676–80.
46. Habib-ur-Rehman, Yasin KA, Choudhary MA, et al. Studies on the chemical constituents of *Phyllanthus emblica*. Nat Prod Res 2007;21(9):775–81.
47. Colucci R, Dragoni F, Conti R, et al. Evaluation of an oral supplement containing *Phyllanthus emblica* fruit extracts, vitamin E, and carotenoids in vitiligo treatment. Dermatol Ther 2015;28(1):17–21.
48. The proposed mechanisms of action for *Ginkgo* [Internet]. Ebmconsult.com. 2016. Available at: http://www.ebmconsult.com/articles/ginkgo-biloba-mechanism-of-action-moa. Accessed June 15, 2016.
49. Parsad D, Pandhi R, Juneja A. Effectiveness of oral *Ginkgo biloba* in treating limited, slowly spreading vitiligo. Clin Exp Dermatol 2003;28(3):285–7.
50. Szczurko O, Shear N, Taddio A, et al. *Ginkgo biloba* for the treatment of vitiligo vulgaris: an open label pilot clinical trial. BMC Complement Altern Med 2011;11(1):21.
51. Middelkamp-Hup MA, Pathak MA, Parrado C, et al. Oral *Polypodium leucotomos* extract decreases ultraviolet-induced damage of human skin. J Am Acad Dermatol 2004;51(6):910–8.
52. Palomino OM. Current knowledge in *Polypodium leucotomos* effect on skin protection. Arch Dermatol Res 2015;307(3):199–209.
53. Winkelmann RR, Del Rosso J, Rigel DS. *Polypodium leucotomos* extract: a status report on clinical efficacy and safety. J Drugs Dermatol 2015;14(3):254–9.
54. Mohammad A. Vitiligo repigmentation with Anapsos *(Polypodium leucotomos*). Int J Dermatol 1989;28(7):479.
55. Reyes E, Jaén P, de las Heras E, et al. Systemic immunomodulatory effects of *Polypodium leucotomos* as an adjuvant to PUVA therapy in generalized vitiligo: a pilot study. J Dermatol Sci 2006;41(3):213–6.
56. Nestor M, Bucay V, Callender V, et al. *Polypodium leucotomos* as an adjunct treatment of pigmentary disorders. J Clin Aesthet Dermatol 2014;7(3):13.
57. Middelkamp-Hup MA, Bos JD, Rius-Diaz F, et al. Treatment of vitiligo vulgaris with narrow-band UVB and oral *Polypodium leucotomos* extract: a randomized double-blind placebo-controlled study. J Eur Acad Dermatol Venereol 2007;21(7):942–50.
58. Soumyanath A, Venkatasamy R, Joshi M, et al. UV irradiation affects melanocyte stimulatory activity and protein binding of piperine. Photochem Photobiol 2006;82(6):1541–8.
59. Lin Z, Hoult JR, Bennett DC, et al. Stimulation of mouse melanocyte proliferation by *Piper nigrum* fruit

extract and its main alkaloid, piperine. Planta Med 1999;65(7):600–3.

60. Venkatasamy R, Faas L, Young AR, et al. Effects of piperine analogues on stimulation of melanocyte proliferation and melanocyte differentiation. Bioorg Med Chem 2004;12(8):1905–20.
61. Faas L, Venkatasamy R, Hider RC, et al. In vivo evaluation of piperine and synthetic analogues as potential treatments for vitiligo using a sparsely pigmented mouse model. Br J Dermatol 2008;158(5):941–50.
62. Wu D, Wang J, Pae M, et al. Green tea EGCG, T cells, and T cell-mediated autoimmune diseases. Mol Aspects Med 2012;33(1):107–18.
63. Zhu Y, Wang S, Lin F, et al. The therapeutic effects of EGCG on vitiligo. Fitoterapia 2014;99:243–51.

Genetics of Vitiligo

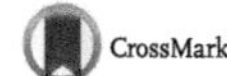

Richard A. Spritz, MD*, Genevieve H.L. Andersen, BS

KEYWORDS

• Vitiligo • Autoimmunity • Gene • Genomewide association study • Genetic linkage
• Genetic epidemiology

KEY POINTS

- Vitiligo is a complex disorder (also termed polygenic and multifactorial), reflecting simultaneous contributions of multiple genetic risk factors and environmental triggers.
- Large-scale genomewide association studies, principally in European-derived whites and in Chinese, have discovered approximately 50 different genetic loci that contribute to vitiligo risk, some of which also contribute to other autoimmune diseases that are epidemiologically associated with vitiligo. At many of these vitiligo susceptibility loci the corresponding relevant genes have now been identified and, for some of these genes, the specific DNA sequence variants that contribute to vitiligo risk are also now known.
- A large fraction of these genes encode proteins involved in immune regulation, several others play roles in cellular apoptosis, and still others are involved in regulating functions of melanocytes.
- Although many of the specific biologic mechanisms through which these genetic factors operate to cause vitiligo remain to be elucidated, it is now clear that vitiligo is an autoimmune disease involving a complex relationship between programming and function of the immune system, aspects of the melanocyte autoimmune target, and dysregulation of the immune response.

INTRODUCTION, BACKGROUND, AND GENETIC EPIDEMIOLOGY

The disorder now known as vitiligo was first described by Claude Nicolas Le Cat in 1765.[1] However, the first specific consideration of a genetic component in vitiligo did not come until 1950, when Stűttgen[2] and Teindel[3] simultaneously reported a total of 8 families with multiple relatives affected by vitiligo. Stűttgen[2] noted that, in his affected family, vitiligo seemed to exhibit dominant inheritance after intermarriage to a family with apparent recessive thyroid disease, a very early recognition of what would now be considered complex (polygenic, multifactorial) inheritance. Mohr,[4] Siemens,[5] and Vogel[6] subsequently reported concordant identical twin-pairs affected by vitiligo, pointing to a major role for genetic factors. Early clinical case series reported a frequency of vitiligo in probands' relatives of 11% to 38%,[7–10] highlighting the importance of genetic factors even in typical vitiligo cases.

Nevertheless, formal genetic epidemiologic studies of vitiligo came much later. Hafez and colleagues,[11] and Das and colleagues,[12] suggested a polygenic, multifactorial mode of inheritance, and estimated vitiligo heritability at 46%[12] to 72%.[11] Subsequent investigations likewise supported a polygenic, multifactorial model,[13–18] with heritability approximately 50%.[18] A twin study of vitiligo in European-derived whites[17] found that the concordance of vitiligo was 23% in monozygotic twins, underscoring the importance of nongenetic factors as well as genetic factors in vitiligo pathogenesis. In this same study, large-scale genetic

The authors have no commercial or financial conflict of interest related to this article. They received no funding for writing this article.
Human Medical Genetics and Genomics Program, University of Colorado School of Medicine, 12800 East 19th Avenue, Room 3100, MS8300, Aurora, CO 80045, USA
* Corresponding author.
E-mail address: richard.spritz@ucdenver.edu

Dermatol Clin 35 (2017) 245–255
http://dx.doi.org/10.1016/j.det.2016.11.013

epidemiologic analyses[17] indicated that in European-derived whites the overall frequency of vitiligo in probands' first-degree relatives was 7%, with the risk 7.8% in probands' parents and 6.1% in siblings, consistent with polygenic, multifactorial inheritance and age-dependency of vitiligo onset. Importantly, among vitiligo probands' affected relatives, the frequency of vitiligo was equal in male and female subjects, eliminating the female sex bias found in most vitiligo clinical case series. Moreover, a careful study of families with multiple relatives affected by vitiligo[19] showed earlier age-of-onset and greater skin surface involvement than in singleton cases,[17] as well as greater frequency of other autoimmune diseases, suggesting that in such multiplex families genes likely contribute more to vitiligo risk than in singleton cases.

RELATIONSHIP TO OTHER AUTOIMMUNE DISEASES

The genetic basis of vitiligo is deeply intertwined with the genetic basis of other autoimmune diseases with which vitiligo is epidemiologically associated. Indeed, the earliest clue to the autoimmune origin of vitiligo came in the original 1855 report of Addison disease,[20] which included a patient with idiopathic adrenal insufficiency, generalized vitiligo, and pernicious anemia, a co-occurrence of autoimmune diseases that suggested shared etiologic factors. Subsequently, the co-occurrence of different autoimmune diseases, including vitiligo, was reported by many investigators, particularly Schmidt,[21] and key combinations of concomitant autoimmune diseases were later codified by Neufeld and Blizzard.[22] Beginning with the vitiligo case series reported by Steve,[23] numerous investigators have since documented prevalent co-occurrence of vitiligo with various other autoimmune diseases, particularly autoimmune thyroid disease (both Hashimoto disease and Graves disease), pernicious anemia, Addison disease, systemic lupus erythematosus,[17] rheumatoid arthritis, adult-onset type 1 diabetes mellitus, and perhaps psoriasis.[19] Of particular importance, these same vitiligo-associated autoimmune diseases also occur at increased frequency in first-degree relatives of vitiligo probands who do not themselves have vitiligo, indicating that these autoimmune diseases share at least some of their genetic underpinnings with vitiligo.[19]

EARLY GENETIC MARKER STUDIES

The earliest attempts to identify genetic markers associated with vitiligo began in the mid-1960s, assaying polymorphic blood proteins, such as the ABO and other blood group antigens[24–30]; secretor status[26,27,31]; and, later, serum alpha 1-antitrypsin and haptoglobin phenotypes,[32] with no positive results. A decade later, numerous investigators reported association studies of vitiligo with human leukocyte antigen (HLA) types, which have also been associated with many other autoimmune diseases. Initial association studies of vitiligo and HLA yielded inconsistent and largely spurious findings due to testing different ethnic groups, inadequate statistical power, and inadequate correction for multiple-testing of many different HLA types.[33–37] Nevertheless, Foley and colleagues[38] correctly identified association of the HLA-DR4 class II serotype with vitiligo, borne out by subsequent studies, the first known genetic association for vitiligo. Importantly, HLA-DR4 is also strongly associated with several other autoimmune diseases.

A large number of additional HLA association studies of vitiligo were published subsequently, again with generally inconsistent findings. Nevertheless, Liu and colleagues[39] conducted a careful meta-analysis of 11 previous studies of HLA class I serotypes and found robust association of vitiligo with HLA-A2 with odds ratio (OR) 2.07, a finding borne out by subsequent studies. Specific associations of vitiligo with the class I and class II gene regions of the major histocompatibility complex (MHC) were subsequently replicated and refined by detailed molecular genetic and genomewide association studies (GWASs), even to the point of identifying apparently causal genetic variation (see later discussion).

NON-MAJOR HISTOCOMPATIBILITY COMPLEX CANDIDATE GENE ASSOCIATION STUDIES

The development of DNA technology in the late 1970s ushered in an era of testing candidate genes for association with a great many diseases, including vitiligo. Unfortunately, numerous retrospective studies have shown that well over 95% of published case-control genetic association studies represent false-positives, due to inadequate sample size and statistical fluctuation, genotyping errors, occult population stratification, inadequate correction for multiple-testing, and publication bias of positive results.[40,41] As the result, this type of study is no longer considered appropriate for primary discovery of genetic association. Accordingly, of the approximately 70 genes for which association with vitiligo has been claimed based on such studies, this article discusses only those 2 non-MHC candidate gene associations that have received widespread independent confirmation, including by unbiased GWASs.

Kemp and colleagues[42] reported the first vitiligo non-MHC candidate gene association with *CTLA4*, which encodes a T-cell coreceptor involved in regulation of T-cell activation and which is associated with several of the other autoimmune diseases that are epidemiologically associated with vitiligo. In fact, *CTLA4* association was strongest in vitiligo patients who also had other concomitant autoimmune diseases,[43] a finding subsequently replicated by another study and meta-analysis.[44] Association of *CTLA4* with vitiligo has been variable among studies of different populations; however, at least in European-derived whites, it has been demonstrated by GWASs.

A second important non-MHC candidate gene association, also reported by Kemp,[45] was with *PTPN22*, encoding LYP protein tyrosine phosphatase, which likewise has been genetically associated with many different autoimmune diseases. Again, this association was replicated in most other studies of European-derived whites[46,47] and by GWASs, but not in most other populations. Thus, along with HLA class II, *CTLA4* and *PTPN22* likely are 2 of the genes that underlie epidemiologic association of vitiligo with other autoimmune diseases, at least in European-derived whites.

GENOMEWIDE STUDIES

Candidate gene analyses carry an intrinsic a priori bias by selection of genes for study. In contrast, genomewide analyses of polygenic, multifactorial diseases are, in principle, unbiased beyond the assumption that genetic factors play some role. There are 3 approaches to genomewide genetic analysis. Genomewide linkage analysis tests for cosegregation of polymorphic markers with disease within families with multiple affected relatives and across such families. Such families are uncommon, the genetic resolution of linkage is low, and the genetic analyses require several important assumptions that may not be correct. GWASs, the current gold standard, require large numbers of cases and controls but are reasonably powerful, can detect many genotyping errors, can provide fine-mapping, can detect population outliers and correct for population stratification, can appropriately account for multiple-testing, and require independent replication and a stringent genomewide significance criterion ($P < 5 \times 10^{-8}$) to declare discovery. For reasons that are not clear, linkage and GWASs often do not detect the same genetic signals. Genomewide or exome DNA sequencing studies can be configured similarly to linkage or GWASs but are far more expensive and have not yet been applied to vitiligo.

Genetic Linkage Studies

Initial linkage studies of vitiligo were not genomewide, focusing on the MHC and other specific candidate regions of the genome, and will not be discussed here. The first genomewide linkage study of vitiligo was indirect. Nath and colleagues[48] mapped a locus on chromosome 17p13 they called *SLEV1* in a subset of lupus families who also had relatives with vitiligo. Spritz and colleagues[49] subsequently confirmed the *SLEV1* linkage signal by genomewide linkage analysis of vitiligo families in which various other autoimmune diseases also occurred. That group eventually fine-mapped and identified the corresponding gene as *NLRP1*,[50] which encodes an inflammasome regulatory protein.

In a unique large European-derived white kindred with near autosomal-dominant vitiligo, Spritz and colleagues[51,52] used genomewide linkage to map a locus they termed Autoimmune Susceptibility 1 (*AIS1*) at chromosome 1p31.3-p32.2. That group subsequently identified the corresponding gene as *FOXD3*,[53] encoding a key regulator of melanoblast differentiation. This vitiligo kindred was found to segregate a private sequence variant in the *FOXD3* promoter that upregulated transcription in vitro, which would be expected to reduce melanoblast differentiation. Recently, Schunter and colleagues[54] identified another *FOXD3* promoter variant associated with vitiligo that also increases transcriptional activity. Spritz and colleagues[49] also mapped 2 additional vitiligo linkage signals in European-derived white vitiligo families, *AIS2* on chromosome 7 and *AIS3* on chromosomes 8.[52,55] Specific genes corresponding to *AIS2* and *AIS3* have not yet been identified.

In parallel linkage studies of Han Chinese vitiligo families, Zhang and colleagues identified 3 loci, *AIS4* on chromosome 4q12-q21[56] and 2 unnamed loci on 6p21-p22 and 22q12.[57] These investigators suggested that *AIS4* might be *PDGFRA*,[58] though this seems much less likely than *KIT*. The chromosome 6 locus may correspond to the MHC. Also, Ren and colleagues[59] found that the chromosome 22 locus may correspond to *XBP1*.

Genomewide Association Studies

The first GWAS of vitiligo was of a unique population isolate in Romania in which there is a very high prevalence of vitiligo and other autoimmune diseases.[60] This study identified association with an

Table 1
Vitiligo susceptibility genes identified by genomewide association studies

Chr.	Locus	Protein	Function
1	*RERE*	Arginine-glutamic acid dipeptide repeats	Regulator of apoptosis
1	*PTPN22*	Protein tyrosine phosphatase, nonreceptor type 22	Alters responsiveness of T-cell receptors
1	*FASLG*	FAS ligand	Regulator of immune apoptosis
1	*PTPRC*	Protein tyrosine phosphatase, receptor type C	Regulator of T- and B-cell antigen receptor signaling
2	*PPP4R3B*	Protein phosphatase 4 regulatory subunit 3B	Unknown
2	*BCL2L11?*	BCL2 like 11	Regulator of apoptosis in thymocyte negative selection
2	*IFIH1*	Interferon induced with helicase C domain 1	Innate immune receptor
2	*CTLA4*	Cytotoxic T-lymphocyte-associated protein 4	T-lymphocyte checkpoint regulator
2	*FARP2-STK25*	?	?
3	*UBE2E2*	Ubiquitin-conjugating enzyme E2 E2	Protein ubiquitination pathway; damage response
3	*FOXP1*	Forkhead box protein P1	Transcriptional regulator of B-cell development
3	*CD80*	T-lymphocyte activation antigen CD80	T-cell costimulatory signal
3	*LPP*	Lipoma-preferred partner	Unknown
3	*FBXO45-NRROS*	?	?
4	*PPP3CA*	Serine/threonine-protein phosphatase 2B catalytic subunit alpha isoform	T-lymphocyte calcium-dependent, calmodulin-stimulated protein phosphatase
6	*IRF4*	Interferon regulatory factor 4	Transcriptional activator in immune cells and melanocytes
6	*SERPINB9*	Serpin B9	Endogenous inhibitor of granzyme B
6	*HLA-A*	HLA class I histocompatibility antigen, A	Presents peptide antigens to the immune system
6	*HLA-DRB1/DQA1*	HLA class II histocompatibility antigens, DRB1 and DQA1	Present peptide antigens to the immune system
6	*BACH2*	BTB domain and CNC homolog 2	Transcriptional activator, regulator of apoptosis
6	*RNASET2-FGFR1OP-CCR6*	?	?
7	*CPVL*	Probable serine carboxypeptidase CPVL	Inflammatory protease; trims antigens for presentation
8	*SLA*	Src-like-adapter	Regulator of T-cell antigen receptor signaling
9	*NEK6*	NIMA-related serine/threonine-protein kinase Nek6	Regulator of apoptosis

(*continued on next page*)

Table 1
(continued)

Chr.	Locus	Protein	Function
10	*IL2RA*	Interleukin-2 receptor subunit alpha	IL2 receptor; regulates regulator T lymphocytes
10	*ARID5B*	AT-rich interactive domain-containing protein 5B	Transcriptional coactivator
10	*ZMIZ1*	Zinc finger MIZ domain-containing protein 1	Possible PIAS-family transcriptional or sumoylation regulator
10	*CASP7*	Caspase-7	Apoptosis executor protein
11	*CD44*	CD44 antigen	Regulator of FOXP3 expression
11	*PPP1R14B-PLCB3-BAD-GPR137-KCNK4-TEX40-ESRRA-TRMT112-PRDX5*	?	?
11	*TYR*	Tyrosinase	Melanocyte melanogenic enzyme; vitiligo autoantigen
11	Gene desert	?	?
12	*PMEL*	Premelanosome protein PMEL	Melanocyte melanosomal type I transmembrane glycoprotein
12	*IKZF4*	Zinc finger protein Eos	Transcriptional repressor; regulates FOXP3 transcription in regulatory T lymphocytes
12	*SH2B3*	SH2B adapter protein 3	Links T-lymphocyte receptor activation signal to phospholipase C-gamma-1, GRB2 and phosphatidylinositol 3-kinase
13	*TNFSF11*	Tumor necrosis factor ligand superfamily member 11	T-lymphocyte cytokine that binds to TNFRSF11A and TNFRSF11B
14	*GZMB*	Granzyme B	Apoptosis executioner protein of cytotoxic T lymphocytes
15	*OCA2-HERC2*	Oculocutaneous albinism 2	Melanocyte melanogenic protein; vitiligo autoantigen
16	*MC1R*	Melanocortin 1 receptor	Melanocyte melanogenic protein; vitiligo autoantigen
17	*KAT2A-HSPB9-RAB5C*	?	?
18	*TNFRSF11A*	Tumor necrosis factor receptor superfamily member 11A	Regulates interactions between T lymphocytes and dendritic cells
19	*TICAM1*	TIR domain-containing adapter molecule 1	TLR3/TLR4 adapter; mediates NF-kappa-B and interferon-regulatory factor (IRF) activation; induces apoptosis
19	*SCAF1-IRF3-BCL2L12*	?	?

(*continued on next page*)

Table 1
(*continued*)

Chr.	Locus	Protein	Function
20	*RALY- ASIP*	Agouti signaling protein	Regulator of melanocytes via MC1R
20	*PTPN1*	Tyrosine-protein phosphatase nonreceptor type 1	Dephosphorylates JAK2 and TYK2 kinases; cellular response to interferon?
21	*UBASH3A*	Ubiquitin-associated and SH3 domain-containing protein A	Promotes accumulation of activated T-cell receptors on surface
22	*C1QTNF6*	Complement C1q tumor necrosis factor-related protein 6	Unknown
22	*ZC3H7B-TEF*	?	?
X	*IL1RAPL1*	Interleukin-1 receptor accessory protein-like 1	Unknown
X	*CCDC22-FOXP3-GAGE*	?	FOXP3 regulates development and inhibitory function of regulatory T-lymphocytes

Note: Questionmarks (?) denote specific gene or function not yet been identified.

SNP within *SMOC2* on chromosome 6q27, in close vicinity to *IDDM8*, a linkage and association signal for type 1 diabetes mellitus and rheumatoid arthritis.[61]

The Spritz group has also carried out 3 successive GWASs of vitiligo of US-derived and European-derived whites.[62–65] As shown in **Table 1**, these analyses have identified confirmed associations of vitiligo with 48 distinct loci, altogether accounting for 22.5% of vitiligo heritability in European-derived whites, as well as several additional loci with suggestive significance.[65] About half of the confirmed vitiligo loci encode immunoregulatory proteins, consistent with the autoimmune nature of vitiligo; several others encode regulators of apoptosis; and at least 6 encode either melanocyte components or regulators of melanocyte function. Of this last group, all have also been implicated in both normal pigmentary variation and risk of melanoma, and all show a remarkable inverse genetic relationship between vitiligo risk and melanoma risk,[62,63,65] suggesting that vitiligo may result from dysregulation of a normal mechanism of immune surveillance for melanoma.[66,67] Many of these proteins encoded by the confirmed vitiligo genes interact directly in functional biological pathways that are key to vitiligo pathogenesis (**Fig. 1**), suggesting that most of the pathways involved in vitiligo susceptibility may have already been discovered.

Fine-mapping and functional analyses of these vitiligo loci identified in European-derived whites indicates that for vitiligo, as for other complex diseases, about half of causal variants seem to affect gene regulatory regions, whereas only about 15% are located within exons, many resulting in missense substitutions. Spritz and colleagues have shown that, for both MHC class I (*HLA-A*)[68,69] and MHC class II (*HLA-DRB1/-DQA1*),[70,71] the vitiligo-associated causal SNPs are located in transcriptional enhancer elements that upregulate expression of the corresponding MHC genes, resulting in gain of function. Interestingly, the MHC class II association signal also constitutes a quantitative trait locus for vitiligo age-of-onset.[72] For *NLRP1*, which encodes an inflammasome regulatory component, the vitiligo-associated causal SNPs constitute haplotypes of missense variants in almost complete linkage disequilibrium, which together synergize to result in constitutive gain of NLRP1 function and thus activation of interleukin-1 beta.[73] For *GZMB*, encoding granzyme B, an apoptotic effector protein used by cytotoxic T-cells to kill their targets, the causal vitiligo-associated SNP is a common missense variant R55Q[74] that alters GZMB function. For *TYR*, encoding tyrosinase, a key melanogenic enzyme and the major vitiligo autoimmune antigen, the vitiligo-associated SNPs are protective, and represent the missense variants S192Y and R402Q that are common in European-derived whites but not in other populations and which reduce thermal stability and catalytic function.[75]

In addition to studies in European-derived whites, there have been several GWASs of vitiligo in Asian populations. Zhang and colleagues carried out a large GWAS of vitiligo in the Han and Uygur populations of China, detecting complex association signals in the class I and class II regions of the MHC and with the *RNASET2-FGFR1OP-CCR6* region of chromosome 6q24.[76] Deeper analysis of this GWAS[77] detected additional association signals in the region of *PMEL*, 10q22.1 and a nearby locus suggested to be *ZMIZ1*,[78] and 11q23.3. Of these associations in Chinese, only that in the *RNASET2-FGFR1OP-CCR6* region corresponds to an association

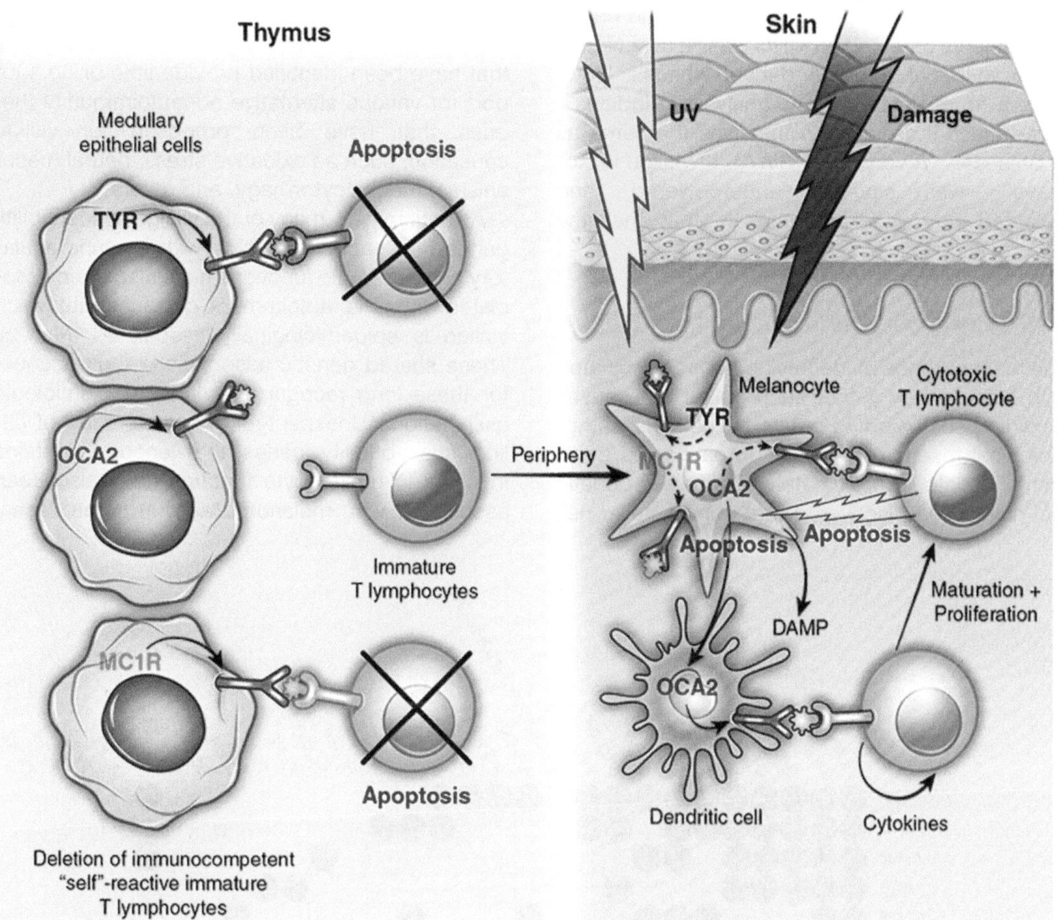

Fig. 1. General framework of vitiligo pathogenesis. During early development, a T-lymphocyte repertoire is selected by positive selection of immunocompetent immature T lymphocytes in the thymic cortex. Immunocompetent T lymphocytes that recognize self-antigens expressed by medullary epithelial cells undergo negative selection and undergo apoptosis. Immunocompetent immature T lymphocytes that do not encounter a cognate self-antigen then exit the thymus to the peripheral circulation. In the skin, many or most cases of vitiligo initiate with skin damage, often ultraviolet (UV) exposure or trauma, a process termed Koebnerization. Damaged melanocytes apoptose and release molecules that act as damage-associated molecular patterns (DAMPs), which stimulate activation of local dendritic cells. Dendritic cells engulf melanosomal proteins, which are degraded in the proteasome, and fragments that act as peptide antigens are presented by HLA class II molecules on the dendritic cell surface. Immature T lymphocytes that express cognate T-cell receptors bind these self-antigens and are activated to express costimulatory molecules that result in cell proliferation and differentiation into CD8+ effector cytotoxic T lymphocytes, with the assistance of CD4+ T-helper cells. The resultant activated cytotoxic T lymphocytes recognize and bind the cognate self-antigen presented by HLA class I molecules on the melanocyte surface, assisted by interaction of FAS ligand on the T cell and FAS on the target melanocyte. The cytotoxic T lymphocyte then elaborates granzyme B and perforin, which induce apoptosis of the target melanocyte. Almost all of these processes involve proteins that are encoded by 1 or more genes associated with genetic susceptibility to vitiligo.

detected in white patients.[63] Indeed, although MHC class I and class II region associations were detected in whites[62,65,68,69,71] and Chinese,[76] the specific underlying associations seem to be somewhat different. This is surprising because a GWAS of vitiligo in Japanese[79] detected an MHC class I association with *HLA-A*02:01* that appears identical to that in European-derived whites, whereas an immunocentric GWAS of vitiligo in Asian Indian and Pakistani subjects detected an MHC class II association similar to that of European-derived whites.[80] However, a more detailed MHC analysis in Indians[81] found class II association that was the same as in Chinese.[76] A very small GWAS of vitiligo in Koreans[82] was severely underpowered, and detected no association signals that met the genomewide significance threshold.

WHERE ARE WE NOW?

The main purpose of identifying genes associated with disease risk is that such genes are causal, providing solid starting points for defining pathobiological mechanisms and approaches to treatment. To date, approximately 50 different genetic loci have been discovered that contribute to risk of vitiligo, most in European-derived whites (see **Table 1**). For most of these loci, specific genes have been identified, which have greatly furthered understanding of the biological causation of vitiligo. Almost all of the identified genes encode proteins involved in immunoregulation, apoptosis, and melanocyte function, underscoring the autoimmune basis of vitiligo, with dysregulated immune programming, cellular activation, and melanocyte target cell recognition and killing (see **Fig. 1**). Thus far, the vitiligo susceptibility genes that have been identified provide little or no support for various alternative nonautoimmunity theories that have been proposed for vitiligo causation, such as oxidative stress, neural mechanisms, melanocytorrhagy, and others.

As anticipated, many of the vitiligo susceptibility genes that encode proteins with immunoregulatory and apoptotic functions have also been associated with other autoimmune diseases with which vitiligo is epidemiologically associated (**Fig. 2**). These shared genetic associations thus account for these long recognized clinical epidemiologic associations. Unexpectedly, however, most of vitiligo susceptibility genes that encode proteins involved in melanocyte function have also been associated with melanoma and, in some cases,

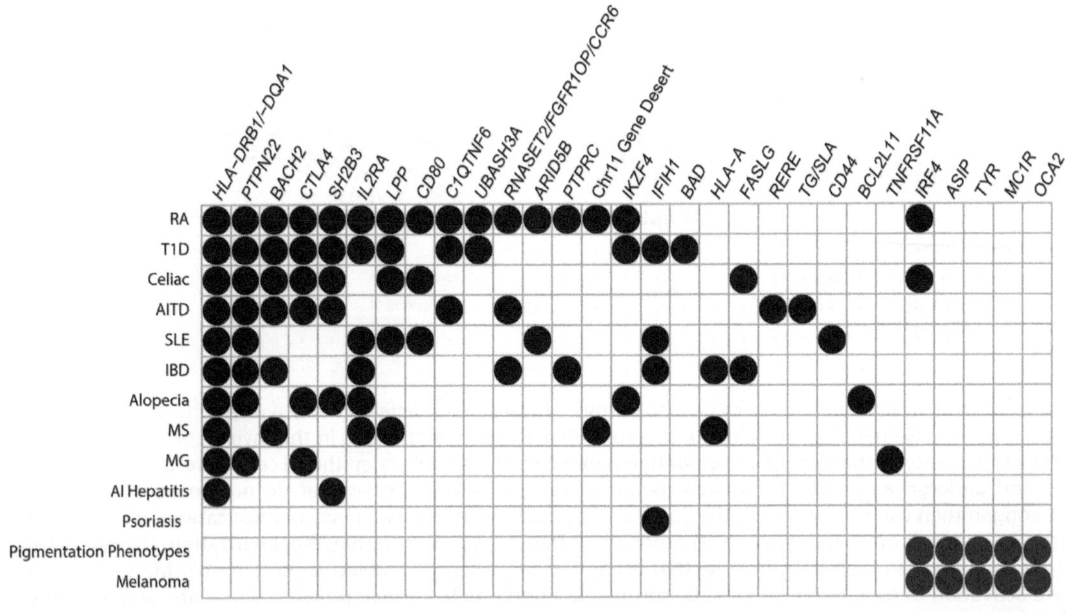

Fig. 2. Shared genetic associations of vitiligo with other autoimmune diseases and with pigmentation and melanoma phenotypes. Blue circles indicate shared genetic associations between vitiligo and other autoimmune diseases. Red circles indicate shared genetic associations between vitiligo and normal pigmentary variation phenotypes and melanoma. Only associations identified by GWASs and meeting the genomewide significance criterion ($P < 5 \times 10^{-8}$) are shown. Associations claimed based on candidate gene case-control studies are not included. AI hepatitis, autoimmune hepatitis; AITD, autoimmune thyroid disease; IBD, inflammatory bowel disease; MG, myasthenia gravis; MS, multiple sclerosis; RA, rheumatoid arthritis; SLE, systemic lupus erythematosus; T1D, type 1 diabetes mellitus.

nonmelanoma skin cancers, in each case involving the same associated SNPs but with opposite effects. Although the precise meaning of this observation is not yet clear, it suggests that vitiligo might involve a dysregulated mechanism that has evolved for immune surveillance for melanoma[66,67] and other skin cancers, consistent with the approximately 3-fold reduced incidence of melanoma and nonmelanoma skin cancers observed in patients with pre-existing vitiligo.[83,84] Alternatively, it might be that gene variants that reduce skin pigmentation elevate risk for all forms of skin cancer, melanoma and nonmelanoma.

Most vitiligo susceptibility genes have been detected in European-derived whites. Some of these genes likewise contribute to vitiligo risk in Asian populations, whereas others apparently do not. In European-derived whites, the identified genes and gene variants altogether account for about 25% of total vitiligo genetic risk. It remains unknown whether the remainder of risk is attributable to additional unknown variation in these same genes, to additional unknown genes that exert smaller effects, to genetic interactions that potentiate gene effects, or to other causes. Understanding this will be essential to achieve personalized medicine for vitiligo, enabling reasonably accurate prediction of risks and classification of patients into genetically based subgroups that may benefit from specialized approaches to vitiligo treatment or even prevention.

REFERENCES

1. Le Cat M. Traité de la Couleur de la Peau Humaine. Amsterdam (Netherlands): 1765.
2. Stűttgen G. Die vitiligo in erbbiologischer betrachtung. Z Haut Geschlechtskr 1950;9(11):451–7.
3. Teindel H. Familiäre vitiligo. Z Haut Geschlechtskr 1950;9(11):457–62.
4. Mohr J. Vitiligo in a pair of monovular twins. Acta Genet Stat Med 1951;2(3):252–5.
5. Siemens HW. Het erfelijkheidsvraagstuk bij vitiligo. Ned Tijdschr Geneeskd 1953;97(38):2449–51.
6. Vogel F. Dermatological observations on uniovular twins: vitiligo, ichthyosis simplex, psoriasis. Z Haut Geschlechtskr 1956;20(1):1–4 [in German].
7. Sidi E, Bourgeois-Gavardin J. The treatment of vitiligo with ammi majus. Presse Med 1953;61(21): 436–40.
8. Behl PN. Leucoderma and its treatment with ammi majus. J Indian Med Assoc 1955;24(16):615–8.
9. Levai M. A study of certain contributory factors in the development of vitiligo in South Indian patients. AMA Arch Derm 1958;78(3):364–71.
10. Lerner AB. Vitiligo. J Invest Dermatol 1959;32(2, Part 2):285–310.
11. Hafez M, Sharaf L, Abd el-Nabi SM. The genetics of vitiligo. Acta Derm Venereol 1983;63(3):249–51.
12. Das SK, Majumder PP, Majumdar TK, et al. Studies on vitiligo. II. Familial aggregation and genetics. Genet Epidemiol 1985;2(3):255–62.
13. Majumder PP, Das SK, Li CC. A genetical model for vitiligo. Am J Hum Genet 1988;43(2):119–25.
14. Bhatia PS, Mohan L, Pandey ON, et al. Genetic nature of vitiligo. J Dermatol Sci 1992;4(3):180–4.
15. Majumder PP, Nordlund JJ, Nath SK. Pattern of familial aggregation of vitiligo. Arch Dermatol 1993; 129(8):994–8.
16. Nath SK, Majumder PP, Nordlund JJ. Genetic epidemiology of vitiligo: multilocus recessivity cross-validated. Am J Hum Genet 1994;55(5):981–90.
17. Alkhateeb A, Fain PR, Thody A, et al. Epidemiology of vitiligo and associated autoimmune diseases in Caucasian probands and their families. Pigment Cell Res 2003;16(3):208–14.
18. Zhang XJ, Liu JZB, Gui JP, et al. Characteristics of genetic epidemiology and genetic models for vitiligo. J Am Acad Dermatol 2004;51(3):383–90.
19. Laberge G, Mailloux CM, Gowan K, et al. Early disease onset and increased risk of other autoimmune diseases in familial generalized vitiligo. Pigment Cell Res 2005;18(4):300–5.
20. Addison T. On the constitutional and local effects of disease of the supra-renal capsules. London: Samuel Highley; 1855.
21. Schmidt M. Eine biglanduiare Erkrankung (Nebennieren und Schilddruse) bei Morbus Addisonii. Verh Dtsch Ges Pathol 1926;21:212–21.
22. Neufeld M, Blizzard RM. Polyglandular autoimmune diseases. In: Pinchera A, Doniach D, Fenzi GF, et al, editors. Symposium on autoimmune aspects of endocrine disorders. New York: Academic Press; 1980. p. 357–65.
23. Steve BF. Further investigations in the treatment of vitiligo. Va Med Mon (1918) 1945;71(1):6–17.
24. Srivistava GN, Shukla RC. ABO blood groups in vitiligo. Indian J Med Res 1965;53(3):221–5.
25. Singh G, Shanker P. Vitiligo and blood groups. Preliminary report. Br J Dermatol 1966;78(2):91–2.
26. Sehgal VN, Dube B. ABO blood groups and vitiligo. J Med Genet 1968;5:308–9.
27. Dutta AK, Mondal SB, Dutta SB. ABO blood group and secretory status in vitiligo. J Indian Med Assoc 1969;53(4):186–9.
28. Oriente Biondi C, Ruocco V. Vitiligo and blood groups. Rass Int Clin Ter 1969;49(22):1395–9 [in Italian].
29. Kareemullah L, Taneja V, Begum S, et al. Association of ABO blood groups and vitiligo. J Med Genet 1977;14(3):211–3.
30. Wasfi AI, Saha N, El Munshid HA, et al. Genetic association in vitiligo: ABO, MNSs, Rhesus, Kell and Duffy blood groups. Clin Genet 1980;17(6):415–7.

31. Sehgal VN, Dube B. Secretory state in vitiligo. Dermatologica 1969;138(2):89–92.
32. Mujahid Ali M, Banu M, Waheed MA, et al. Serum alpha 1-antitrypsin and haptoglobin phenotypes in vitiligo. Arch Dermatol Res 1990;282(3):206–7.
33. Retornaz G, Betuel H, Ortonne JP, et al. HL-A antigens and vitiligo. Br J Dermatol 1976;95(2):173–5.
34. Kachru RB, Telischi M, Mittal KK. HLA antigens and vitiligo in an American black population. Tissue Antigens 1978;12(5):396–7.
35. Metzker A, Zamir R, Gazit E, et al. Vitiligo and the HLA system. Dermatologica 1980;160(2):100–5.
36. Nakagawa H, Otuka F, Kukita A, et al. Histocompatible antigens in vitiligo vulgaris II. Nihon Hifuka Gakkai Zasshi 1980;90(10):939–41 [in Japanese].
37. Minev N, Tonkin N, Martinova F. Association of the HLA system with vitiligo. Vestn Dermatol Venerol 1985;(5):41–2 [in Russian].
38. Foley LM, Lowe NJ, Misheloff E, et al. Association of HLA-DR4 with vitiligo. J Am Acad Dermatol 1983; 8(1):39–40.
39. Liu J-B, Li M, Chen H, et al. Association of vitiligo with HLA-A2: a meta-analysis. J Eur Acad Dermatol Venereol 2007;21(2):205–13.
40. Hirschhorn JN, Lohmueller K, Byrne E, et al. A comprehensive review of genetic association studies. Genet Med 2002;4(2):45–61.
41. Ioannidis JPA, Tarone R, McLaughlin JK. The false-positive to false-negative ratio in epidemiologic studies. Epidemiology 2011;22(4):450–6.
42. Kemp EH, Ajjan RA, Waterman EA, et al. Analysis of a microsatellite polymorphism of the cytotoxic T-lymphocyte antigen-4 gene in patents with vitiligo. Br J Dermatol 1999;140(1):73–8.
43. Blomhoff A, Kemp EH, Gawkrodger DJ, et al. CTLA4 polymorphisms are associated with vitiligo, in patients with concomitant autoimmune diseases. Pigment Cell Res 2004;18(1):55–8.
44. Birlea SA, LaBerge GS, Procopciuc LM, et al. *CTLA4* and generalized vitiligo: two genetic association studies and a meta-analysis of published data. Pigment Cell Melanoma Res 2009;22(2):230–4.
45. Cantón I, Akhtar S, Gavalas NG, et al. A single-nucleotide polymorphism in the gene encoding lymphoid protein tyrosine phosphatase (*PTPN22*) confers susceptibility to generalised vitiligo. Genes Immun 2005;6:584–7.
46. LaBerge GS, Bennett DC, Fain PR, et al. *PTPN22* is genetically associated with risk of generalized vitiligo, but *CTLA4* is not. J Invest Dermatol 2008;128: 1757–62.
47. LaBerge GS, Birlea SA, Fain PR, et al. The *PTPN22* -1858C>T (R620W) functional polymorphism is associated with generalized vitiligo in the Romanian population. Pigment Cell Melanoma Res 2008;21(2):206–8.
48. Nath SK, Kelly JA, Namjou B, et al. Evidence for a susceptibility gene, *SLEV1*, on chromosome 17p13 in families with vitiligo-related systemic lupus erythematosus. Am J Hum Genet 2001;69(6):1401–6.
49. Spritz RA, Gowan K, Bennett DC, et al. Novel vitiligo susceptibility loci on chromosomes 7 (*AIS2*) and 8 (*AIS3*), confirmation of *SLEV1* on chromosome 17, and their roles in an autoimmune diathesis. Am J Hum Genet 2004;74(1):188–91.
50. Jin Y, Mailloux CM, Gowan K, et al. *NALP1* in vitiligo-associated multiple autoimmune disease. N Engl J Med 2007;356(12):1216–25.
51. Alkhateeb A, Stetler GL, Old W, et al. Mapping of an autoimmunity susceptibility locus (*AIS1*) to chromosome 1p31.3p32.2. Hum Mol Genet 2002;11(6): 661–7.
52. Fain PR, Gowan K, LaBerge GS, et al. A genomewide screen for generalized vitiligo: confirmation of *AIS1* on chromosome 1p31 and evidence for additional susceptibility loci. Am J Hum Genet 2003;72(6):1560–4.
53. Alkhateeb A, Fain P, Spritz RA. Candidate functional promoter variant in the *FOXD3* melanoblast developmental regulator gene in autosomal dominant vitiligo. J Invest Dermatol 2005;125:388–91.
54. Schunter JA, Löffler D, Wiesner T, et al. A novel *FoxD3* variant is associated with vitiligo and elevated thyroid auto-antibodies. J Clin Endocrinol Metab 2015;100(10):E1335–42.
55. Jin Y, Riccardi SL, Gowan K, et al. Fine-mapping of vitiligo susceptibility loci on chromosomes 7 and 9 and interactions with *NLRP1 (NALP1)*. J Invest Dermatol 2010;130(3):774–83.
56. Chen JJ, Huang W, Gui JP, et al. A novel linkage to generalized vitiligo on 4q13-q21 identified in a genomewide linkage analysis of Chinese families. Am J Hum Genet 2005;76(6):1057–65.
57. Liang Y, Yang S, Zhou Y, et al. Evidence for two susceptibility loci on chromosomes 22q12 and 6p21-p22 in Chinese generalized vitiligo families. J Invest Dermatol 2007;127(11):2552–7.
58. Xu S, Zhou Y, Yang S, et al. Platelet-derived growth factor receptor alpha gene mutations in vitiligo vulgaris. Acta Derm Venereol 2010;90(2):131–5.
59. Ren Y, Yang S, Xu S, et al. Genetic variation of promoter sequence modulates *XBP1* expression and genetic risk for vitiligo. PLoS Genet 2009;5(6): e1000523.
60. Birlea SA, Fain PR, Spritz RA. A Romanian population isolate with high frequency of vitiligo and associated autoimmune diseases. Arch Dermatol 2008; 144(3):310–6.
61. Birlea SA, Gowan K, Fain PR, et al. Genome-wide association study of generalized vitiligo in an isolated European founder population identifies *SMOC2*, in close proximity to *IDDM8*. J Invest Dermatol 2010;130(3):798–803.
62. Jin Y, Birlea SA, Fain PR, et al. Variant of *TYR* and autoimmunity susceptibility loci in generalized vitiligo. N Engl J Med 2010;362(18):1686–97.

63. Jin Y, Birlea SA, Fain PR, et al. Common variants in *FOXP1* are associated with generalized vitiligo. Nat Genet 2010;42(7):576–8.
64. Jin Y, Birlea SA, Fain PR, et al. Genome-wide association analyses identify 13 new susceptibility loci for generalized vitiligo. Nat Genet 2012;44(6):676–80.
65. Jin Y, Andersen G, Yorgov D, et al. Genome-wide association studies of autoimmune vitiligo identify 23 new risk loci and highlight key pathways and regulatory variants. Nat Genet 2016;48(11):1418–24.
66. Spritz RA. The genetics of generalized vitiligo: autoimmune pathways and an inverse relationship with malignant melanoma. Genome Med 2010;2(10):78.
67. Das PK, van den Wijngaard RMJGJ, Wankowicz-Kalinska A, et al. A symbiotic concept of autoimmunity and tumour immunity: lessons from vitiligo. Trends Immunol 2001;22:130–6.
68. Hayashi M, Jin Y, Yorgov D, et al. Autoimmune vitiligo is associated with gain-of-function by a transcriptional regulator that elevates expression of *HLA-A*02:01 in vivo.* Proc Natl Acad Sci U S A 2016;113(5):1357–62.
69. Jin Y, Ferrara T, Gowan K, et al. Next-generation DNA re-sequencing identifies common variants of *TYR* and *HLA-A* that modulate the risk of generalized vitiligo via antigen presentation. J Invest Dermatol 2012;132(6):1730–3.
70. Fain PR, Babu SR, Bennett DC, et al. HLA class II haplotype DRB1*04-DQB1*0301 contributes to risk of familial generalized vitiligo and early disease onset. Pigment Cell Res 2005;19:51–7.
71. Cavalli G, Hayashi M, Jin Y, et al. MHC class II super-enhancer increases surface expression of HLA-DR and HLA-DQ and affects cytokine production in autoimmune vitiligo. Proc Natl Acad Sci U S A 2016;113(5):1363–8.
72. Jin Y, Birlea SA, Fain PR, et al. Genome-wide analysis identifies a quantitative trait locus in the MHC class II region associated with generalized vitiligo age of onset. J Invest Dermatol 2011;131(6):1308–12.
73. Levandowski CB, Mailloux CM, Ferrara TM, et al. *NLRP1* haplotypes associated with vitiligo and autoimmunity increase interleukin-1β processing via the NLRP1 inflammasome. Proc Natl Acad Sci U S A 2013;110(8):2952–6.
74. Ferrara TM, Jin Y, Gowan K, et al. Risk of generalized vitiligo is associated with the common 55R-94A-247H variant haplotype of *GZMB* (encoding granzyme B). J Invest Dermatol 2013;133(6):1677–9.
75. Tripathi RK, Giebel LB, Strunk KM, et al. A polymorphism of the human tyrosinase gene is associated with temperature-sensitive enzymatic activity. Gene Expr 1991;1(2):103–10.
76. Quan C, Ren YQ, Xiang LH, et al. Genome-wide association study for vitiligo identifies susceptibility loci at 6q27 and the MHC. Nat Genet 2010;42(7):614–8.
77. Tang XF, Zhang Z, Hu DY, et al. Association analyses identify three susceptibility Loci for vitiligo in the Chinese Han population. J Invest Dermatol 2013;133(2):403–10.
78. Sun Y, Zuo X, Zheng X, et al. A comprehensive association analysis confirms *ZMIZ1* to be a susceptibility gene for vitiligo in Chinese population. J Med Genet 2014;51(5):345–53.
79. Jin Y, Hayashi M, Fain PR, et al. Major association of vitiligo with *HLA-A*02:01* in Japanese. Pigment Cell Melanoma Res 2015;28(3):360–2.
80. Birlea SA, Ahmad FJ, Uddin RM, et al. Association of generalized vitiligo with MHC class II loci in patients from the Indian subcontinent. J Invest Dermatol 2013;133(5):1369–72.
81. Singh A, Sharma P, Kar HK, et al, Indian Genome Variation Consortium. HLA alleles and amino-acid signatures of the peptide-binding pockets of HLA molecules in vitiligo. J Invest Dermatol 2012;132(1):124–34.
82. Cheong KA, Kim NH, Noh M, et al. Three new single nucleotide polymorphisms identified by a genome-wide association study in Korean patients with vitiligo. J Korean Med Sci 2013;28(5):775–9.
83. Teulings HE, Overkamp M, Ceylan E, et al. Decreased risk of melanoma in patients with vitiligo: a survey among 1307 patients and their partners. Br J Dermatol 2013;168:162–71.
84. Paradisi A, Tabolli S, Didona B, et al. Markedly reduced incidence of melanoma and nonmelanoma skin cancer in a nonconcurrent cohort of 10,040 patients with vitiligo. J Am Acad Dermatol 2014;71(6):1110–6.

Vitiligo Pathogenesis and Emerging Treatments

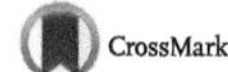

Mehdi Rashighi, MD[a,b], John E. Harris, MD, PhD[a,*]

KEYWORDS

• Vitiligo • Cellular stress • Autoimmunity • Chemokines • Targeted therapy • Melanogenesis

KEY POINTS

- Vitiligo results from the destruction of epidermal melanocytes by autoreactive cytotoxic T cells.
- Melanocyte-specific autoimmunity in vitiligo is a result of interplay among multiple factors, including genetic predisposition, environmental triggers, melanocyte stress, and innate and adaptive immune responses.
- An optimal treatment strategy in vitiligo would stabilize melanocytes, suppress the autoimmune response, and restore immune tolerance as well as stimulate melanocyte regeneration, proliferation, and migration to lesional skin.
- A better understanding of the key pathways involved in vitiligo onset and progression will enable developing treatments that have greater efficacy and a good safety profile.

INTRODUCTION

Vitiligo is a common, disfiguring autoimmune disease that negatively affects patients' self-esteem and quality of life.[1,2] Existing vitiligo treatments, which are used off-label, are general, nontargeted immunosuppressants that provide only modest efficacy. Developing safe and effective treatments requires a better understanding of disease pathogenesis to identify new therapeutic targets.[3] Vitiligo is caused by a dynamic interplay between genetic and environmental risks that initiates an autoimmune attack on melanocytes in the skin.

VITILIGO PATHOGENESIS

Genetics

The observation that vitiligo was more prevalent in the immediate relatives of patients with vitiligo provided early evidence of its heritability. Although vitiligo affects approximately 1% of the general population,[4] the risk of a patient's sibling developing the disease is 6% and for an identical twin it is 23%.[5] In addition, patients with vitiligo and their relatives have an increased risk of developing other autoimmune diseases, including autoimmune thyroiditis, type 1 diabetes mellitus, pernicious anemia, and Addison disease, suggesting that vitiligo is also an autoimmune disease.[6] These early observations were later confirmed by genome-wide association studies, which identified numerous common genetic variants in vitiligo patients encoding for components of both the innate immune system (NLRP1, IFIH1, CASP7, C1QTNF6, and TRIF) and adaptive immune system (FOXP3, BACH2, CD80, CCR6, PTPN22, interleukin [IL]-2R, α-GZMB, and HLA classes I and II)[7–9] (see also Richard Spritz and Genevieve Andersen's article, "Genetics of Vitiligo," in this issue).

Oxidative Stress

Accumulating evidence suggests that melanocytes from vitiligo patients have intrinsic defects that reduce their capacity to manage cellular stress (reviewed by Harris[10]). Epidermal cells,

Funding: Funded by NIH; Grant number AR069114.

[a] Department of Dermatology, University of Massachusetts Medical School, Worcester, MA 01605, USA; [b] Department of Dermatology, Tehran University of Medical Sciences, 415 Taleqani Avenue, Tehran 1416613675, Iran
* Corresponding author. 364 Plantation Street, LRB 325, Worcester, MA 01605.
E-mail address: John.Harris@umassmed.edu

Dermatol Clin 35 (2017) 257–265
http://dx.doi.org/10.1016/j.det.2016.11.014
0733-8635/17/

including melanocytes, are constantly exposed to environmental stressors, such as ultraviolet (UV) radiation and various chemicals, which can increase production of reactive oxygen species (ROS). Although healthy melanocytes are capable of mitigating these stressors, melanocytes from vitiligo patients seem more vulnerable. For example, melanocytes from perilesional vitiligo skin demonstrate a dilated endoplasmic reticulum and abnormalities in their mitochondria and melanosome structure, all of which are characteristic of elevated cellular stress. High concentrations of epidermal H_2O_2 level and a decreased level of catalase, a critical enzyme that protects cells from oxidative damage, have been observed in skin of patients with vitiligo.[11–17]

Environment

The earliest triggering events that lead to vitiligo are not fully understood. Multiple studies suggest that a combination of melanocyte intrinsic defects and exposure to specific environmental factors may play a central role in disease onset. This was evident in a group of factory workers who developed vitiligo after exposure to monobenzone, an organic chemical phenol, in their gloves.[18] Later studies confirmed that a history of exposure to other phenolic and catecholic chemicals found in dyes (especially hair dyes), resins/adhesives, and leather was associated with vitiligo.[19,20]

Melanogenesis is a multistep process through which the melanocyte produces melanin. Tyrosinase is a rate-limiting enzyme in this process that controls the production of melanin through oxidation of the amino acid tyrosine, a naturally occurring phenol (reviewed by d'Ischia and colleagues[21] and discussed further by John E. Harris's article, "Chemical-Induced Vitiligo," in this issue). In vitro studies demonstrated that chemical phenols can act as tyrosine analogs within the melanocyte, precipitating high levels of cellular stress. This stress may include increased production of ROS and triggering of the unfolded protein response, which in turn activates innate inflammation.[22,23]

Innate Immunity

As discussed previously, genome-wide association studies in vitiligo patients implicated multiple susceptibility loci related to the genes that control the innate immunity.[7–9] This likely causes dysregulated innate activation in response to melanocyte stress, demonstrated through recruitment of innate populations like natural killer cells and production and release of high levels of proinflammatory proteins and cytokines, including heat shock proteins (HSPs), IL-1β, IL-6, and IL-8[22–28] (reviewed in Refs.[10,29]). Among larger HSP molecules, inducible HSP70 (HSP70i) is unique, because it can be secreted to chaperone peptides specific to the originating host cells.[30] Recently, HSP70i has been shown to be important for vitiligo pathogenesis in a mouse model through induction of inflammatory dendritic cells, which themselves may be cytotoxic or carry and present melanocyte-specific antigens to T cells in lymphoid tissues.[24,25] This has been proposed to be a key cross-talk step between innate and adaptive immunity, leading to the T-cell–mediated autoimmune destruction of melanocytes.[31]

Adaptive Immunity

Ultimately, cytotoxic $CD8^+$ T cells are responsible for the destruction of melanocytes.[32] Cytokines secreted within the skin act as an early signal to help these autoreactive T cells locate stressed melanocytes. This is probably important because the epidermis is not vascularized, so active mechanisms are required to help them efficiently locate melanocytes.[33] Chemokines are small, secreted proteins that act as chemoattractants to guide T-cell migration. Interferon (IFN)-γ and IFN-γ–induced chemokines (CXCL9 and C-X-C Motif Chemokine Ligand 10 [CXCL 10]) are highly expressed in the skin and blood of patients with vitiligo as well as in a mouse model.[34–36] In addition, IFN-γ and CXCL10 are required for both disease progression and maintenance in a mouse model of the disease.[34,37] Recently, a separate study demonstrated not only that serum CXCL10 was higher in patients with vitiligo compared with healthy controls but also that its level was associated with disease activity and significantly decreased after successful treatment, suggesting it may be used as a biomarker to monitor the disease activity and treatment response.[36]

EMERGING TREATMENTS

Based on current understanding of vitiligo pathogenesis, a successful strategy to treat vitiligo should incorporate 3 distinct approaches: reducing melanocyte stress, regulating the autoimmune response, and stimulating melanocyte regeneration. Existing treatments partially address these needs; however, emerging therapies may do this in a more targeted way, and combination therapies may synergize to produce a better overall response (**Fig. 1**).

Reducing Melanocyte Stress

The apparent reduction of catalase enzyme in the epidermis of vitiligo patients as well as elevated

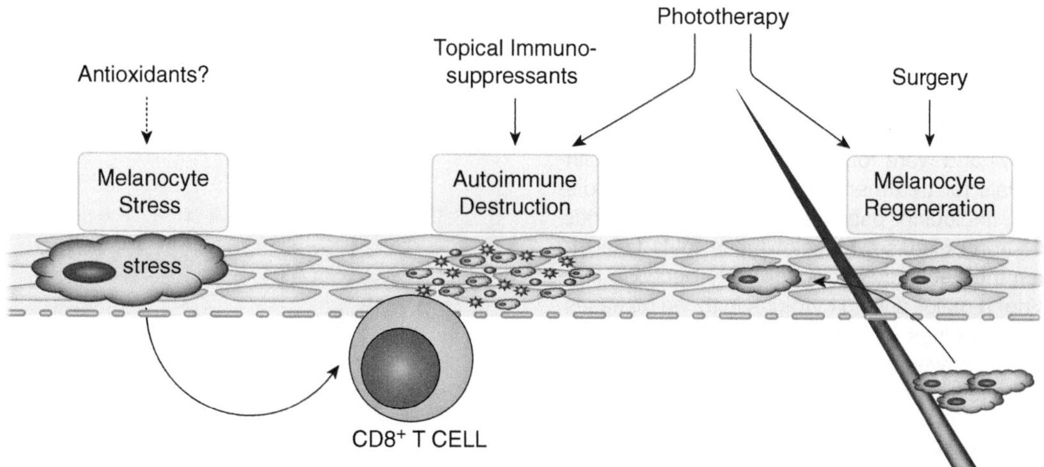

Fig. 1. Vitiligo pathogenesis begins with altered melanocytes that exhibit an elevated cellular stress response. This triggers autoimmunity, which targets melanocytes for destruction, resulting in focal depigmentation. Repigmentation requires the growth and migration of melanocytes, typically from hair follicles. Thus, there are 3 goals to consider during the treatment of vitiligo: (1) reducing melanocyte stress, (2) suppressing autoimmune targeting of melanocytes, and (3) promoting melanocyte regeneration. Current treatments, including topical immunosuppressants, phototherapy, and surgical approaches, partially address these goals in overall nontargeted ways.

levels of ROS in lesional skin prompted the hypothesis that treating patients with antioxidants or otherwise controlling ROS might be an effective treatment strategy.[38] Pseudocatalase describes a treatment cream comprised of any number of metal ions capable of converting H_2O_2, a common ROS, into water and oxygen. Early studies using pseudocatalase combined with phototherapy for vitiligo patients seemed promising[38–40]; however, they were either not controlled or not blinded, and subsequent studies have not reproduced positive results.[41–43] It is unclear if this strategy could be optimized or otherwise improved for the development of future therapies.

Oral or topical natural health products, vitamins, and supplements have been suggested as possible therapies based on their antioxidant and anti-inflammatory properties[44] (reviewed by Pearl E. Grimes and Rama Nashawati's article, "The Role of Diet and Supplements in Vitiligo Management," in this issue). The herbal supplement *Gingko biloba* has been tested in 2 small trials and reported to promote some improvement.[45,46] The plant extract *Polypodium leucotomos* reportedly improved responses to narrow band (NB)-UVB in a small group of vitiligo patients compared with placebo.[47] One group tested NB-UVB with or without supplementation by an antioxidant pool that included α-lipoic acid, vitamin C, vitamin E, and polyunsaturated fatty acids. They reported greater efficacy in patients who received a combination of NB-UVB plus antioxidants.[48] Larger, controlled trials need to be conducted to determine if adding antioxidants is a beneficial strategy to add to patient management.

Regulating Autoimmunity

Over the past decade, significant progress has been made in the development of immunomodulators to treat inflammatory skin disease, including more targeted treatments. Recent advances in understanding of the immunopathogenesis of vitiligo have helped identify novel immune targets to develop and test new vitiligo treatments.

Inducible heat shock protein 70

One group reported a role for HSP70i in vitiligo pathogenesis, suggesting that it was released by stressed melanocytes and initiated innate inflammation within the skin.[49] They then found that mutating the protein made it less immunogenic and seemed to even induce tolerance when expressed in the skin of a mouse model, preventing the onset of disease. They proposed future testing this as a new treatment of vitiligo,[25] although DNA delivery of a mutant protein in patient skin may take some time to develop and demonstrate safety.

Interferon-γ/CXCL10

The authors previously reported that the IFN-γ/CXCL10 axis is a critical signaling pathway required for both the progression and maintenance of vitiligo and hypothesized that targeting this pathway could be an effective treatment strategy.[34,37] A variety of antibodies and small molecule inhibitors have already been developed to target components of this pathway (including IFN-γ, CXCL10, and the CXCL10 receptor CXCR3) and were found safe in early-phase clinical trials for treatment of other autoimmune diseases, including psoriasis, rheumatoid arthritis, and Crohn disease. Most of these trials failed to reach their efficacy endpoint, likely because IFN-γ is not a major driving cytokine in those diseases. Recent findings in patients and a mouse model suggest, however, that vitiligo is an optimal disease to test those investigational drugs.[3]

Janus kinase–signal transducer and activator of transcription signaling

Janus kinase (JAK)–signal transducer and activator of transcription (STAT) signaling is essential to transmit extracellular signals of many cytokines, including IFN-γ, to the nucleus. After ligation of the cytokine receptor, JAKs phosphorylate STAT proteins, which become activated and induce transcription of target genes. There are 4 members of the JAK family, including JAK1, JAK2, JAK3, and tyrosine kinase 2. Among these, JAK1 and JAK2 are directly involved in IFN-γ signaling, which activate STAT1 and thus induce the transcription of IFN-γ–induced genes, including CXCL10 (**Fig. 2**) (reviewed by Villarino and colleagues[50]).

Several small molecule JAK inhibitors with distinct selectivity have been tested in patients or are under development. A patient with generalized vitiligo was reported to respond to treatment with oral tofacitinib, a JAK 1/3 inhibitor approved for the treatment of moderate to severe rheumatoid arthritis.[51] Ruxolitinib, another JAK inhibitor with JAK 1/2 selectivity, is currently approved by the Food and Drug Administration (FDA) for the treatment of intermediate-risk or high-risk myelofibrosis and polycythemia vera.[52,53] The authors and colleagues reported that a patient with vitiligo developed rapid repigmentation on his face and trunk after initiating oral ruxolitinib.[54] The treatment response from these inhibitors did not seem durable, because patients lost the repigmentation after discontinuing treatment[54] (Dr B. King, personal communication, April, 2016).

Similar to all other immunosuppressive drugs, tofacitinib and ruxolitinib may have adverse effects, including opportunistic infections and rare malignancies. In addition, ruxolitinib may induce blood abnormalities, including thrombocytopenia, anemia, and neutropenia.[55] Topical formulation of these drugs may provide therapeutic benefit without increasing the risk of adverse events.[56]

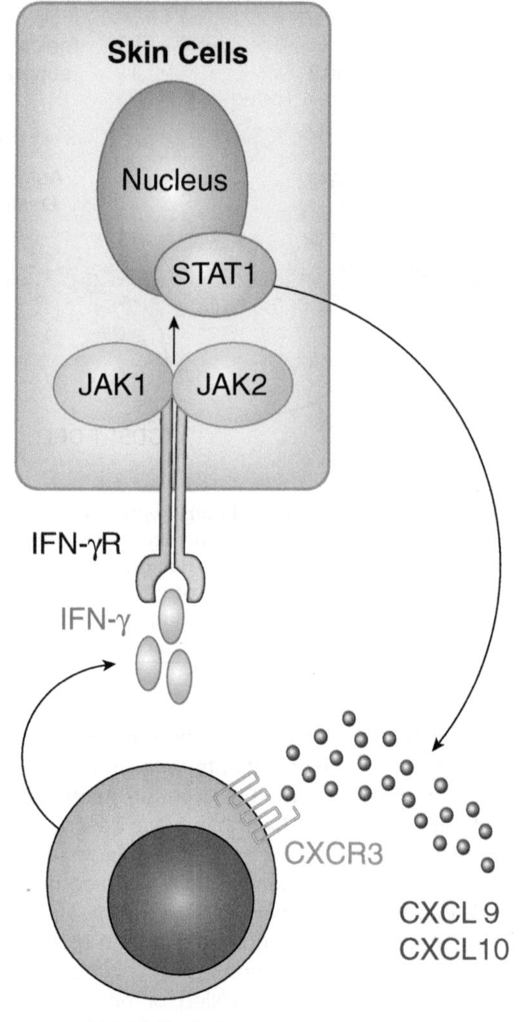

Fig. 2. Autoimmunity in vitiligo is driven by the IFN-γ–CXCL10 cytokine signaling pathway. Activated melanocyte-specific CD8+ T cells secrete IFN-γ, which signals through the IFN-γ receptor (IFN-γR) to activate JAK1/2 and STAT1. This JAK/STAT activation induces the production of CXCL9 and CXCL10, which signal through their receptor CXCR3 to recruit more autoreactive T cells to the epidermis, resulting in widespread melanocyte destruction. Targeting this cytokine pathway represents an emerging treatment strategy for vitiligo.

Currently, an open-label, phase 2, proof-of-concept clinical trial is recruiting participants to test the efficacy of topical ruxolitinib 1.5% in the treatment of vitiligo.[57]

In addition to JAK inhibitors, STAT inhibitors could potentially have similar effects. So far, 7 members have been identified in this family; however, only STAT1 as a homodimer has been implicated in IFN-γ signaling (reviewed by Villarino and colleagues[50]). A previous in vitro study reported that statins, which lower cholesterol via inhibition of 3-hydroxy-3-methylglutaryl-coenzyme A (HMG-CoA) reductase, inhibited STAT1 function.[58] In addition, a vitiligo patient was reported to improve after taking oral simvastatin.[59] A recent study tested systemic simvastatin in a mouse model of vitiligo and found it effective in both preventing and reversing disease.[60] A small pilot clinical trial the authors conducted to test the efficacy of high-dose (80 mg daily) oral simvastatin in patients with generalized vitiligo did not reach its primary efficacy endpoint.[61] Adverse effects of simvastatin limit dosing in humans, which may be responsible for the disparate results between the mouse model and vitiligo patients. An ongoing study is currently recruiting patients to evaluate the benefits of combining atorvastatin and UVB for the treatment of active vitiligo,[62] and future studies could test topical simvastatin as a way to increase local concentrations without toxicity.

Immune checkpoints

Successful application of immunotherapy to treat metastatic melanoma via blockade of inhibitory checkpoints has gained recent attention. Immune checkpoints are molecules that modulate T-cell responses to inflammation and include cytotoxic T-lymphocyte–associated protein 4 (CTLA-4) and programmed cell death protein 1 (PD-1), among others.[63] The treatment response of melanoma patients to immune checkpoint inhibitors correlates with the development of vitiligo.[64] Some investigators have hypothesized that activating these surface receptors could restore tolerance in vitiligo patients.[65]

Abatacept is a fusion protein composed of the fragment crystallizable (Fc) region of the immunoglobulin IgG1 fused to the extracellular domain of CTLA-4. It is currently approved by the FDA for the treatment of moderate to severe rheumatoid arthritis.[66] Recently, an open-label, single-arm, pilot study was initiated to test the efficacy of abatacept in patients with vitiligo.[67] Additionally, PD-1 ligand (a PD-1 agonist) is currently under development and is being tested in preclinical phases of inflammatory bowel disease and psoriasis.[68]

Stimulating Melanocyte Regeneration

α-Melanocyte–stimulating hormone

Phototherapy is currently first-line therapy for vitiligo, especially in patients with widespread disease[1,2] (reviewed by Samia Esmat and colleagues' article, "Phototherapy and Combination Therapies for Vitiligo," in this issue). Although the mechanism of its therapeutic effects are not completely understood, repigmentation from phototherapy is probably due to its ability to induce immunosuppression and also to the induction of melanocyte stem cell differentiation and proliferation.[69] α-Melanocyte–stimulating hormone (α-MSH) is a naturally occurring hormone that stimulates melanogenesis (reviewed by Videira and colleagues[70]). Afamelanotide, a synthetic analog of α-MSH, is currently approved by the European Medicines Agency to mitigate photosensitivity in erythropoietic protoporphyria[71] and thus may also improve the efficacy of phototherapy for vitiligo.[72] Recently, a randomized comparative multicenter trial was conducted to test the safety and efficacy of an afamelanotide subcutaneous implant in combination with NB-UVB in adults with generalized vitiligo. The combination therapy was somewhat well tolerated, although side effects included nausea and skin hyperpigmentation, which led some subjects to withdraw from the trial. The treatment resulted in faster and increased total repigmentation compared with NB-UVB monotherapy. This response was most evident in patients with darker skin (Fitzpatrick skin types IV to VI).[73] It is currently unknown whether afamelanotide monotherapy would have any benefit in the treatment of vitiligo.

Wnt signaling

A recent study reported that melanocytes from vitiligo patients had defective Wnt signaling, a pathway that promotes the differentiation of melanocyte precursors in skin. The investigators hypothesized that this impaired signaling contributed to disease pathogenesis and, in particular, inhibited melanocyte regeneration and repigmentation during treatment. Studies using explanted human skin ex vivo suggested that Wnt activators could enhance melanocyte differentiation.[35] Thus, therapeutic Wnt activation could potentially serve as an adjunctive therapy for vitiligo that supports melanocyte regeneration.[74]

Selective sunscreen

Despite being the most effective current treatment of vitiligo, patient access to phototherapy is a challenge. To receive therapy, patients typically attend a specialized clinic 2 to 3 times weekly for up to 1 to 2 years to achieve a satisfactory response. Although sun exposure is an inexpensive alternative to phototherapy, it is difficult to monitor exposure, and nontherapeutic wavelengths of light can be erythematogenic and dose limiting. Recently, a topical formulation of dimethicone 1% was reported to selectively block wavelengths of sunlight below 300 nm, permitting therapeutic wavelengths in the NB-UVB range (approximately 311–312 nm)

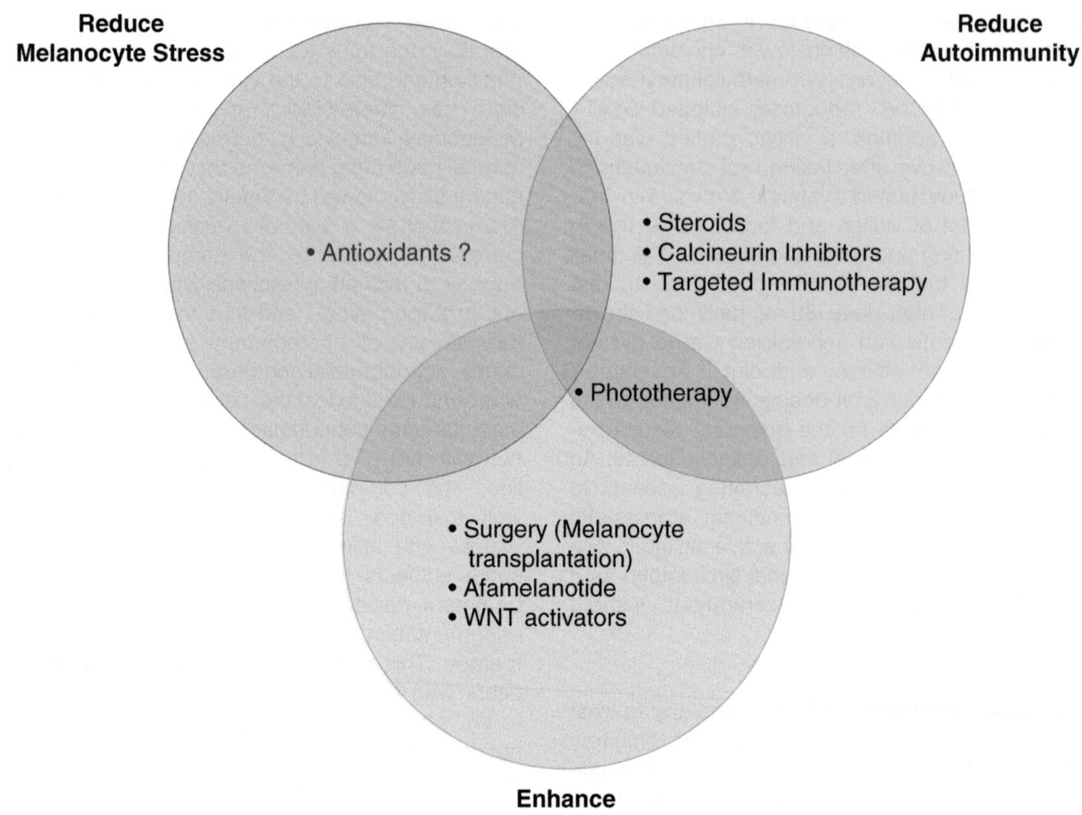

Fig. 3. Current and emerging treatments address 3 major goals in vitiligo treatment. Current treatments are listed in black and emerging treatments in red.

to penetrate. A small double-blind placebo-controlled study found that application of this cream followed by sun exposure was safe and effective at inducing repigmentation in lesional skin.[75] This needs to be confirmed in larger clinical trials, however, and, as the investigators acknowledged, its use would be limited by inadequate sunlight during certain times of the year or involvement of body areas that cannot be exposed in public. In addition, potentially harmful UVA light is not blocked by this cream; thus, this approach may not be as safe as NB-UVB phototherapy.

SUMMARY

Research to better understand the pathogenesis of vitiligo has revealed that an optimal treatment strategy should consider 3 key aspects of the disease: (1) normalizing melanocyte stress, (2) inhibiting autoimmunity, and (3) promoting melanocyte regeneration. Although current therapies, such as phototherapy, topical immunomodulators, and surgical approaches, exert their effects through these mechanisms, they do so in a general, untargeted way, resulting in suboptimal responses and potential side effects. Emerging therapies seek to target specific pathways identified through basic, translational, and clinical research studies in vitiligo to improve both efficacy and safety for patients (**Fig. 3**). Although this is a hopeful and exciting time for vitiligo patients and their physicians, this excitement should be balanced with caution, particularly because melanoma may take advantage of these same pathways to avoid immunesurveillance or promote their growth. As with most medical treatments, however, careful patient selection and monitoring should enable normalizing pathogenic responses in vitiligo to achieve homeostasis as in healthy individuals.

REFERENCES

1. Ezzedine K, Eleftheriadou V, Whitton M, et al. Vitiligo. Lancet 2015;386(9988):74–84.
2. Picardo M, Dell'Anna ML, Ezzedine K, et al. Vitiligo. Nat Rev Dis Primers 2015;1(1):1–16.
3. Rashighi M, Harris JE. Interfering with the IFN-gamma/CXCL10 pathway to develop new targeted treatments for vitiligo. Ann Transl Med 2015;3(21):343.

4. Taieb A, Picardo M. Clinical practice. Vitiligo. N Engl J Med 2009;360(2):160–9.
5. Alkhateeb A, Fain PR, Thody A, et al. Epidemiology of vitiligo and associated autoimmune diseases in Caucasian probands and their families. Pigment Cell Res 2003;16(3):208–14.
6. Gill L, Zarbo A, Isedeh P, et al. Comorbid autoimmune diseases in patients with vitiligo: a cross-sectional study. J Am Acad Dermatol 2016;74(2):295–302.
7. Jin Y, Birlea SA, Fain PR, et al. Genome-wide association analyses identify 13 new susceptibility loci for generalized vitiligo. Nat Genet 2012;44(6):676–80.
8. Shen C, Gao J, Sheng Y, et al. Genetic susceptibility to vitiligo: GWAS approaches for identifying vitiligo susceptibility genes and loci. Front Genet 2016;7:3.
9. Spritz RA. Six decades of vitiligo genetics: genome-wide studies provide insights into autoimmune pathogenesis. J Invest Dermatol 2012;132(2):268–73.
10. Harris JE. Cellular stress and innate inflammation in organ-specific autoimmunity: lessons learned from vitiligo. Immunol Rev 2016;269(1):11–25.
11. Boissy RE, Liu YY, Medrano EE, et al. Structural aberration of the rough endoplasmic reticulum and melanosome compartmentalization in long-term cultures of melanocytes from vitiligo patients. J Invest Dermatol 1991;97(3):395–404.
12. Schallreuter KU, Moore J, Wood JM, et al. In vivo and in vitro evidence for hydrogen peroxide (H2O2) accumulation in the epidermis of patients with vitiligo and its successful removal by a UVB-activated pseudocatalase. J Investig Dermatol Symp Proc 1999;4(1):91–6.
13. Shalbaf M, Gibbons NC, Wood JM, et al. Presence of epidermal allantoin further supports oxidative stress in vitiligo. Exp Dermatol 2008;17(9):761–70.
14. Koca R, Armutcu F, Altinyazar HC, et al. Oxidant-antioxidant enzymes and lipid peroxidation in generalized vitiligo. Clin Exp Dermatol 2004;29(4):406–9.
15. Dell'Anna ML, Ottaviani M, Albanesi V, et al. Membrane lipid alterations as a possible basis for melanocyte degeneration in vitiligo. J Invest Dermatol 2007;127(5):1226–33.
16. Schallreuter KU, Wood JM, Berger J. Low catalase levels in the epidermis of patients with vitiligo. J Invest Dermatol 1991;97(6):1081–5.
17. Gibbons NC, Wood JM, Rokos H, et al. Computer simulation of native epidermal enzyme structures in the presence and absence of hydrogen peroxide (H2O2): potential and pitfalls. J Invest Dermatol 2006;126(12):2576–82.
18. Oliver E, Schwartz L, Warren L. Occupational leukoderma preliminary report. JAMA 1939;113:927–8.
19. Fisher AA. Differential diagnosis of idiopathic vitiligo. Part III: occupational leukoderma. Cutis 1994;53(6):278–80.
20. Wu S, Li WQ, Cho E, et al. Use of permanent hair dyes and risk of vitiligo in women. Pigment Cell Melanoma Res 2015;28(6):744–6.
21. d'Ischia M, Wakamatsu K, Cicoira F, et al. Melanins and melanogenesis: from pigment cells to human health and technological applications. Pigment Cell Melanoma Res 2015;28(5):520–44.
22. Toosi S, Orlow SJ, Manga P. Vitiligo-inducing phenols activate the unfolded protein response in melanocytes resulting in upregulation of IL6 and IL8. J Invest Dermatol 2012;132(11):2601–9.
23. van den Boorn JG, Picavet DI, van Swieten PF, et al. Skin-depigmenting agent monobenzone induces potent T-cell autoimmunity toward pigmented cells by tyrosinase haptenation and melanosome autophagy. J Invest Dermatol 2011;131(6):1240–51.
24. Kroll TM, Bommiasamy H, Boissy RE, et al. 4-Tertiary butyl phenol exposure sensitizes human melanocytes to dendritic cell-mediated killing: relevance to vitiligo. J Invest Dermatol 2005;124(4):798–806.
25. Mosenson JA, Zloza A, Nieland JD, et al. Mutant HSP70 reverses autoimmune depigmentation in vitiligo. Sci Transl Med 2013;5(174):174ra28.
26. Levandowski CB, Mailloux CM, Ferrara TM, et al. NLRP1 haplotypes associated with vitiligo and autoimmunity increase interleukin-1beta processing via the NLRP1 inflammasome. Proc Natl Acad Sci U S A 2013;110(8):2952–6.
27. Yu R, Broady R, Huang Y, et al. Transcriptome analysis reveals markers of aberrantly activated innate immunity in vitiligo lesional and non-lesional skin. PLoS One 2012;7(12):e51040.
28. van den Boorn JG, Jakobs C, Hagen C, et al. Inflammasome-dependent induction of adaptive NK cell memory. Immunity 2016;44(6):1406–21.
29. Richmond JM, Frisoli ML, Harris JE. Innate immune mechanisms in vitiligo: danger from within. Curr Opin Immunol 2013;25(6):676–82.
30. Vega VL, Rodriguez-Silva M, Frey T, et al. Hsp70 translocates into the plasma membrane after stress and is released into the extracellular environment in a membrane-associated form that activates macrophages. J Immunol 2008;180(6):4299–307.
31. Mosenson JA, Eby JM, Hernandez C, et al. A central role for inducible heat-shock protein 70 in autoimmune vitiligo. Exp Dermatol 2013;22(9):566–9.
32. van den Boorn JG, Konijnenberg D, Dellemijn TA, et al. Autoimmune destruction of skin melanocytes by perilesional T cells from vitiligo patients. J Invest Dermatol 2009;129(9):2220–32.
33. Rork JF, Rashighi M, Harris JE. Understanding autoimmunity of vitiligo and alopecia areata. Curr Opin Pediatr 2016;28(4):463–9.
34. Rashighi M, Agarwal P, Richmond JM, et al. CXCL10 is critical for the progression and maintenance of depigmentation in a mouse model of vitiligo. Sci translational Med 2014;6(223):223ra23.

35. Regazzetti C, Joly F, Marty C, et al. Transcriptional analysis of vitiligo skin reveals the alteration of WNT pathway: a promising target for repigmenting vitiligo patients. J Invest Dermatol 2015;135(12):3105–14.
36. Wang X, Wang Q, Wu J, et al. Increased expression of CXCR3 and its ligands in vitiligo patients and CXCL10 as a potential clinical marker for vitiligo. Br J Dermatol 2016;174(6):1318–26.
37. Harris JE, Harris TH, Weninger W, et al. A mouse model of vitiligo with focused epidermal depigmentation requires IFN-gamma for autoreactive CD8(+) T-cell accumulation in the skin. J Invest Dermatol 2012;132(7):1869–76.
38. Schallreuter KU, Wood JM, Lemke KR, et al. Treatment of vitiligo with a topical application of pseudocatalase and calcium in combination with short-term UVB exposure: a case study on 33 patients. Dermatology 1995;190(3):223–9.
39. Schallreuter KU, Moore J, Behrens-Williams S, et al. Rapid initiation of repigmentation in vitiligo with Dead Sea climatotherapy in combination with pseudocatalase (PC-KUS). Int J Dermatol 2002;41(8):482–7.
40. Schallreuter KU, Kruger C, Wurfel BA, et al. From basic research to the bedside: efficacy of topical treatment with pseudocatalase PC-KUS in 71 children with vitiligo. Int J Dermatol 2008;47(7):743–53.
41. Patel DC, Evans AV, Hawk JL. Topical pseudocatalase mousse and narrowband UVB phototherapy is not effective for vitiligo: an open, single-centre study. Clin Exp Dermatol 2002;27(8):641–4.
42. Bakis-Petsoglou S, Le Guay JL, Wittal R. A randomized, double-blinded, placebo-controlled trial of pseudocatalase cream and narrowband ultraviolet B in the treatment of vitiligo. Br J Dermatol 2009;161(4):910–7.
43. Gawkrodger DJ. Pseudocatalase and narrowband ultraviolet B for vitiligo: clearing the picture. Br J Dermatol 2009;161(4):721–2.
44. Cohen BE, Elbuluk N, Mu EW, et al. Alternative systemic treatments for vitiligo: a review. Am J Clin Dermatol 2015;16(6):463–74.
45. Szczurko O, Shear N, Taddio A, et al. Ginkgo biloba for the treatment of vitilgo vulgaris: an open label pilot clinical trial. BMC Complement Altern Med 2011;11:21.
46. Parsad D, Pandhi R, Juneja A. Effectiveness of oral Ginkgo biloba in treating limited, slowly spreading vitiligo. Clin Exp Dermatol 2003;28(3):285–7.
47. Middelkamp-Hup MA, Bos JD, Rius-Diaz F, et al. Treatment of vitiligo vulgaris with narrow-band UVB and oral Polypodium leucotomos extract: a randomized double-blind placebo-controlled study. J Eur Acad Dermatol Venereol 2007;21(7):942–50.
48. Dell'Anna ML, Mastrofrancesco A, Sala R, et al. Antioxidants and narrow band-UVB in the treatment of vitiligo: a double-blind placebo controlled trial. Clin Exp Dermatol 2007;32(6):631–6.
49. Mosenson JA, Zloza A, Klarquist J, et al. HSP70i is a critical component of the immune response leading to vitiligo. Pigment Cell Melanoma Res 2012;25(1):88–98.
50. Villarino AV, Kanno Y, Ferdinand JR, et al. Mechanisms of Jak/STAT signaling in immunity and disease. J Immunol 2015;194(1):21–7.
51. Craiglow BG, King BA. Tofacitinib citrate for the treatment of vitiligo: a pathogenesis-directed therapy. JAMA Dermatol 2015;151(10):1110–2.
52. Mesa RA, Yasothan U, Kirkpatrick P. Ruxolitinib. Nat Rev Drug Discov 2012;11(2):103–4.
53. Vannucchi AM, Kiladjian JJ, Griesshammer M, et al. Ruxolitinib versus standard therapy for the treatment of polycythemia vera. N Engl J Med 2015;372(5):426–35.
54. Harris JE, Rashighi M, Nguyen N, et al. Rapid skin repigmentation on oral ruxolitinib in a patient with coexistent vitiligo and alopecia areata (AA). J Am Acad Dermatol 2016;74(2):370–1.
55. Galli S, McLornan D, Harrison C. Safety evaluation of ruxolitinib for treating myelofibrosis. Expert Opin Drug Saf 2014;13(7):967–76.
56. Craiglow BG, Tavares D, King BA. Topical ruxolitinib for the treatment of alopecia universalis. JAMA Dermatol 2016;152(4):490–1.
57. Tufts Medical Center. Topical ruxolitinib for the treatment of vitiligo. ClinicalTrials.gov [Internet]. Bethesda (MD): National Library of Medicine (US); 2000. Available at: https://clinicaltrials.gov/ct2/show/NCT02809976. Accessed June 29, 2016.
58. Zhao Y, Gartner U, Smith FJ, et al. Statins downregulate K6a promoter activity: a possible therapeutic avenue for pachyonychia congenita. J Invest Dermatol 2011;131(5):1045–52.
59. Noel M, Gagne C, Bergeron J, et al. Positive pleiotropic effects of HMG-CoA reductase inhibitor on vitiligo. Lipids Health Dis 2004;3:7.
60. Agarwal P, Rashighi M, Essien KI, et al. Simvastatin prevents and reverses depigmentation in a mouse model of vitiligo. J Invest Dermatol 2015;135(4):1080–8.
61. Vanderweil SG, Amano S, KoW, et al. A small doubleblind, placebo-controlled, phase-II, proof-of-concept clinical trial to evaluate oral simvastatin as a treatment for vitiligo. J Am Acad Dermatol 2017;76(1):150–1.
62. Centre Hospitalier Universitaire de Nice. Atorvastatin in active vitiligo. ClinicalTrials.gov [Internet]. Bethesda (MD): National Library of Medicine (US); 2000. Available at: https://clinicaltrials.gov/ct2/show/NCT02432534. Accessed January 19, 2016.
63. Weber J. Immune checkpoint proteins: a new therapeutic paradigm for cancer–preclinical background: CTLA-4 and PD-1 blockade. Semin Oncol 2010;37(5):430–9.

64. Macdonald JB, Macdonald B, Golitz LE, et al. Cutaneous adverse effects of targeted therapies: part II: inhibitors of intracellular molecular signaling pathways. J Am Acad Dermatol 2015;72(2):221–36 [quiz: 37–8].
65. Speeckaert R, van Geel N. Targeting CTLA-4, PD-L1 and IDO to modulate immune responses in vitiligo. Exp Dermatol 2016. [Epub ahead of print].
66. Moreland L, Bate G, Kirkpatrick P. Abatacept. Nat Rev Drug Discov 2006;5(3):185–6.
67. Brigham and Women's Hospital. Open-label pilot study of abatacept for the treatment of vitiligo. ClinicalTrials.gov [Internet]. Bethesda (MD): National Library of Medicine (US); 2000. Available at: https://clinicaltrials.gov/ct2/show/NCT02281058. Accessed June 29, 2016.
68. Genexin.com [Internet]. Available at: http://www.genexine.com/m31.php. Accessed June 30, 2016.
69. Bulat V, Situm M, Dediol I, et al. The mechanisms of action of phototherapy in the treatment of the most common dermatoses. Coll Antropol 2011; 35(Suppl 2):147–51.
70. Videira IF, Moura DF, Magina S. Mechanisms regulating melanogenesis. An Bras Dermatol 2013; 88(1):76–83.
71. Fabrikant J, Touloei K, Brown SM. A review and update on melanocyte stimulating hormone therapy: afamelanotide. J Drugs Dermatol 2013;12(7):775–9.
72. Grimes PE, Hamzavi I, Lebwohl M, et al. The efficacy of afamelanotide and narrowband UV-B phototherapy for repigmentation of vitiligo. JAMA Dermatol 2013;149(1):68–73.
73. Lim HW, Grimes PE, Agbai O, et al. Afamelanotide and narrowband UV-B phototherapy for the treatment of vitiligo: a randomized multicenter trial. JAMA Dermatol 2015;151(1):42–50.
74. Harris JE. Melanocyte regeneration in vitiligo requires WNT beneath their Wings. J Invest Dermatol 2015;135(12):2921–3.
75. Goren A, Salafia A, McCoy J, et al. Novel topical cream delivers safe and effective sunlight therapy for vitiligo by selectively filtering damaging ultraviolet radiation. Dermatol Ther 2014;27(4):195–7.

Index

Note: Page numbers of article titles are in **boldface** type.

Dermatol Clin 35 (2017) 267–273
http://dx.doi.org/10.1016/S0733-8635(17)30020-7
0733-8635/17

J

K

L

M

N

O

P

Q

R

W

Z

Printed and bound by CPI Group (UK) Ltd, Croydon, CR0 4YY
03/10/2024
01040304-0012